OUR
DAILY
MEDS

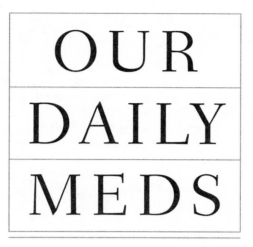

OUR
DAILY
MEDS

How the Pharmaceutical Companies Transformed
Themselves into Slick Marketing Machines
and Hooked the Nation on Prescription Drugs

MELODY PETERSEN

SARAH CRICHTON BOOKS
Farrar, Straus and Giroux
New York

Sarah Crichton Books
Farrar, Straus and Giroux
18 West 18th Street, New York 10011

Library of Congress Cataloging-in-Publication Data
Petersen, Melody, 1964–
    Our daily meds : how the pharmaceutical companies transformed
themselves into slick marketing machines and hooked the nation on
prescription drugs / Melody Petersen.— 1st ed.
        p.   cm.
    "Sarah Crichton books."
    Includes bibliographical references and index.
    ISBN-13: 978-0-374-22827-9 (hardcover : alk. paper)
    ISBN-10: 0-374-22827-2 (hardcover : alk. paper)
    1.   Drugs—United States—Marketing.   I.   Title.
    [DNLM: 1. Drug Industry—economics—United States.   2. Drug
Industry—ethics—United States.   3. Biomedical Research—economics—
United States.   4. Marketing—ethics—United States.   5. Physician's
Practice Patterns—ethics—United States.   6. Prescriptions, Drug—
economics—United States.   QV 736 P484o 2008]
HD9666.5.P415 2008
338.4'761510973—dc22
                                                                2008002097

Designed by Cassandra J. Pappas

www.fsgbooks.com

1   3   5   7   9   10   8   6   4   2

For Michael

CONTENTS

OUR
DAILY
MEDS

Introduction

DOCTORS CALL IT the resurrection drug. They have watched as it freed patients from what seemed an inescapable death.

The medicine treats sleeping sickness, a disease far more lethal and terrifying than its name implies. Opportunistic tsetse flies spread the disease through much of Africa, devastating villages and killing tens of thousands of people a year. The jewel-eyed yellowish brown flies thrive in thickets along rivers where women and children go to collect water. With a bite, the bloodsuckers inject deadly parasites into their human victims. As the parasites multiply, their human hosts appear to go mad. The victims grow agitated and confused, slur their speech, and stumble. Finally come coma and death.

The pharmaceutical company that manufactured the medicine, a failed cancer drug with the tongue-twisting name eflornithine, abandoned it in 1995, seeing no profit in selling it in poor countries.

But the resurrection drug made its own revival a few years later—not in Africa, but in the United States, a land free of tsetse flies but with fourteen million women worried about unwanted facial hair. Another company began selling it in the form of a depilatory cream to minimize female mustaches. With its lavender-colored logo resembling a graceful swan and advertisements sporting young, beautiful models, eflornithine became another prescription drug marketing success.

The company christened its product Vaniqa.

THIS IS A book about a great transformation in the prescription drug industry over the last twenty-five years. Once the most successful pharmaceutical companies were those with the brightest scientists searching for cures. Now the most profitable and powerful drugmakers are those with the most creative and aggressive marketers. The drug companies have become marketing machines, selling antidepressants like Paxil, pain pills like Celebrex, and heart medications like Lipitor with the same methods that Coca-Cola uses to sell Sprite and Procter & Gamble uses to sell Tide.

Selling prescription drugs—rather than *discovering* them—has become the pharmaceutical industry's obsession.

Prescription drug marketing now permeates every corner of American society—from *Sesame Street* to nursing homes to the nightly news. Medicine ads sprout from billboards, scoreboards, the hoods of race cars, and the back covers of magazines—all once venues of the similarly ubiquitous cigarette ads of the 1960s and 1970s. Imitating neighborhood grocers, the drugmakers offer coupons, free gifts, and deals to buy six prescriptions and get one free. They hold sweepstakes and scholarship contests. They pay to sponsor rock concerts, movie premieres, and baseball's major leagues.

The marketers make the use of their dangerous medicines look attractive and easy. Fentanyl, an addictive narcotic eighty times more potent than morphine, comes in a berry-flavored lollipop. Syringes used to inject children with growth hormone look like kaleidoscope-colored writing pens and PlaySkool toys. In 2006 drug companies gained approval to coat their pills with "pearlescent pigments" to enhance them with a shimmery satin luster and make them look as precious as their price.

During New York's 2003 Fashion Week, swimsuit models shimmied down the catwalk, showing off Johnson & Johnson's new contraceptive, a white-colored patch that was glued to the skin. By wearing the drug as a fashion accessory, one company executive explained, women "can look beautiful and feel confident."

Men attending professional golf tournaments in 2004 heard a different pitch. Step right up for free tips on your golf game, offered marketers working in a tent promoting Cialis, a drug for erectile dysfunction. Step right up for a free video lesson from a sports psychologist, the salesmen invited. By the way, they added, do we have the perfect drug for you!

America has become the world's greatest medicine show.

The marketing works. Never have Americans taken so many prescription drugs.

Americans spent $250 billion in 2005 on prescription drugs, more than the combined gross domestic product of Argentina and Peru. Americans spent more on prescription drugs in 2004 than they did on gasoline or fast food. They paid *twice* as much for their prescription medicines that year as they spent on either higher education or new automobiles.

The American prescription drug market is so lucrative that many foreign drug companies have moved in and now depend on Americans for most of their profits. For foreign executives, the math is simple. Americans spend more on medicines than do all the people of Japan, Germany, France, Italy, Spain, the United Kingdom, Australia, New Zealand, Canada, Mexico, Brazil, and Argentina *combined*.

As the medicine merchants have poured billions of dollars into selling their wares, they have become America's most powerful industry. In the process, they have transformed American life. The small white-capped whiskey-colored bottles that once took up a corner of the bathroom cabinet now play a role in lives that few products can match. Almost 65 percent of the nation now takes a drug available only by prescription. Children line up in the dining hall of their summer camps to get their daily doses. Pharmacies stay open twenty-four hours to meet America's demand. Even the dogs get Prozac if they howl too much at the moon.

The pharmaceutical companies build their laboratories on the campuses of public universities. They recruit patients for clinical trials at shopping malls and county fairs. On network television, the plots of prime-time shows revolve around brand name prescription drugs, at times at the suggestion of marketers at a pharmaceutical company.

The medicine promoters have turned what were once normal life events—menopause, despair from a divorce, anxiety caused by a workaholic boss—into maladies that can be treated with a pill. After all, when patients are customers and medicines are commodities, the industry thrives when people are ill—or believe they are.

The companies have found the United States, with its consumer-driven culture, a perfect medicine market. We expect instant gratification of our desires and a quick fix for whatever bothers or distracts. Americans are eager to believe in the panaceas offered in the six drug commercials that regularly accompany each evening's news. We are told—and want to believe—that we can swallow a pill and soon be dancing on a dinner cruise, running on the beach, or playing football like John Elway, the former NFL quarterback and promoter of Prevacid, a heartburn pill. If we eat too many cheeseburgers and fries, there is comfort knowing one pill will settle our stomachs while another brings our cholesterol back down.

In the condos of Palm Beach, the bungalows of Los Angeles, and the farmhouses of Iowa, people are taking more and more pills. The average American collected more than twelve prescriptions from his pharmacy in 2006, up from eight prescriptions in 1994. Older Americans take home even more—an average of thirty prescriptions each year.

In 2003 Secretary of State Colin Powell explained the nation's new prescription habit to a journalist for the Arabic newspaper *Asharq Al-Awsat*.

"So do you use sleeping tablets to organize yourself?" asked the writer, Abdul Rahman Al-Rashed.

"Yes. Well, I wouldn't call them that," Powell replied. "They're a wonderful medication—not medication. How would you call it? They're called Ambien, which is very good. You don't use Ambien? Everybody here uses Ambien."

There is a problem, however, with the new American way, one that the drug companies and doctors prescribing the medicines do not like to talk about. Experts estimate that more than a hundred thousand Americans die each year not from illness but from their prescription drugs. Those deaths, occurring quietly, almost without notice in hospitals, emergency rooms, and homes, make medicines one of the leading causes of death in the United States.

On a daily basis, prescription pills are estimated to kill more than 270 Americans—more than twice as many as are killed in automobile accidents. Prescription medicines, taken according to doctors' instructions, kill more Americans than either diabetes or Alzheimer's disease.

America has become "a grossly overprescribed nation," says Dr. Arnold Relman, professor emeritus at Harvard Medical School and the former editor of *The New England Journal of Medicine*. "Again and again you see examples where patients get far more medication than they need. The average senior in America is probably taking twice or three times the medications they require."

Doctors prescribe one drug only to create new problems for the patient with the pill's side effects. Rather than realize the medicine is making them ill, patients believe they are just getting old and ask for even more pills. Arthritis patients get pain relievers, which raise their blood pressure. At their next visit, doctors prescribe medicines for hypertension, which come with a whole new set of adverse effects.

It is estimated that the nation may now pay as much to care for patients who were harmed by their prescriptions as it spends on those medicines in the first place.

Despite these injuries and deaths, the medicine merchants have not stopped with adults. They are now targeting the increasingly profitable and fast-growing medicine market for children. The companies' marketers have created storybooks, video games, and soft, cuddly toys to attract children's attention. They have also learned to aim their appeals at parents' desire to have the perfect child. Parents of short children are told that daily injections of human growth hormone can help their son grow inches and be better accepted by his peers. They are told that Ritalin will help their daughter get higher grades. An antidepressant, they learn, may help their shy child play with other kids. In 2002 and 2003 prescription spending rose faster for children than for seniors, baby boomers, or any other group.

But so far scientists know little about the long-term effects of using powerful adult drugs in children, making the booming pediatric market a grand American experiment. The drugs have already harmed thousands of children. Federal regulators received more than seven thousand reports of drugs harming infants and toddlers under age two between 1997 and 2000, according to a university study. More than 750 of those children died.

THE VAST MAJORITY of the industry's marketing dollars is directed not at consumers but at physicians, the gatekeepers whom patients trust. In 2004 the industry employed an army of 101,000 sales representatives to call on those doctors—two and a half times the size of its sales force in 1995. There is now one drug salesperson for every six physicians, each with an expense account that lets him shower doctors with gifts and cash. Surveys show that virtually every American physician now takes these handouts.

Sales representatives at a company called Tap Pharmaceutical Products gave frequent prescribers of its medicine Lupron television sets and VCRs for their offices and tickets to Broadway's *Phantom of the Opera*. When a doctor asked the drug company to pay to relocate his office, Tap's executives wrote a check. When physicians wished they could earn more money, Tap paid up to $25,000 for consultants to guide them on how to be better businessmen.

A training manual for Tap's salespeople explained they should expect doctors and hospitals to ask them for cash. The sales reps could deliver the money, the manual directed, as long as they remembered that "the primary factor" was "what will the grant do for you and your company." The company expected doctors receiving the gifts to return the favor by writing more prescriptions. "If a non-user physician asks for money," the manual instructed, referring to doctors who did not prescribe Tap's products, "ask for scripts."

By the beginning of the twenty-first century, doctors had come to count on the industry's handouts. "It's nice after an exhausting day at work to go to a dinner, sporting event or spa where we can discuss with our peers and learn more about treatments for various diseases," wrote Dr. Nancy Sika and Dr. Colleen Heniff in a letter to federal officials in 2002 when the government proposed restricting some of the gifts. "Why are we singled out by the government not to have the same perks as other businesses?

"As physicians we are a very ethical, intelligent group," they wrote. "I have not seen us be swayed to use a product just because we were taken out."

But patients tell stories of how their doctors gave in to the sales pitches. Mrs. Albert F. Rust of Kirtland Hills, Ohio, said she was horrified as she watched a doctor switch her elderly mother to a new drug that was heavily promoted from one that seemed to be helping her. "The representative of the company has been after me to switch my patients," the doctor had explained.

"We were helpless," Mrs. Rust said. "I cried and so did Mom. She was 87 years old and a timid elderly person. I won't forget her confusion and sadness."

BECAUSE ONLY ABOUT 10 percent of the price of most brand name pills goes to cover the cost of the raw chemicals and manufacturing, the industry has plenty left even after paying for advertisements, research, and the high salaries and expensive perks of its executives. While patients and taxpayers have been left with emptied pockets, the drugmakers have been flush with cash. From 1995 to 2002 they were the nation's most profitable industry. In 2004 the pharmaceutical companies turned nearly sixteen cents of each dollar of revenue into profit, according to *Fortune* magazine. That compares with the median profit earned by America's five hundred largest public companies that year of a little more than five cents.

With their hoards of cash, the companies have readily handed money to patient groups, hospitals, universities, medical schools, physician societies, government agencies, and just about any organization they want on their side. Harvard, for one, has a lecture hall named for Pfizer in a building named for Mallinckrodt, another company.

The industry's cash-filled coffers have given it a stranglehold on medical science. Most of the nation's best academic medical minds have at some time been on the industry's payroll as consultants. As the drug

companies' influence has grown inside our universities, research priori-
ties have abruptly shifted to hurt the public's interest. Professors see more
money in working on the next blockbuster heartburn medicine than in
studying the environmental causes of cancer. They and the companies
that financially support them are more interested in developing hair loss
treatments and other lifestyle drugs for rich Americans than in discovering cures for diseases like malaria, which is devastating poor countries
and killing a child every thirty seconds.

The drug companies' chain of influence is so complete that there are
few people left to look objectively at the effects of their products on the
nation's health or at the consequences of their power for society.

Washington is the axis of the industry's power. The pharmaceutical
companies spent more on lobbying between 1998 and 2004 than any
other industry. By 2004 the companies employed a legion of lobbyists so
large there were more than two for each member of Congress. By using
their wealth to buy influence, the drug companies have repeatedly
squelched attempts to regulate their prices and promotional practices.
The United States is the only developed country in the world that does
not control prescription drug prices. Only the United States and one
other country, New Zealand, allow drugmakers to advertise to consumers. The industry has also won new laws that have added years to the
average length of time their products are protected from competition by
patents. Another law allowed the companies to profit from medical discoveries made by taxpayer-funded scientists. And when these new measures boosted the drug companies' profits, other laws gave them tax
credits so lucrative that as a group they pay far lower taxes on average
than other major industries.

Overall, the pharmaceutical industry has created a market for its
products in the United States in which ordinary economics no longer
apply. Patients do not get the best medicines for their ailments at the
best prices. Instead, America's medicine market is one where more
competition can mean prices will rise rather than fall. It is also a market in which patients suffer when they get the wrong drug because
the industry's powerful promotional forces have distorted the available

medical information. No one knows how many people are swallowing expensive new pills when older, far cheaper drugs that are not promoted would be best.

MEDICINES CAN AND do save lives. Antibiotics, first sold in the 1940s, have saved millions of people from infections that otherwise would have been fatal. Vaccines have virtually wiped out diseases like polio. Children with leukemia can now survive into adulthood because of medicines discovered in the decades following World War II. In the 1990s protease inhibitors and other antiviral drugs sharply reduced the death rate from AIDS. The drug marketers have told us these stories over and over.

The tragedy lies not with the medicines but with the marketing and the unprecedented power these companies now have over the practice of medicine. We've come to a time when decisions on how to treat a disease have as great a chance of being hatched in a corporate marketing department as by a group of independent doctors working to improve the public's health. In too many cases, whether a medicine helps or harms a patient has become secondary to how much it will bring shareholders in profits. That is the story of this book, the one that doesn't get told.

In its broadest terms, this book is about how America's for-profit medical system—filled with incentives to make money and disincentives for good care—has failed. While we are swallowing too many pills, we are also undergoing unneeded surgeries, X-rays, and CT scans. The companies striving to sell us as many pills, medical devices, and hospital stays as possible have goals that conflict with a basic tenet of medical intervention: do not overtreat.

Instead, the medical marketers of the twenty-first century work by the advice given to displaymen employed by the nation's department stores in the early 1900s as they learned to seduce the masses into buying more shirts, dresses, and toys.

"Sell them their dreams," a radio announcer urged a convention of displaymen in 1923. "Sell them what they longed for and hoped for and almost despaired of having . . . Sell them this hope and you won't have to worry about selling them goods."

Like the displaymen before them, the medicine merchants have learned to sell us our hopes and dreams, a pill for our every desire. Too few of us realize the dangers.

Part I

RX REPUBLIC

ONE

Creating Disease

ONCE I THOUGHT I knew what disease was. It had seemed black and white. A person was either healthy or sick. Just the sound of the words of disease—cancer, diabetes, heart failure—could instill a sense of dread. Then I listened to the drug marketers and learned that the definition of disease was less certain. It was malleable, even slippery, in fact. A disease could be invented if one had the money, the power, and an adman's knack for salesmanship.

In January 2003 Neil Wolf, the vice president of a large drug manufacturer called Pharmacia, stood before dozens of pharmaceutical executives gathered at the Crowne Plaza Hotel in Philadelphia and explained the simple formula his company had used to create a disease. The public first heard word of this malady in 1998. News reports that year said it was a serious affliction, an epidemic, affecting as many as one in every four American adults. Mysteriously, the reports began just weeks before pharmacies were stocked with a new medicine for the disease, some white-colored tablets called Detrol. Now, five years later, in a hotel ballroom reserved for the Pharmaceutical Marketing Global Summit, Wolf was preparing to reveal the company's secrets and explain just how he and his colleagues had conceived and packaged this new ailment and sold it to the American public as if it were introducing a new car.

The Global Summit was one of the biggest annual events for pharmaceutical marketers. Outside the ballroom, dozens of vendors of drug marketing services were waiting in sales booths for their chance to woo the corporate executives. The creativity of these vendors had few limits. One firm offered the big pharmaceutical companies the chance to build tents shaped like giant pill capsules on the midways of auto races like the Indianapolis 500, where nurses would screen fans for whatever ills the drug company desired. In a booth farther down the aisle, another firm offered to promote prescription pills at the shopping malls it owned in thirty-six states. "The mall is the medium," the company proclaimed.

Many of the pharmaceutical executives attending the Global Summit were young, perhaps still in their twenties and not long out of college or an M.B.A. program. They had come to the conference to network and learn the secrets that would propel their careers. Many of them already knew part of the story of Detrol and eagerly waited to learn more.

As Wolf, a bearded man with graying hair, took the stage inside the ballroom, the audience quieted. The first slide of his presentation appeared on the large screen. It held the title he had selected for his speech: "Positioning Detrol (Creating a Disease)."

"We wanted people to see something in *Reader's Digest*," he said, "and go to the doctor and say, 'I have this condition.'"

WHEN I BEGAN writing about pharmaceutical companies for *The New York Times* in early 2000, it was a time of exuberance and easy money on Wall Street. Stay-at-home mothers watched the cheery announcers on CNBC, the financial cable channel, keeping track of hot investment opportunities while hurrying their children off to school. Grandfathers withdrew money from savings accounts and bought stocks to boost their pensions. Middle managers quit their jobs to become day traders, buying and selling stocks using their home computers. Many start-up companies, with little more than a business plan of how they would make money through the Internet, saw their share prices rise by twenty to thirty times, even though they had never recorded a profit.

During this American boom it was the pharmaceutical manufacturers that most consistently excited market-crazed investors looking for fast growth with little risk. While the hot-selling technology companies held little more than a promise of sales in the future, the drug companies were succeeding in real time, making profits at more than twice the rate of the broader market, a feat they had accomplished for two decades. They weren't the high-risk technology companies they claimed to be. They made money even when the economy turned sour.

Selling medicines was an odd business. Disease meant money. Suffering brought profit. When I interviewed the pharmaceutical executives, I often heard something like this: "Our respiratory business is doing extremely well, as is our cholesterol business. The depression business has performed better than expected. Parts of that business are really growing strongly. It is the migraine market that is the problem."

The executives talked about their companies' medicines as if they were Hollywood producers about to release a new film. They spoke of "launching their next blockbuster," which they defined as a medicine that could bring in sales of one billion dollars or more in a single year. It was astounding to learn a company could earn so much from chemicals pressed into tablets. A billion dollars was enough in 2004 to send more than eighty-eight thousand American students to a public university, covering not only their tuition, but also their fees, room, and board.

My editors at the *Times* told me they wanted stories about the amazing new medicines these companies were discovering. But most of the products the executives boasted about were little different from those already being sold. AstraZeneca was developing a new cholesterol-lowering medicine, which would be the seventh entry in the class of drugs called statins. Executives at GlaxoSmithKline were talking about the company's new asthma drug called Advair, which was nothing more than a combination of two of the company's older medicines. The drugs had a new name and a fresh marketing campaign, but patients still had the same two drugs.

Then there were the companies that tried to extend their rich monopolies by introducing what they said were new and improved versions of products that had become wildly successful. Schering-Plough was preparing to sell Clarinex, which it said was even better than its best-selling allergy drug Claritin. Forest Laboratories brought out Lexapro, claiming it had beaten its star product, the antidepressant Celexa, in clinical trials. And AstraZeneca began selling its new "purple pill."

AstraZeneca had created pharmaceutical marketing history by focusing its promotion on the color of its product rather than on its name or even what it did. The pill's color had become a marketing tool, with the deep violet color giving it the feel of royalty and instilling loyalty in those who took it. According to industry consultants at IMS Health, AstraZeneca was one of the first drug companies to give their medicines unique shades to strengthen the value of their brand and public identity, just as Coca-Cola had done with the color red and the United Parcel Service with brown. Marketers were giving the pill a personality.

"Pink is perceived as calming, and may be suitable for heart drugs or tranquilizers, while bold colors such as red suggest rapid action and stimulation, and may therefore be appropriate for a painkiller or antidepressant," the IMS consultants wrote in an article in 2001. "On the other hand, it is difficult to imagine a pill in black, a color associated with death and morbidity."

If some patients did not realize their purple heartburn pill was actually AstraZeneca's Prilosec, then they did not notice as their doctors switched them to the "new" drug of the same shade but with the turn-of-the-century name Nexium.

The introduction of products like Clarinex, Lexapro, and Nexium followed a pattern. The government approved them, and the first boxes left the loading docks just months before the patent protecting the company's older product expired. Once a drug's patent expires, generic manufacturers can sell the pills, and prices plummet. Scientists who were independent from the makers of these drugs published reports saying they could find no evidence that the new products were better than the old. The independent scientists urged patients to save money by taking the generic, but their advice was drowned out by the din of the new advertising campaigns.

In this profit-driven world of medicine, I did not often hear the executives talk of cures. The companies seemed to have little interest in getting to the bottom of what was actually causing cancer, heart failure, or diabetes. Instead, they focused like honeybees circling a picnic cake on products for what they called chronic disorders. These were drugs that did not cure but "managed" diseases as patients took them once a day for the rest of their lives.

It was investors who drove the companies' push to medicate America on a daily basis. Wall Street analysts grilled the pharmaceutical executives about their marketing campaigns during conference calls held every three months. Were they hiring more sales reps? When would that new advertising campaign that executives had promised begin? How many dinners had the company hosted for doctors? The financial analysts ranked the companies by the number of drugs they sold that had reached that golden benchmark of one billion dollars in sales in a single year.

One day I asked Daniel Vasella, the chairman of Novartis, how his company went about creating the blockbusters that investors demanded. He talked about how a company must first have a product that satisfied "an unmet need."

"Much of it is data-driven, information-driven," Vasella explained. "You create a desire."

PHARMACIA CALLED ITS new disease "overactive bladder."

Neil Wolf told the audience in Philadelphia that as the company was developing Detrol in the mid-1990s, executives decided they were not satisfied with their original plan to promote the drug as a treatment for incontinence. The market for drugs for people who accidentally wet themselves was small, he said. Many doctors believed incontinence was not a disease that should be treated with prescription medications but a normal part of aging that could be managed by changing one's habits. They suggested patients avoid caffeine and drink less fluid before bed or a trip to the store. Patients who nevertheless wanted a prescription drug could choose from an array of cheap medicines that had been on the market for decades and worked in a similar way to Detrol. With such low-priced drugs and doctors hesitant to prescribe them, the market for medicines for incontinence was worth just forty million dollars a year in the United States, hardly significant to the major pharmaceutical firms looking for their next big hit. This did not sway Pharmacia executives, however, who were determined to enter the market and shake it up.

At the time the executives were planning how to sell Detrol, the company had just gone through a difficult merger. Pharmacia AB of Sweden and the Upjohn Company of Kalamazoo, Michigan, had joined to form one company called Pharmacia & Upjohn. A bitter battle over turf and power still raged between executives on the two continents. Exhilarated by his appointment as chief executive, Fred Hassan, a Pakistan-born, Harvard-schooled chemical engineer, set out to show Wall Street that Pharmacia & Upjohn could create global markets for prescription drugs just like its much larger rivals. Detrol would be the new company's first test.

According to Wolf, the Detrol marketers were determined to take a drug that was considered "a niche product" and turn it into "a mass market opportunity." They decided they would not stop with their original plan to promote Detrol to the twelve million Americans believed to be incontinent. They dreamed of nearly tripling the size of the market. To do this, they planned to promote the drug to people annoyed by their frequent urges to use the bathroom. To expand the number of potential customers even more, the marketers said they would also tout Detrol to those who frequently acted on those urges and found themselves in the toilet nine or more times a day.

Wolf explained that people stricken with these overactive bladders were hindered by what he called "toilet mapping" and "defensive voiding." People who "mapped toilets" would not leave their homes, he said, until they knew the location of every clean facility in the vicinity of their planned travels. A person who used "defensive voiding," Wolf said, never passed a restroom without stopping in. Pharmacia hoped to make these frequent restroom users into its longtime customers by spurring an idea in their minds. Too much of their lives revolved around the toilet. Detrol, taken every day, would set them free.

HER HALLUCINATIONS BEGAN soon after she started taking Detrol. They came only at night. She would wake up and talk with the apparitions, all of them family members who had long been dead.

Her memory also failed. After an examination, her doctor suspected the worst. He diagnosed Alzheimer's disease, an illness that means the beginning of the end. Alzheimer's horrifies patients and their families because it slowly robs people of their memories and their very souls. It can take a brilliant mind and reduce it to that of a helpless child. The woman's doctor reached for his prescription pad, giving her yet another medicine, this one called Aricept, which was supposed to slow the mental decline.

But the woman did not have Alzheimer's at all. Instead, Detrol had brought on the hallucinations and begun to steal her mind.

PHARMACIA WAS HARDLY the first drug company to use marketing to create a disease. By the beginning of the twenty-first century, the process of expanding markets by creating new maladies had become almost mechanized within the pharmaceutical industry.

In 2003 Vince Parry, a pharmaceutical branding expert, wrote in the industry magazine *Medical Marketing & Media* that marketers were taking their ability to create new disorders "to new levels of sophistication." He called this process "the art of branding a condition."

Parry knew what worked to sell prescription drugs. He was the chief branding officer at inChord Communications, Inc., a network of medical marketing companies with hundreds of employees.

"The idea behind 'condition branding' is relatively simple," he wrote. "If you can define a particular condition and its associated symptoms in the minds of physicians and patients, you can also predicate the best treatment for that condition."

Parry traced marketers' use of this technique back to the early twentieth century. He pointed to how the Lambert Company, which eventually became the drug giant Warner-Lambert, had greatly expanded the market for Listerine in the 1920s by creating public anxiety about a serious-sounding condition called halitosis. The word, which was first used around 1874, comes from the Latin word *halitus*. While it sounds like a dreadful malady that might cause death and suffering, it simply means having bad breath. In 1921 Gerald Lambert, the son of the company's founder, began a mass advertising campaign based on the word. The ads blamed halitosis for troubles ranging from a stagnant career to the failure to find a mate. The medical historian James Harvey Young wrote that Lambert increased Listerine's net earnings forty-fold through the ad campaign. The advertisements, he said, raised worries in readers' minds with slogans like this one: "You 5,000,000 women who want to get married: How's Your Breath Today?"

"This coined word frightened the continent," Young wrote, "not because bad breath was a fatal malady but because it was a social disaster."

Of all the categories of medical disorders, none is better suited for "condition branding," Parry explained, than the field of anxiety and depression. Because mental disorders are rarely based on measurable physical symptoms, he said, they are "open to conceptual definition." Many of the growing number of psychiatric conditions listed in the *Diagnostic and Statistical Manual of Mental Disorders*, the primary reference for psychiatrists, were brought to light through funding by the pharmaceutical companies, Parry wrote. For example, few Americans had heard of an illness called panic disorder, he said, before Upjohn began marketing a drug called Xanax to treat it in the 1970s. Likewise, few people knew they could be suffering from something called generalized anxiety disorder if they worried too much until GlaxoSmithKline told them that a pill called Paxil would ease its symptoms. And in 2000 millions of women learned they might suffer from something called premenstrual dysphoric disorder, or simply PMDD. News reports of the disorder began just as marketers at Eli Lilly repackaged Prozac in a lavender and pink capsule, renamed it the sweeter-sounding Sarafem, and began selling it to treat this new disease. Lilly's television ads promoting the "new" drug showed a frustrated woman trying to untangle a shopping cart from a messy lineup of carts in front of a store. "Think it's PMS?" the announcer asked. "It could be PMDD."

Lilly's marketing methods did not work as well in Europe. In December 2003 European regulators forced Lilly to stop selling Prozac, also known as fluoxetine, for the premenstrual disorder, saying it was "not a well-established disease."

"There was considerable concern that women with less severe premenstrual symptoms might erroneously receive a diagnosis of PMDD resulting in widespread inappropriate use of fluoxetine," wrote Lilly executives in a letter announcing the regulators' decision to British doctors.

MEDICAL MARKETERS OWE much of their success at creating new disorders to the fact that there is no real definition of disease. The word is nearly ubiquitous in everyday discussions about health, but scholars have never come to an agreement on its meaning.

"The word 'disease' is in general use without formal definition, most of those using it allowing themselves the comfortable delusion that everyone knows what it means," wrote J. G. Scadding, a professor of medicine at the University of London and a leading philosopher of diagnosis, in 1967.

Webster's defines disease as any deviation of a body from its normal or healthy state. But what is normal? And how does one define health, for that matter?

With these concepts so obscure, with hundreds of diagnostic tests available to determine whether we are sick, but no such test to confirm we are well, the possibilities for companies aiming to expand medicine markets are vast.

After listening to the marketers, Americans now ask for prescriptions to treat baldness, low sex drive, and menopause, all once considered a normal part of aging. Problems like heartburn and constipation, which are uncomfortable but hardly life-threatening, now demand a trip to the doctor. If a patient is said to benefit when his cholesterol level is less than 130, why can't he be helped more by taking additional pills to get it even lower? We now have clinical names and treatment guidelines for unhappiness, loneliness, and shyness, as if it were no longer okay to feel the emotions that make a life.

In 1992, years before the emergence of diseases like erectile dysfunction and overactive bladder, the journalist Lynn Payer warned that
medical marketers of all types—drug companies, doctors, hospitals, manufacturers of diagnostic tests, medical writers, and even patient advocacy groups—were convincing millions of healthy people that they were
ill. Medical marketing would be beneficial, she argued, if the amount of
disease were finite. Then medical providers would compete with one another to give patients the best treatment for their disease at the best possible price. But disease is a fluid and political concept, she said, which
means the marketers can create their own demand by concocting disorders and broadening the definition of disease to include more and more
people. The marketers "gnaw away at our self-confidence," she wrote.
"And that makes us really sick."

Perform enough tests and even the healthiest person will eventually
fail. The medical marketers say the three-step process of testing, diagnosis, and treatment helps lengthen lives. Often forgotten or not disclosed,
however, is the fact that the remedy of pills, injections, or surgeries might
be worse than the disease. Even the tests needed to find the disease—
the needles, the probing endoscopes, the radiation-emitting CT scans—
can harm. Unnecessary procedures also waste billions of dollars every
year. One study found that almost 40 percent of tests ordered by hospital physicians were not needed. More important, doctors can become so
distracted with finding disease that they no longer have enough time for
those who truly are sick.

In 1924, before the discovery of antibiotics and most of our modern-
day medicines, the French writer Jules Romains wrote a three-act play
titled *Knock* that was a telling portrait of America's future. Romains's
satire, which is still read by French schoolchildren, is the story of an am-
bitious doctor who comes to the sleepy town of Saint-Maurice. Dr. Knock
buys the practice of the town's longtime physician, who was known for
telling patients that time would heal their afflictions. Dr. Knock decides
he is not satisfied with the meager financial rewards that come from offering such medical advice. He vows to bring medical progress to Saint-
Maurice, while producing riches for himself.

Quickly, Dr. Knock makes use of the schoolmaster, asking him to instruct his students about the dangers of germs. He asks the town crier to tell the villagers that he is offering free consultations, although his services are not to remain free for long.

Soon Dr. Knock has diagnosed most of the townspeople with maladies, which he describes using big words and frightening terms that give him the voice of apparent authority. He also prescribes costly medicines and makes the town pharmacist his partner in the battle against disease, promising that his income will be tripled. The innkeeper also becomes wealthy as he transforms his hotel into a hospital.

By the end of the play, most of the townspeople are getting up at the same time each night to take their rectal temperatures, showing the power that Dr. Knock now has over them. Dr. Knock's underlying maxim: well people are sick people who simply don't know it—yet.

To CREATE A disease for Detrol, Pharmacia needed a regiment. It found its recruits among the world's physicians.

By the mid-1990s, many American doctors had grown frustrated with the financial limits imposed on them by health maintenance organizations and the other forms of managed care that became popular in the 1980s and 1990s as a way of restraining medical costs. Watching their salaries stall, the doctors were easily seduced by the welcoming arms of the drug industry, where the money still flowed. They found they could significantly boost their bank accounts and upgrade their lifestyles by winning favor with a pharmaceutical sales representative and joining a company's payroll as a speaker, consultant, researcher, or adviser or by serving in all these functions at the same time.

The doctors most in demand could boost their incomes by hundreds of thousands of dollars a year. Dr. Martin Keller, the chief of the psychiatry department at Brown University, earned more than $500,000 in consulting fees in 1998, mostly from companies whose drugs he touted at medical conferences and in published reports. In 2004 the written contract between Dr. Arnold Klein, a Beverly Hills dermatologist, and

Allergan, the company that makes Botox, became public when he was sued by a patient. The contract paid him $25,000 every three months for consulting and as much as $10,000 a day for meetings, plus expenses for airfare, hotel, and meals. By 2003 the drug companies had even re-cruited and hired many of the physicians and scientists at the federal government's esteemed National Institutes of Health. For instance, Pfizer paid Dr. P. Trey Sunderland, an expert on Alzheimer's disease, more than $500,000 between 1998 and 2004 for dozens of speaking appearances all over the world.

The industry had so many physicians on its payrolls that some drug companies created special services that allowed doctors to get paid or re-serve air travel and hotels with a simple call or click on a website. At a website created by Merck, doctors could find out when their checks from the company would arrive in the mail and make travel reservations twenty-four hours a day. Merck even let the doctors it was flying around the world select their "first choice" and "second choice" of hotels.

Most doctors saw nothing wrong with this.

"They are making a lot of hay about nothing," said Dr. Charles B. Nemeroff, the chairman of the department of psychiatry at Emory School of Medicine, after two scientists raised concerns about how he had fa-vorably described some experimental treatments for depression without disclosing his financial ties to the corporate developers. At the time, Dr. Nemeroff was a paid speaker for ten drugmakers and a consultant to twenty-three pharmaceutical companies.

But marketing experts working for the industry know better. They say drug companies make far more money by using their promotional budg-ets to hire physicians to vouch for their products than by spending the same amount on either advertising or sales representatives.

"Your entire sales force making calls for an entire year may not be as effective as one trusted expert recommending your product at a con-ference," wrote George Silverman, a marketing consultant, in 2000. Silverman's expertise was in what he called word-of-mouth marketing. Companies can spur prescriptions by getting a physician to tell his peers about the benefits of a new drug, he said, as long as the message is de-livered in a way that makes it appear to be independent. These messages are now delivered at hundreds of thousands of dinner meetings, expert roundtables, conferences, educational courses, focus groups, and advisory boards that the companies organize and pay for every year.

Silverman was a former psychologist who founded Market Navigation, a consulting firm in Orangeburg, New York, in 1979. He claimed to have worked on some of the most successful product launches in the pharmaceutical industry's history. In his free time, Silverman performed as an illusionist and was a member of the Academy of Magical Arts, a private club in Hollywood. He used his illusions in seminars, he explained, to show the parallels between marketing and magic.

"I just like to remind people that things are not always as they seem," he said, "[that] there's more than meets the eye, that you have to examine conventional wisdom because much of it is just very realistic-looking illusion."

By the late 1990s, the industry's method of paying doctors to market their products was so successful that many Madison Avenue advertising firms had created internal divisions that specialized in organizing the events where the industry-hired physicians lectured. Employees working in these divisions hired and trained doctors to speak at the dinners and meetings, created colorful presentations of slides and written materials, and often wrote the text of speeches to be delivered.

A marketing firm called Thomson Physicians World said in a 2002 brochure that it had signed up more than twenty thousand physicians to speak on behalf of the drug industry. These doctors, Physicians World promised, would "become critical linchpins in product positioning."

At the Pharmaceutical Marketing Congress in 2002, corporate drug executives provided more details on how they selected their physicians. Eric Pauwels, an executive from Bayer, led a panel discussion on "Prelaunch Marketing Strategies" before a room packed with pharmaceutical marketers. Among the panelists were Andrea P. Bruell, the director and global commercial leader at Johnson & Johnson, and Libby Keating, U.S. marketing director at AstraZeneca. The panelists agreed that a key to creating a blockbuster seller was getting doctors on the company's payroll early—months, if not years, before the drug was expected to be approved.

"How many times do we get close to launch and say, 'We have to have someone talk about our product?'" Pauwels asked.

To find these doctors, Keating said she attended medical meetings and listened to the speakers. She also searched the medical literature to see what doctors' names came up again and again.

Bruell said that Johnson & Johnson often did not pick the most vocal and popular experts that Keating had described. Instead, she said, Johnson & Johnson selected some physicians who "are not well known, but have potential."

"We can build their reputation in the community," she explained.

Pauwels agreed with Bruell. He said Bayer also did not stop at the top-level experts. "We work with the second-tier or the rising stars," he said. These doctors, he said, "are probably more willing to say Product X is better than Product Y."

PHARMACIA PAID TO gather its physicians at several large meetings, including two symposia held in London, the first in 1997 and the second in 1999.

Marketers like Neil Wolf referred to the physicians they recruited as "thought leaders," "key opinion leaders," or simply "KOLs."

"We used KOLs to change the way urologists spoke about the condition," Wolf told the audience as he continued his presentation.

Pharmacia covered most, if not all, of the expenses of these symposia in London and also paid many of the doctors who attended. Some of the physicians became the company's longtime consultants. Some went on to make many speeches for Pharmacia before their peers. Others were paid to perform clinical trials or write medical journal articles.

At the symposia, Pharmacia's urologists discussed how overactive bladder should be defined. They eventually agreed with the drug company that a patient did not have to be incontinent to have the disease of overactive bladder. Instead, frequently running to the toilet or having sudden, overwhelming feelings that one needed to urinate was enough to be diagnosed with the disease. The doctors talked about how they believed, just as Pharmacia's executives believed, that this new disease could have a "profound" effect on a patient's quality of life. An overactive bladder, they said, could cause sexual dysfunction, emotional problems, and withdrawal from social activities. They also talked about Detrol and how clinical trials (paid for by Pharmacia) had found the drug was not only safe and effective but one of the best medicines to treat the disease.

Pharmacia then paid to have the proceedings of the two London meetings published in supplements to the prominent medical journal *Urology* and distributed to physicians around the world. The first supplement in December 1997 had thirty articles, many of them written by doctors whom Pharmacia had put on its payroll. The articles showed how Pharmacia's wagon could get in front of its pony. One article said that "generally accepted definitions" of overactive bladder had not yet been established, although it was "highly desirable" to do so. Another article, appearing deeper in the supplement, concluded that Detrol had been found to be a "safe and long-term effective treatment" for the disease that the previous author had explained was not yet defined.

Some may wonder why a highly regarded scientific journal like *Urology* would allow its pages to be used for such blatant commercial purposes. Yet it is only one example of how even the publishers of prominent medical journals became part of the vast enterprise of marketing prescription drugs during the 1990s. *Urology* is published by Reed Elsevier, a global publisher of journals, books, and other information. According to the company's website in 2004, it had a "pharmaceutical division" that offered drugmakers "the opportunity to use the brand name of one of Elsevier's distinguished biomedical journals to publish and disseminate your conference material or scientific findings to as wide or as targeted an audience as appropriate."

"Our aim," Elsevier said, "is to ensure that we are the first choice marketing and education solutions provider for the pharmaceutical industry throughout the world."

One could argue that it was not Pharmacia but the physicians it had hired as consultants who created the disease of overactive bladder. The names of these doctors are in the medical journal articles that laid out the definition of the disease. But Wolf gave Pharmacia the credit. Industry marketing experts went further. They credited Wolf himself.

"Neil Wolf isn't embarrassed to talk about overactive bladder," explained an article in *Advertising Age* magazine in June 1999. "In fact, he helped coin the term."

Indeed, Wolf and other Pharmacia executives had aimed to control the debate each step of the way. Pharmacia paid for the meetings where the physicians it had hired as consultants urged the attendees, who included even more doctors on the drugmaker's payroll, to come to a consensus on how to define and treat this new disease. When one is being paid by a company that is also hosting your party—perhaps even paying your airfare, putting you up in a four-star hotel, and treating you to exquisite meals and wine—and you hear another Pharmacia-paid physician say he has patients who have been disabled by the nine visits they make to the restroom each day, how much incentive is there to stand up and say, "You must be crazy! How can using the toilet nine times a day mean you have a disease? Couldn't treating these patients with a powerful drug bring more harm than good?"

If any doctors had the courage to raise their hands and question the company that was paying the bills, their comments never made it into the dozens of articles on the new disease that Pharmacia paid to have written, published, and dispersed.

And another disease was born.

IT WAS TIME for Pharmacia to switch targets and sell its new disorder to the American public. The company's goal, Wolf said, was to convince frequent restroom users that their overactive bladders were not just an annoyance or an inconvenience but a serious condition requiring professional medical care. Pharmacia set out to generate some buzz.

In the last two decades, the pharmaceutical industry had become adept at working behind the scenes to get people talking about their products. Executives found this tactic appealing because they could avoid government regulations that limited what could be promised in advertisements. In ads, companies cannot overstate the benefits of a drug or understate the harm that can come from taking it. But if covert corporate marketers are clever, if they create a buzz-generating event that looks real and unplanned, neither the public nor the regulators may discover what is really going on.

For instance, the actress Lauren Bacall told Matt Lauer in an interview on NBC's *Today* show in 2002 about a drug called Visudyne, which she claimed would have stopped her friend from going blind. The actress urged viewers to go to their doctors and find out if they also needed the drug. She did not mention she was on the payroll of Novartis, the medicine's maker.

On an episode of *ER*, the NBC television series, a patient with Alzheimer's disease is treated with a medicine called Aricept. Writers put the pill into the script at the urging of the public relations firm working for Pfizer. The firm later boasted that twenty-five million Americans had learned about Pfizer's medicine from the television show.

And in a video paid for by Wyeth-Ayerst, the maker of the hormone replacement therapy Prempro, Lauren Hutton boasted she "started looking a lot better" after she began taking the drug. "I can go into a room and pretty much tell who is and who isn't taking estrogen," the supermodel said. The pills, she added, even helped her sex life. With menopause, "you get irritable so you don't feel like doing anything," she said. "You don't even want to go to the movies, much less have sex. But once I got it all worked out, I sometimes go to the movies two or three times a day."

Six months after that December 2000 video, government researchers announced they had shut down a study of Prempro after finding it caused a higher risk of breast cancer, heart disease, and stroke. While the drug would remain on the market, the news startled millions of women who had believed the daily pills would keep them vigorous, sexy, and young.

Robert Chandler and Gianfranco Chicco were two of the industry's top experts on producing buzz about pharmaceutical products. They operated a global public relations firm from an office in the heart of Manhattan's meatpacking district. While the two men agreed that doctors had long been among the industry's most powerful "buzz drivers," they said they had found that just about anyone—from politicians to the president of the local PTA—could be employed to generate positive twitter about a pill.

"While buzz should always appear to be spontaneous," they wrote in 2002, "it should, in fact, be scientifically crafted and controlled as tightly as advertising in *The New England Journal of Medicine*."

Done in the right way, they explained, these events could generate conversations and excitement for a drug that increased demand for it "virtually overnight."

The "ultimate goal," they said, was for the company to "sell the consumer a message or product without the consumer even being aware that a 'sell' is taking place."

PATRICK PERRY, A writer for *The Saturday Evening Post*, caught up with Debbie Reynolds during her tour through Canada. The aging star of *Singin' in the Rain* was as sunny and feisty as ever.

"I love the road, greasepaint and the roar of the crowd," Reynolds exclaimed. "I love performing live." Yet there was a reason she was still singing and dancing after reaching the age of seventy. Her variety shows would not be possible, she said, without a medicine called Detrol.

"Overactive bladder affects you because it defects you," she explained to Perry. She had been forced to plan her life around her overactive bladder, she said, avoiding long car trips and making sure she knew the location of the restroom everywhere she went. Reynolds added a bit of reassurance to any reader horrified to realize that he or she had these defects too. "People do not need to be frightened."

Anyone who believes that he is suffering, she said, should call his doctor. "Effective treatment is available," she advised. "Years ago, there wasn't any help."

Perry's article featuring Reynolds appeared in January 2003. He wrote that the movie star had launched Standing Ovations, a campaign to raise awareness of the condition called overactive bladder. He did not mention that the actress was actually working for Pharmacia, which had created Standing Ovations to help sell its new bladder pills.

The Saturday Evening Post was hardly the only media outlet to help Pharmacia spread word of the strange new bladder affliction. Dozens of journalists at newspapers and television stations across the country wrote stories about the disorder said to be destroying the lives of millions of Americans. Editors and television news directors loved these reports. Silly stories of people running to the toilet brightened the day's news. And the journalists did not have to work hard. Pharmacia's public relations staff offered the reporters all they needed for a good read: suffering patients, concerned doctors, and a new miracle drug to help make the troubles disappear. Mr. Wolf told the audience in Philadelphia that he was especially pleased by an article written by Jane Brody, which appeared in *The New York Times* in 1998. It began, "For the last decade, Susan, a Long Island businesswoman who recently turned 50, has been plagued by an annoying and potentially humiliating problem: She has to empty her bladder a dozen or more times a day."

Pharmacia made sure that no journalist needed to track down statistics. The company created them by paying for opinion polls and surveys. Knowing that romance sells in America, Pharmacia's poll in 2001 quizzed people on their bladder problems and sex lives. The survey's result: half the Americans surveyed who said they were not in a sexual relationship blamed their empty lives on their overactive bladders.

While many journalists used these statistics in their news reports, federal regulators were less than pleased when the company used results from one of its surveys in a sales brochure. The brochure featured photos of smiling men and women and claimed that patients taking Detrol had reported "an improved sense of well being." According to the brochure, 74 percent of the patients taking the pill "felt more confident when going out," while 73 percent "felt free from concern about their overactive bladder." The FDA sent a warning letter to Pharmacia in December 2000, insisting it stop using the brochure and the statistics. The numbers were not supported by evidence, the regulators said, and came from nothing more than a market research survey of patients taking Detrol. On top of that, Pharmacia appeared to have biased the survey results to favor Detrol, the regulators said, by questioning only patients who were satisfied with their pills. The pollsters had not included patients who started to take Detrol only to find the drug did not work or had side effects they could not tolerate.

Yet the statistics kept coming. In 2003 a group of researchers published a survey saying they had found that more than 16 percent of the

American population suffered from overactive bladders. The survey, called the National Overactive Bladder Evaluation program, included some fine print. It had been paid for by Pharmacia, and its authors included a Pharmacia executive and several of the company's longtime physician consultants.

Pharmacia's marketers had created the disease and a new medicine market, and now they were expanding it, making it even more lucrative. And drug companies of all sizes began funneling more of their research dollars into developing medicines aimed at keeping busy Americans away from the toilet. In 2003 the Swiss drugmaker Novartis, flush with cash from selling the antifungal drug Lamisil and other medicines to Americans, plunked down $225 million for an experimental bladder pill that was being considered for approval by the FDA. The Novartis chairman, Daniel Vasella, estimated then that the market for overactive bladder medicines was growing by 30 percent a year.

Competitors tried to imitate Pharmacia's proven sales techniques. After Pharmacia paid to have the American Society of Travel Agents hand out advice to travelers on medical conditions including overactive bladder, Alza Corporation, the maker of a pill called Ditropan, turned to professional golfers and female executives. In 2001 Alza used Bruce Devlin, a professional golfer and television sports analyst, to tell the public about his frequent bathroom visits. Four years later, the maker of Ditropan paid for a campaign where the National Association of Female Executives warned women that there was a 20 percent chance that they might be suffering from an overactive bladder.

At the same time, Pharmacia began spending millions of dollars on television advertisements. The commercials showed scenes of a juror in a courtroom and a school crossing guard struggling to control their bladders, while a jingle played "Gotta go, gotta go, gotta go right now." Pharmacia also created a five-question screening guide that doctors could use to diagnose their patients swiftly. "Do you go to the bathroom so often that it interferes with the things you do (more than 8 times in 24 hours)?" the questionnaire asked. "Do you always have to know where the bathroom is because of frequent, strong, sudden urges to urinate?" To let consumers diagnose themselves, Pharmacia published these questions in ads in publications like *Reader's Digest*. One inventive sales representative taped the questionnaire inside the bathroom stalls in physicians' offices.

Pharmacia's marketing skills and its fast-rising sales soon attracted a suitor. Pfizer, the world's largest drug company, bought Pharmacia in 2002. Marketers at Pfizer, considered among the most aggressive in the industry, quickly found a way to expand the market for Detrol even more. The Pfizer marketers replaced the aging Debbie Reynolds with a younger, more athletic star to show Americans that overactive bladder was not just a problem for the older set. Twenty years after she had won an Olympic gold medal, gymnast Mary Lou Retton was traveling to shopping malls across the country and being paid by Pfizer to tell people they did not need to be dashing for the toilet.

One of Retton's first stops on her Pfizer tour was the Cincinnati Mills Mall in Ohio, where she spoke to shoppers about "taking charge of your own success" and about how Detrol was keeping her out of the bathroom. Shoppers posed for photos with the gymnast and signed up to win a new Ford pickup truck. "I wish I hadn't waited so long to talk to my doctor," Retton said, "but I didn't realize this was a health problem that could happen to anyone, even someone my age."

Over the years, federal regulators tried to police all the promotional noise created by Pharmacia and its competitors. Between 1999 and 2001, the FDA repeatedly sent letters to both Pharmacia and Alza, warning them that their promotion was illegal because it described the pills as safer and more effective than they really were. The regulators found that the companies were making claims that were not backed by scientific studies.

In 1999, for instance, Pharmacia claimed in an ad aimed at physicians that Detrol worked more selectively on a patient's bladder than on her salivary glands. To doctors, this claim was important. It implied that Detrol was better at causing a dry bladder than a dry mouth, which is a frequent side effect of the pill. But the FDA pointed out that Pharmacia's study on selectivity was not even done on humans. Instead, it was a study on cats.

The FDA said Alza had broken the law by claiming in a promotional letter sent to consumers that a study had shown that Ditropan reduced

wetting accidents by up to 90 percent. The FDA said Alza had manipulated the study in a way that made Ditropan look more effective than it
really was. To do that, the company had chosen only patients it knew
would benefit from the pill. These patients had already taken a similar
drug with the same active ingredient as Ditropan and had shown success. In essence, the study had been rigged.

But the FDA's actions had little effect. The agency's small staff
charged with monitoring the industry's marketing campaigns, which
were growing ever more sophisticated and secretive and so extensive
they could cost hundreds of millions of dollars for a single drug, were
like a couple of cops trying to enforce the NO HONKING signs posted on
street corners in Manhattan.

By early 2006, Detrol was selling at a rate that would bring Pfizer an
expected one billion dollars for the year, earning it a place among the
industry's coveted blockbusters.

Said Neil Wolf, the man behind it all: "Overactive bladder has now
become part of the American lexicon."

SHE WAS ONLY forty-six, but her memories fell away as if her mind
were riddled with holes. She forgot meetings at work and outings with her
family. She coped by trying to write things down. Remembering numbers was almost impossible. Sometimes, when she spoke, the words came
out in the wrong order.

Another woman, age seventy-three, suffered a similar swift decline.
At first, she had vivid hallucinations of dead relatives. Then she began to
forget. Her husband brought her to the doctor, who diagnosed Alzheimer's disease.

Neurologists at the University of Florida studied the women's cases.
They questioned whether the diagnosis of Alzheimer's disease had been
too swift. They went over the clues and began to understand what connected the two women: they both had lost their memories after beginning to take Detrol.

Both women regained much of their memories after they stopped
taking the pills. But for the older woman, it took many weeks. The neurol-

ogists, who had been working in a clinic directed by Dr. Kenneth Heilman, wrote up reports about the women and published them in prominent medical journals to warn doctors that Detrol could cause dementia.

"Some people have a mild impairment," said Dr. Jack Tsao, one of the neurologists, "and this pushes them over the edge."

The cases of the two Florida women were some of the early reports of how Detrol could harm the memories of those who take it. In 2005 academic researchers at Emory University in Atlanta reported similar problems. They found that the cognition of patients with Alzheimer's disease grew worse when they took either Detrol or Ditropan.

Both bladder drugs have what doctors call anticholinergic effects, which means they block the action of acetylcholine, a neurotransmitter. Nerve cells release neurotransmitters to send signals to neighboring cells. The anticholinergic medicines block some of these signals. Many drugs, including some used to treat allergies, anxiety, blood pressure, convulsions, depression, Parkinson's disease, and psychosis, have been found to have anticholinergic effects. So many medicines have anticholinergic effects that some people may be taking two or more of these drugs at the same time.

Scientists have found what they believe is physical evidence of harm from these anticholinergic drugs in the brain. In 2003 British researchers studied the brains of patients who had died from Parkinson's disease. They found that the brains of the patients who had taken anticholinergic drugs for two years or longer had more than twice the level of abnormal clumps of amyloid plaque and tangled bundles of fibers as those who had not taken the drugs or had taken them for a short time. Such plaque and tangled fibers in the brain are considered the hallmarks of Alzheimer's disease.

Doctors have found that this medication-induced dementia often reverses if it is found and the patient stops taking the offending drug. But how many people never learn that it was their medicine that took their minds away?

Pharmacia had created a disease, but its remedy was harming some people in ways not worth fewer visits to the bathroom.

TWO

Midwestern Medicine Show

OF THE FIFTY states, there was one I believed the medicine merchants might find the least alluring. Sitting in the heart of Middle America, Iowa is a place where change takes time to happen. In the state's towns and cities, parking lots are full of roomy American-made cars. Men wear flannel shirts and caps printed with their brand of seed corn. Radio stations play songs by REO Speedwagon and the Doobie Brothers decades after they have fallen off the charts. In many parts, cows outnumber the human residents. Out there one is struck by how far the eye can see. Travelers on a county road might see a silver grain elevator rise up like the wizard's castle in the Land of Oz, marking the location of a town still miles away. There is a good chance that the one-stoplight town of twenty years ago is still a one-stoplight town today.

I grew up in Iowa, lived there for twenty-one years. In the place I remembered, people had a no-nonsense way of getting around their troubles without a lot of complaints. It was a state, for example, where few people were all that surprised by stories like that of seventy-three-year-old Alvin Straight. Unable to drive a car because of worsening vision, Straight drove his '66 John Deere lawn mower some 240 miles to Wisconsin in 1994 to see an ailing brother. At the mower's top speed of five miles per hour, the trip took six weeks.

Like Straight, the Iowans I knew were people who seemed determined to make it on their own. They were not the sort to put blind faith in a chemical remedy for the woes of modern life, not the type to swear that a pill would, according to the ad for Paxil, "let the world say hello to the real you."

Certainly, I thought, the drug marketers would face resistance in my home state. And so, on the last day of spring 2005, I flew back to Iowa to talk to people, listen to stories, and just hang around to see who might turn up.

HER EYES WERE closed, and her lips formed a gentle smile. A beautiful woman with long dark hair and flawless olive-colored skin, she seemed to be dreaming as she floated among the clouds. She slept peacefully even though the pharmaceutical sales representative had set her down next to the ham sandwiches and cans of pop chilling on ice. The angelic woman, a model featured in a large poster advertising the sleeping pill Ambien, served as a suggestive centerpiece as twenty Iowa women filed by the table to pick up their free lunches. The women chatted about the sudden bout of hot, humid June weather before settling into their seats to listen to the drug saleswoman tell them how they too could fall into blissful slumber.

The staff at the sand-colored brick medical center in Storm Lake, a town of twenty thousand people nestled among the cornfields of northwestern Iowa, had invited the public to learn about insomnia from Rebecca Hillmer, a sales rep for Sanofi-Aventis, a French drug company with extensive and expanding operations in the United States.

The women who had come to lunch and learn did not look like the type that might be losing sleep by spending too much time at Malarky's, the purple-painted place for food and spirits just down the street. Many of the women were older residents of the town built at the edge of the windy blue lake it was named for. Other women in the audience were nurses, who could take whatever they learned from Ms. Hillmer back to their patients. The woman in the well-tailored pantsuit sitting next to me whispered in my ear that she believed it was her antidepressant medication that was keeping her up.

Sanofi's aggressive marketing of Ambien had Americans taking sleeping pills at a pace not seen before. Even a small but fast-growing number of children were now settling down for the night with the help of an Ambien tablet. Between 2000 and 2004 the number of children ages ten to nineteen taking prescription sleeping pills had increased by 85 percent.

Now, however, a new pill called Lunesta was raising anxiety among the Sanofi executives. A competing company had announced it would be spending as much money to promote Lunesta as McDonald's was paying to promote its fast food. The Lunesta ads appearing on television and in magazines featured an evanescent luna moth quietly fluttering in a deep purple starry night and offered slogans like "For refreshing sleep—night after night after night." It was this "night after night" part that had the French company's executives particularly stewing. When Sanofi's product, Ambien, was approved, the FDA required the company to warn doctors it should rarely be prescribed for more than ten days. The company's pill was so dangerous that the Drug Enforcement Administration controlled its use as tightly as potent tranquilizers like Halcion, Valium, and Miltown. Many doctors hesitated to prescribe it.

Sanofi executives had decided to go around those physicians and push their product directly to an overworked, stressed-out public, including the women of Storm Lake. Ms. Hillmer, a middle-aged saleswoman with silver wire-rim glasses and short graying hair, stood before the women in a black business suit in the hospital's Education Center. She told the women she had gone to Buena Vista University, a centerpiece of this town of quiet, leafy neighborhoods and more than a dozen churches. Ms. Hillmer also told them she knew so much about insomnia that her colleagues had dubbed her "the sleep queen."

"I work for a pharmaceutical company," she said, "but I'm not here to push any medication."

She did not mention Ms. Ambien, who was sleeping in the poster back by the soda pop.

As the women munched their potato chips and oatmeal raisin cookies, Ms. Hillmer spoke of the ills that could befall them if they did not get their sleep. Insomnia, she said, could hurt their memories, increase their moodiness, and lead to heart disease. Missing sleep might make them obese, she said, and lead to "some severe psychotic issues." And it can cause automobile crashes, she said, when insomniacs doze off behind the wheel.

To illustrate this last point, Ms. Hillmer invited a silver-haired woman wearing a bright blue gingham jacket to try on a pair of goggles. Schoolteachers used the eyewear, she said, to show kids how blurred their vision would be if they tried to drive drunk. The woman reluctantly pulled on the glasses and tried to walk. "Do I look drunk?" she mumbled as she stumbled down the aisle.

Ms. Hillmer waved her hands in the air, gesturing at her volunteer. "I don't mean to scare you," she told the women, "but it's just something we don't think about." Her message in short: insomnia threatened the nation's health and could kill you on the drive home.

She then told the women what might help them sleep. She talked about what she called sleep hygiene, which included steps like avoiding caffeine and not exercising just before bed. And if these measures fail, she said, "see your physician" for medications "that work."

"Some of the sleep medications—the newer ones—they work right away," she said. They'll knock you out so fast, she said, that you had just "better have your pajamas on and your teeth brushed" before swallowing one.

She asked if the women had questions. One by one, the women began admitting to their sleepless nights the way one might admit to alcoholism at an AA meeting.

"I have this problem," said a fortyish woman in T-shirt and jeans. She explained how she dozed for a couple hours and then woke up for two hours, a cycle that left her with little more than four hours of sleep each night. "I have like no energy on Saturday," she said.

"Talk to your physician," Ms. Hillmer said helpfully. "There are medications that can help with that." She told the woman that it was probably her anxiety or depression that was keeping her up. "There's no shame in that," the saleswoman said.

"I think it's hormones," the woman muttered.

Ms. Hillmer thanked the women for listening, urging each one to pick up one of the "sleep kits" she had placed in a stack by Ms. Ambien on their way out. The sleep kit was a black plastic case etched with the pink and aqua Ambien logo. Inside were a deck of playing cards embossed with the Ambien brand name, a compact disc with soothing music, and a card to send away for a free Ambien sleep mask, as long as one also provided the drug company with her name, address, and a description of her personal sleep problems. The *All About Ambien* brochure inside the kit boasted that the company's pill was "the #1 prescribed sleep aid in the U.S."

In the end, Ms. Hillmer never actually spoke the word "Ambien," but I can't say that mattered. She also never told the women about the possible dangers of those newer medications that "work right away." According to the information that the government requires Sanofi to tell doctors and patients about its drug, Ambien's risks do not end with its high potential for addictiveness. Because the sedative can make one dizzy and sleepy during the day, patients must be warned against driving, operating heavy machinery, or piloting a plane. In other words, Ambien can cause the very accidents that Ms. Hillmer suggested could happen without adequate sleep. Patients who stop taking Ambien can suffer from "withdrawal insomnia" and have even more trouble falling asleep. Some people who have taken Ambien have woken up and not remembered events from the previous day, according to the drug's written warnings. Others have said that Ambien caused them to sleepwalk and do other strange things while they were sleeping, including eating an entire loaf of bread. Some have said they got into their cars and drove while they were asleep. Still other Ambien users have hallucinated, acted aggressively, or contemplated suicide. People over the age of sixty-five, who made up about half the women at the luncheon, are particularly susceptible to suffering harm from sleeping pills, including Ambien. The pills can cause older people to lose their memories or to fall if they become dizzy. The elderly take sleeping pills at the highest rate of any age-group, but on average they gain only twenty-five minutes of extra sleep a night.

Ms. Hillmer's sales tactics had not been aggressive like those of a promoter of vacation time shares. Instead, her approach had been far more subtle but quite effective.

After Sanofi's insomnia class, I stopped at the local Hy-Vee supermarket for a soft drink for the drive back to my parents' farm, which was two hours south. I parked next to a large sign that said, FILL YOUR PRESCRIPTIONS AT YOUR FRIENDLY HY-VEE. Inside, I walked down the liquor aisle to get to the pharmacy, where employees had laid out free copies of a glossy magazine. The publication was filled with pharmaceutical ads, including one from Sanofi that said I could try Ambien, the pill so tightly controlled by the DEA, for free.

Late that afternoon, I watched the national news on NBC. In between reports of what the network reporter called an amazing new treatment for Alzheimer's, even though it still had years of testing before possibly being considered for government approval, and a cheerily delivered report entitled "Life-saving Medicine: What's Our Future?" was an ad for Ambien, the pill that "works like a dream."

THE FREE LUNCH of ham sandwiches in Storm Lake was just the beginning of the trail of promotion and hype that I found as I followed the drug marketers through my home state. You can't buy health, but the pharmaceutical companies were everywhere, trying to sell it.

Over the weeks I spent in Iowa, I found prescription drug advertisements on scoreboards at a golf tournament, in bass fishing magazines, and in the small weekly newspaper of my hometown, population 810. The marketers' announcements came over the radio, the television, and the loudspeaker in a drugstore in Des Moines. Even if Iowans turned off their television sets and threw away their magazines, the pharmaceutical companies had ways of reaching them. I found the medicine promoters at the mall, on college campuses, and sitting on the board of a local chapter of the American Heart Association. In a library used by the public schools I stumbled upon a storybook created by a company to promote its antidepressant. I discovered the drug companies screening Iowans for diseases, while their salespeople stood nearby, handing out brochures touting the product that just happened to treat the malady they were being tested for. The companies had moved far beyond being merely the providers of medicines. They seemed to be omnipresent, carefully controlling the flow of information.

And like Big Brother, the drug companies were quietly collecting information on the public, accumulating it in corporate databases, which they could then use to make personal appeals to those they hoped would become their lifelong customers. This was part of a promotional tactic the marketers called compliance, which was aimed at keeping Iowans on their daily meds.

MANY OF THE marketers' ads were written with words meant to create fear that disease was just around the corner. Iowans opened magazines to read ads with taglines like "What you don't know could kill you" and the ominous "All it may take is the formation of one clot."

Take this quick test, the ads urged. Monitor your numbers. Talk to your doctor. Do it for your children's sake.

The advertisements sold not only medicines but youth, happiness, friends, beauty, and sex. Implicitly, they promised a utopia of endless days of leisure, romance that was sweet or searing, and even a perfect family, as if those who medicated together stayed together.

The brown-eyed boy beamed in an ad for Adderall, an amphetamine drug for children diagnosed with attention deficit hyperactivity disorder, in the August 2005 issue of *Good Housekeeping* magazine. "Finally! Family hours that last for hours. Friends that ask him to join a group. Schoolwork that matches his intelligence. A trusted solution for ADHD."

An underlying message in the ads was that the medicine would bring about a sort of personal transformation. Those who swallowed the pills would enjoy the good life. They would be more lovable. They would be envied by their neighbors. These tacit promises made by the drug ads were not unlike those made by the promoters of any other consumer product.

"The purpose of publicity is to make the spectator marginally dissatisfied with his present way of life. Not with the way of life of society, but with his own within it," explained John Berger, the art critic, in a classic essay on advertising in 1972. "It suggests that if he buys what it is offering, his life will become better. It offers him an improved alternative to what he is."

"Experience Life," proclaimed the promotional brochure for the antidepressant Wellbutrin that I picked up at an Iowa pharmacy. The brochure showed a scene that could have been the cover of a romance novel. A handsome man swept a young, slender woman off her high heels, just as she stepped off a train.

A television ad on the 5:30 p.m. news used tactics more like those employed by Victoria's Secret, the retailer of women's lingerie. This ad, for a drug called Levitra, promised improved "erectile quality." The ad had nothing to do with treating an illness. It was all about using pills for recreation.

"Strong. Lasting. When he wants it," said the raven-haired actress in a seductive, husky voice. "That's what Levitra is all about."

The language of the advertisements for many pills described the products as powerful and precise, claims that could not always be supported. WORKS FAST. RAISES YOUR PROTECTION. DRAMATICALLY CLEARS SKIN. DRAMATICALLY REDUCES THE PAIN. HEALS THE DAMAGE. HELPS YOU SLEEP.

IT'S NOT MAGIC, said one ad. IT'S BOTOX COSMETIC.

The chirpy slogans for medicines like Zelnorm (Be Yourself Again), Levitra (Stay in the Game), and Restylane (Natural Beauty. It's Yours for the Asking) were hard to distinguish from those for Burger King (Have It Your Way), Wheaties (The Breakfast of Champions), and Eve cigarettes (The first truly feminine cigarette—almost as pretty as you are).

In 1946, George Orwell observed that language can corrupt our thoughts. The "invasion of one's mind by ready-made phrases . . . can only be prevented if one is constantly on guard against them, and every such phrase anaesthetizes a portion of one's brain."

There was no question that the drug companies were attempting such an invasion. In 2005 the pharmaceutical companies were among the biggest spenders on advertising in the United States. In the eleven months leading up to April 2005, seven of the ten biggest advertisers on

46 OUR DAILY MEDS

the *CBS Evening News* were pharmaceutical companies. There were eight pages of prescription drug ads in the twenty-four-page *Parade* magazine tucked inside the newspapers of three hundred American cities on Sunday, February 12, 2006, including Mason City, Iowa's *Globe Gazette*.

The ads in newspapers and magazines included lengthy warnings about the medicine's dangers to satisfy federal rules. But the marketers wrote these sections using complicated medical language that the common American could not understand. The warnings were often printed in type so small that many readers would need a magnifying glass.

The promotions promised magic for patients, but they worked miracles for the pharmaceutical companies. According to one survey, 35 percent of American adults said an ad had prompted them to ask their doctors about a drug or a health condition. More often than not doctors gave these patients the prescriptions they asked about—even when the patients did not actually have the disease. In a study in 2005, doctors prescribed antidepressants to more than half the patients who specifically asked for Paxil, even though these patients did not meet the symptoms of depression and instead had mild, temporary problems, like stress caused by accepting an offer for voluntary retirement.

Some Iowa doctors aided the drug marketers by placing their own ads in the Sunday edition of *The Des Moines Register*. "Erection problems?" asked an advertisement on June 26, 2005, by the Lakeview Center for Urology. "You are not alone." The ad urged Iowans to "call now" and "get your love life back." The clinic's ad helped sell drugs like Viagra and Levitra. But these entrepreneurial doctors were using the language of the pharmaceutical marketers to boost their personal incomes. Each Iowan who responded meant new revenue from office exams, diagnostic tests, and procedures. The doctors had learned they could imitate the pharmaceutical industry's marketing techniques and join in the financial bonanza.

WHY DO THE pharmaceutical companies need to spend 25 percent or more of their revenues on promotion? Because for one thing, the drugs don't work for large numbers of people who take them. The industry's own scientists, executives, and clinical studies confirm this.

"The vast majority of drugs—more than 90 percent—only work in 30 or 50 percent of the people," Dr. Allen Roses, a top executive at Glaxo-SmithKline, said at a meeting in London in December 2003. Dr. Roses was referring to the work of one of his peers, Dr. Brian B. Spear, a scientist at Abbott Laboratories. In 2001 Dr. Spear reviewed the effectiveness of drugs prescribed for fourteen diseases. He and his colleagues found that the medicines worked in as few as 25 percent of patients who took them. Drugs prescribed to strengthen bones worked in only 48 percent of patients taking them for osteoporosis. Pills swallowed to ease migraines succeeded only about 50 percent of the time. Medicines taken to stop incontinence were even less effective, easing bladder problems for only 40 percent of patients.

Dr. Spear and Dr. Roses are experts in pharmacogenetics, an evolving science that is trying to make drugs work better and have fewer side effects by tailoring them to an individual's genes. The hope is that one day doctors will be able to administer simple genetic tests to each patient to determine what medicine will best help him or her. But such frank disclosures about the ineffectiveness of our current medicines lead one to the realization that for decades marketers have been spending heavily to sell their pills to as many patients as possible when they actually work for only a fraction of them.

"If you look across all drug categories today," said Mara G. Aspinall, the president of Genzyme Genetics, "an average of 50 percent of people treated with individual drugs are receiving treatments that are not efficacious for them."

In a discussion with academics in 2006, Ms. Aspinall explained that 30 to 70 percent of patients get no benefit from taking statins, which are designed to reduce cholesterol. As many as 50 percent of patients, she said, are not helped by antidepressants.

Often it is the most heavily marketed drugs that perform the worst.

For example, researchers have struggled to see any improvement at all in patients with Alzheimer's disease who take drugs like Aricept, which was promoted in 2005 with an ad showing a healthy grandmother playing and laughing with her grandchild. The ad's tagline: "Helping people be more like themselves longer." That claim did not match what a group of scientists found in 2006 after analyzing eighteen clinical trials of Aricept and two similar drugs, Razadyne and Exelon. The researchers found that patients taking the pills showed an average improvement of just 2.7 points on a 70-point scale measuring their cognitive function.

This problem can be far more tragic than a waste of money on expensive drugs that do not work. Even an ineffective drug can have side effects, especially for frail and elderly Alzheimer's patients.

Johnson & Johnson warned doctors in 2005 that thirteen patients had died while taking Razadyne in a clinical trial. Among the patients taking the sugar pill in that same trial, only one patient had died. In another trial, eleven patients taking Aricept died, while there were no deaths among those patients taking the placebo. Eisai, the Japanese company that sold Aricept in a partnership with Pfizer, dismissed the deaths of the Aricept patients as a fluke, saying those assigned to take the sugar pill had been healthier than those taking the drug.

The nation's medicines do not perform as promised by the advertisements because federal regulators demand little proof of their effectiveness before approving them for sale. In most cases, a company must show only that its product can outperform a sugar pill to some small degree. That is, it must show that its medicine is better than nothing.

This can be understood by listening to a conversation between an FDA physician who was considering whether to approve the allergy drug Claritin and a scientist who was working for Schering-Plough, the drug's maker. The FDA medical officer, Dr. Sherwin D. Straus, was not convinced that Claritin actually worked at the very low dose of ten milligrams that Schering planned to sell. The company had kept the dose low because it wanted to advertise Claritin as the first "nonsedating" antihistamine. As patients took higher amounts of Claritin, they became drowsy just like patients who used the other allergy drugs already being sold. At a public meeting in 1987, Dr. Straus asked Dr. Anthony Nicholson, the scientist who was helping Schering, why the company had not focused on comparing the effectiveness of Claritin with other antihistamines.

"We are not actually in the business of saying one drug is better than the other," Dr. Nicholson told Dr. Straus. "We are in the business of saying whether a drug is acceptable in terms of its performance profile."

"But how can you say it is acceptable in terms of its performance pro-file," Dr. Straus asked, "without comparing it to what else is out there?"

"We compare it to placebo," Dr. Nicholson answered.

"So you compare it to nothing?"

"Yes."

"And it is better than nothing?"

"Yes."

"All right," Dr. Straus replied. "I can't argue with that."

At the same time, the FDA gives the companies many chances to show their products are better than that tablet of sugar. For example, Pfizer did several studies that failed to show that its antidepressant Zoloft worked better than a placebo before finally completing two trials that the government accepted as good enough for approval. This situation perplexed Dr. Paul Leber, one of the FDA physicians reviewing Pfizer's application.

"How do we interpret . . . two positive results in the context of several more studies that fail to demonstrate that effect?" Dr. Leber asked at a 1990 meeting at which a committee was considering Zoloft's approval. "I am not sure I have an answer to that, but I am not sure that the law requires me to have an answer to that—fortunately or unfortunately. That would mean, in a sense, that the sponsor could just do studies until the cows come home until he gets two of them that are statistically significant by chance alone, walks them out and says he had met the criteria."

And that appears to be what most of the manufacturers of antidepressants have done. In 2002 Dr. Arif Khan, a psychiatrist in Bellevue, Washington, reviewed the data from the dozens of clinical trials that companies had performed to prove that Zoloft, Prozac, Paxil, and six other antidepressants actually worked. These drugs are now some of the most prescribed medicines in America. Dr. Khan and his colleagues found fifty-two completed trials of these drugs, which involved more than ten thousand patients.

In more than half these studies, the sugar tablet relieved the patients' depression just as well as, or better than, the antidepressant.

JUST INSIDE THE main gate to the Iowa State Fair, families were lined up for a ride on the Ferris wheel, "Free Bird" blared over the loudspeaker, and the carnival's pitchmen were just getting warmed up.

A guy in a Cubs T-shirt had just stepped up to the dunk tank. He grabbed a baseball and took aim at a small target that, when hit, would send a loud-mouthed clown sitting at the tank's edge into the drink. "Hey, buddy," heckled the clown as the man went into his windup and threw. He missed. "Why don't you take a couple of Viagra?" the clown taunted.

Farther down the midway, a female barker beckoned passersby to stop and play her game of chance. "Today's the day," she shouted. "I can feel it."

Billboards posted outside the freak show promised six-legged sheep "born alive," a two-headed turtle, and "the Fiji Mermaid" caught off the coast of Mexico. REAL, said the sign. The bearded carny waiting to sell tickets to the curiosities looked bored. Hundreds of his potential customers had already wandered down the street to where a beady-eyed critter named Digger was prancing and waving and creeping up to children behind their backs.

Digger was a five-and-a-half-foot-tall devilish creature with pointy ears, yellow fur, purple claws, and a single tooth that showed when he grinned. Marketers at Novartis had created him to portray a dermatophyte, a type of fungus that can grow under toenails and turn them yellow. The animated menace with his twitching yellow tail had made the company's pill called Lamisil a smash hit, worth seven hundred million dollars a year, in the United States. The Swiss drugmaker had spent tens of millions of dollars on television commercials showing Digger lifting the nail on a large toe, the way one would hoist the hood of a car, and climbing in. After Digger and his friends make themselves comfortable inside the toe, a huge white Lamisil tablet rolls toward them, causing them to flee. A Novartis marketing executive told *The Wall Street Journal* in 2004 that the company's goal for the ads was a serious one aimed at getting Americans to consult their doctor. "We didn't want to create a cute character," he said, "and show happy people at a picnic."

Now, on a hot, muggy August afternoon, the "Lamisil on the Road Tour" had pulled into Des Moines and become an official sponsor of the state fair, along with Miller Brewing, Taco John's, and Terrible's Lakeside Casino. With offerings like tractor pulls, fried Twinkies, and a contest for the fattest boar, the Iowa State Fair attracts more than a million people a year. Thousands walked by that day as Digger paced and growled not far from where Iowa children waited for camel and pony rides.

"Oh, that's that toe fungus," said a man in shorts walking by Novartis's yellow and blue tent. "Oh, yeah," replied the blond-haired teenage girl by his side.

An elderly trio waited in line to meet Digger. When their turn arrived, they gathered around him, put their arms about his shoulders, and smiled as a Novartis salesperson snapped a Polaroid. One of the women, her hair gray and tightly curled, tucked the souvenir photo into her shopping bag, along with a pedometer, engraved with the Lamisil logo, and a toenail file, all gifts from the company's amiable agents.

Novartis had even hired a doctor to examine feet, not an enviable job that day given the sultry weather. The burly podiatrist invited Iowans to step behind a blue curtain for a toenail checkup and a confidential discussion. When they emerged from the room, a salesperson handed them a brochure that said in large blue type, "Ask your doctor how Lamisil Tablets get your nail infection where it grows." The brochure said Lamisil worked by traveling through the bloodstream to the infected area under the toenail. A person had to read closely to learn that the drug traveled to other parts of the body as well with unfortunate effects. In small print near the back of the eighteen-page brochure, it said a person might need a liver test before getting a prescription. There had been "rare cases" in which Lamisil users needed liver transplants or even died.

Left out of the brochure was the fact that in the studies the government relied on to approve Lamisil only 38 percent of patients were cured after taking it for months. And even in that successful group, 15 percent found their nail infections came back after about a year.

The scene Novartis had created—with a character in funny costume and free giveaways—had the playfulness of the opening of a Disney movie.

It held much appeal for children, who learned that prescriptions could bring them a good time. There appeared to be no dark side.

Novartis was using this same approach in 2005 to sell a prescription cream to kids and adults with itchy skin caused by eczema. Ads for the drug called Elidel featured an animated Superman-like character wearing thick eyeglasses and a tight-fitting blue suit with a large yellow *E* fixed upon his burly chest. Mr. Elidel's cape billowed behind him when he flew. When he landed, he flexed his arm to show his bulging bicep.

Not to be outdone, a company with a similar prescription cream called Protopic had invented an orange-colored, growling Eczema Beast. A television commercial showed the pudgy beast being knocked on his back by looming alphabetic letters that spelled "Protopic." The animated letters then crushed the groaning beast, and he dissolved into a pile of orange mud, just as an announcer listed some dangers of using the cream. With the pile of mud now alive and grumbling, few viewers would even hear the announcer's warnings, which he delivered without expression. I watched the commercial three times before I heard and understood that the cream could cause "stinging, burning, and itching" and increase the risk of skin infections.

To delight children more, Fujisawa, the maker of Protopic, offered a phone number where kids could call to receive their own furry stuffed toy beast. Or children could grab their crayons and spend an hour with the company's Eczema Beast coloring book.

Both Novartis and Fujisawa had continued these animated promotional antics in the weeks following an announcement by federal regulators in the spring of 2005 that the prescription creams, which worked by suppressing the immune system, could cause cancer. The regulators said the creams had been shown to cause cancer in monkeys and mice and that they had received thirteen reports of skin cancer and lymphoma in humans, including children.

Other drug companies also targeted children and teens with free games, storybooks, and toys. These companies had moved beyond the practice of selling pediatric medicines to parents and were now promoting them to kids. For toddlers, Abbott Laboratories created a plush hand puppet of a bulldog named Bix to promote Biaxin, an antibiotic for ear infections. A company called Celltech gave away seven-inch superhero dolls, designed with rippled muscles and clothed in blue tights, to promote its medicine for attention deficit disorders. Galderma Laboratories was giving teens seven free music downloads for their first prescription of an acne medicine called Differin and ten more songs when they got a refill, which the company called the "levels of cool." And Wyeth was letting teenage girls create their own melodic ring tones and download them to their cell phones at a website promoting birth control pills called Alesse.

James U. McNeal, an expert on the marketing of all types of products to children, explained in his 1999 book *The Kids Market* that companies had learned to give away toys and other fun prizes because play is a child's number one need. At the same time, children like those who give them things and are fondest of the biggest givers.

"My research suggests that children begin to relate to brands—names, symbols, characters, colors—during infancy when parents introduce them to the concept," McNeal writes. "Hence, when children begin talking, they begin asking for things by brand name . . . Brands that make them cool, make them stand out in a crowd, and give them definition may be sought at any price."

Among the most aggressive promoters of pediatric drugs were those selling growth hormone to short children. These drugs can cost more than twenty thousand dollars a year. The company Genentech was giving away a video game titled *Growth City*. The ad firm that created the game for Genentech said it worked better than an advertisement. "This ad works wonders because, well, it's not an ad," explained the staff at GSW Worldwide. The goal of the video game, they said, was to get "toddlers to teens . . . immersed in the right solutions."

Not to be outdone, Pfizer, the maker of another brand of growth hormone, had created a storybook featuring a puppy called Max, as well as a cuddly toy version of the dog, which children could use to practice injecting themselves with the drug.

Serono, another seller of growth hormone, was giving away a storybook in which the main character was a magic dragon named Spot. The company's advertising firm said it created Spot to be the embodiment of the company's product called Saizen.

In the story, a boy who is Spot's friend gets stuck at the top of the climbing bars on the playground and yells for help. "Spot, his funny green friend, knows just what to do," the book's author writes. "He flaps his wings and shouts, 'Spot to the rescue!'"

THE DRUG COMPANIES could be everywhere and nowhere at the same time. By this I mean that I found them working in every region of Iowa, from the towns on the Missouri River on the state's western border to the river cities on the muddy Mississippi in the east. Yet the companies were adept at hiding when it was in their best interest. To do this, they got out their checkbooks and paid others who appeared to be independent to deliver messages for them, making the promotion all the more powerful and effective. Audiences subject to these covert marketing campaigns did not realize they needed to be just as skeptical of the information as they would of that in a drug ad. They did not even know a marketing effort was under way. These underground marketing operations targeted Iowans of all ages, starting with those in preschool.

For example, Iowa doctors sometimes referred their young patients to a nonprofit group called the Magic Foundation, which was started by mothers with children with rare growth disorders in 1989. Over the years, the foundation had accepted hundreds of thousands of dollars from the companies selling prescription growth hormone products. In a campaign in the early 1990s the Magic Foundation, as well as another group, the Human Growth Foundation, had measured the height of children in public schools. The screeners suggested that the shortest children visit their doctors for medical treatment. Most of the schools and parents did not learn that the two foundations had received most of their funding for the school screenings from Genentech and another hormone manufacturer. The foundations said they were not promoting the drugs, but only trying to get children treatment.

Since then, the Magic Foundation had continued to accept money from Genentech and other corporate sellers of hormones to supplement the membership dues and donations from the public that it receives. The foundation also had continued to recommend hormone injections to short

children and their parents and describe the drugs in ways the manufacturers could not do without breaking the law. A story published in the
foundation's glossy magazine that I picked up at a pediatricians' conference in 2005 was entitled "Me and My Growth Hormone." The story began, "I was short. My little sister was taller than me. Kids at school picked
on me and called me names." The tale continued with the child getting
growth hormone injections and growing so much his pants got too short.
"I'm almost grown now," the story ended. "I'm in the normal range on a
growth chart. Growth hormone is like a miracle drug."

Other clandestine pharmaceutical marketing occurred on Iowa's university campuses. In October 2003, college students all over Iowa were
tested for mental illness on an autumn morning that had been deemed
National Depression Screening Day. This national campaign was organized by a nonprofit group called Screening for Mental Health, Inc.,
which was funded by companies selling antidepressants, including Eli
Lilly, Pfizer, Wyeth, Forest Laboratories, and GlaxoSmithKline. But few
of the college students learned that fact. During the screenings at Iowa
State University, therapists played videos for the students to watch, including *Life After Trauma: What Every Person Should Know*, which was
produced by Pfizer, the maker of Zoloft.

"When I began taking the questionnaire, I got more anxious because
I wondered if I would have symptoms of having an emotional condition,"
wrote Katie Melson of her experience in an article in the *Iowa State Daily*,
the student newspaper. "I could feel the stress building as mid-term
week approached. Two tests, two quizzes and three journalism articles
due, not to mention working around 20 hours a week into the early morning hours as a bartender. Was I feeling disconnected, anxious, irritable or
out of control?" The university's staff told Katie that on the basis of her
answers to the test she might have anxiety. She declined the therapist's
offer to schedule an appointment.

The next year, Central College, in Pella, Iowa, published the results
from its testing for mental illness on National Depression Screening Day.
Almost half the 190 students who took the test had a score that indicated
"diagnosis likely, further evaluation needed." Of those students, two-thirds
were said to have depression, and 58 percent were said to have generalized

anxiety disorder, which is defined as excessive worrying. The Central College officials who announced the results said they did not know how many of the screenings resulted in a false negative, where it missed someone with a mental illness, or a false positive, where it wrongly claimed someone had a mental illness.

With insurance companies quick to pay for antidepressant prescriptions, but often unwilling to pay for more expensive talk therapy, the drug companies easily found hundreds of new customers through these campus screenings, which have been performed across the country. In 2002 Wyeth, the maker of the antidepressant Effexor, hired Cara Kahn, the twenty-three-year-old star of the MTV show *Real World Chicago*, to urge college kids to be screened. Those working with the actress put up posters to attract students with slogans like "Stressed? Come find out how much" and "Come test your mood."

The depression screenings expanded from campuses to the general public. Iowans of any age were invited to dozens of screening sites set up across the state on Thursday, October 6, the official National Depression Screening Day of 2005. In Mason City, screeners erected a table at the South Bridge Mall. In Fort Dodge, screeners worked in the Trinity United Methodist Church. A few years earlier, Iowans living in Des Moines had been offered screenings at their local Hy-Vee supermarket, each with its own pharmacy. The pharmacies may have noticed a boom in their prescription business. A survey estimated that more than 25 percent of those quizzed at the thousands of sites set up for National Depression Screening Day in the United States and Canada in 1996 later started taking prescription antidepressants.

The nonprofit health groups Screening for Mental Health, Inc., and the Magic Foundation were just two of the dozens of organizations collecting money from the pharmaceutical industry each year. By 2006 most nonprofit groups representing patients in the United States had received funding from the industry. The American Heart Association, the American Cancer Society, and the Alzheimer's Association each received significant sums of corporate cash. It was hard to find a patient group that did not take the money. Some nonprofit organizations aggressively solicited the industry's cash. The Crohn's & Colitis Foundation of America had an executive in 2005 with the title of Director of Pharmaceutical Relations.

The payments were not given in generosity. The money came from the companies' marketing departments. Jeffrey Winton, the vice president of global public relations at Pharmacia, explained the industry's motivation in funding these groups in 2002. "Gone are the days when companies just handed out big checks to groups with no discussion afterward," he said. "Now, we see opportunities with groups that not only help them achieve their goals and objectives, but also help us move our business along."

And when some companies failed to find an organization to help with promotion, they simply ordered their marketers to create one. In 2002, Americans learned of the nation's "thrombosis crisis" from a group of physicians called the Council for Leadership on Thrombosis Awareness and Management. The council's leaders urged people to go to their local hospitals and be screened for blood clots. The "council" was little more than the creation of a marketing team at Aventis Pharmaceuticals, the manufacturer of a blood thinner called Lovenox.

In Iowa it had gotten to the point that if there was a conference involving health care, there was a better than even chance that the pharmaceutical industry would be footing at least some of the bill. In December 2003 Pfizer helped pay for a conference for high school girls at the University of Iowa, at which the keynote speaker was Kate Shindle, the former Miss America who had become a Broadway star. A main topic of discussion at the event was girls who suffered from eating disorders, a group Pfizer was interested in. The company was trying to show in studies that these girls could be treated with Zoloft, its antidepressant.

MISS AMERICA WORKED with teenage girls, but the marketers required a more masculine approach when it came to men, a group not generally susceptible to messages that claimed they were sick. "We know that men don't like to go to the doctor as much as women," one Pfizer marketing executive explained in 2003. "How can we best reach men in a way where they're receptive?"

By 2005 it was clear that Pfizer and its competitors had found their answer. They were spending tens of millions of dollars to mimic the marketers of Buicks and Budweisers and hustle fans at professional sporting events, from football and baseball to yacht racing and golf.

Consider, for example, the professional golf tournament known as the John Deere Classic, which takes place in the Iowa and Illinois towns known as the Quad Cities each July. When I went in 2005, I found the blue and white MetLife blimp circling overhead, Michelob flowing from the taps at a fake bar erected as an advertisement near the eighth hole, and a dozen electronic scoreboards scattered over the course listing far more than the players' scores. Each of them included a four-by-six-foot sign that advertised sex, or more specifically, the by-prescription-only sexual aid known as Cialis.

The thousands of golf fans from Iowa and Illinois attending the tournament that Saturday had no choice but to gaze up at the green and yellow Cialis signs again and again as they tracked the performance of their favorite PGA players. There was no description on these signs of what Cialis was or even what it did. It was impossible to know how many children in the crowd asked their parents about the strange name they saw on the scoreboards or how many got a straight answer.

Many of these young golf fans already knew that Cialis was something that men got from the doctor when they wanted to have sex. Eli Lilly and ICOS, the two companies that had joined together to sell Cialis, had jump-started the promotion of their new sex pill on February 1, 2004, by spending millions of dollars on ads during the Super Bowl, one of America's most watched television events of the year. Ads for Cialis, with scenes of a couple sitting outdoors in separate bathtubs, had been a fixture on television ever since.

The Iowa kids may have also learned about Cialis if they were fans of another fast-growing professional sport. Eli Lilly had paid heavily in 2005 to sponsor the nation's major bass fishing competitions. As part of the deal, ads for Cialis played during the popular fishing lessons that aired each Sunday on ESPN in the show *Bassmaster University*. Lilly also put promotions for Cialis on the national Bassmaster website, as well as on similar websites used by local groups of fishing enthusiasts in many states. In Tennessee, when kids went online in 2005 to see who among their young friends had won the Junior Bassmaster contests, they found a promotion for the erectile enhancement drug and with a click could be transported to a site where Lilly was giving away free Cialis pills. That website included a photo of a couple kissing on a dock by a lake as well as lessons on "sexual health." There was a lengthy how-to guide on sex, including lines like "Continuous sexual stimulation is indispensable in order to be able to reach the ultimate pleasure of orgasm/ejaculation and relief." With the help of Eli Lilly, the young anglers were learning everything they needed to catch the big fish and then relax, like the pros.

Back at the Quad Cities golf tournament, Cialis was not the only prescription drug being promoted. At the eighteenth hole, men and women sat behind a white picket fence, sipped their Bud Lights (a tournament sponsor), and watched J. S. Lewis sink his last putt of the day to win the Crestor Charity Challenge. Drugmaker AstraZeneca had created the contest to promote its new cholesterol pill, Crestor. The name of the contest was brilliant. The Crestor Charity Challenge evoked recollections of the Pepsi Challenge, a promotional gimmick that the soda pop manufacturer had used repeatedly in ads to create the impression that cola drinkers preferred the taste of its product to that of Coke. The Crestor Charity Challenge, which AstraZeneca was paying to sponsor at thirty-five professional golf tournaments around the country in 2005, sent an implicit message that Crestor was better and safer than any of the other cholesterol-lowering pills. This was not the case.

In fact, in all the pharmaceutical marketing on the golf course that day, there was not one mention of the risks of these pills, which were not insignificant. Studies had shown that Crestor appeared to be more toxic to the muscles than other cholesterol drugs. Some Americans taking a high dose had suffered from a condition known as rhabdomyolysis, in which muscles are liquefied. "Physicians must tell their patients the truth" about Crestor, the influential British medical journal *The Lancet* had stated in 2003. Compared with its competitors, the journal said, Crestor has "an inferior evidence base supporting its safe use."

The erectile enhancement drug Cialis, on the other hand, could cause dangerous drops in blood pressure. A small number of patients taking it had mysteriously gone blind.

By marketing on the golf course, the drugmakers avoided federal rules that required them to tell consumers of the dangers. They also happened to be taking a page from the marketing manuals of R. J. Reynolds and other tobacco companies. The cigarette makers had learned that even when Congress stops you from advertising on television, there were ways to get your products in front of viewers.

In the early 1970s, R. J. Reynolds had paid millions of dollars to become a top sponsor of NASCAR racing, about the same time a new law banned cigarette commercials on television or radio. For the next thirty years NASCAR's premier event was the Winston Cup series of races, where the track was awash with the red and white colors of the Winston brand and even young children could be seen clad in cigarette-branded caps and T-shirts. A fan watching the race on television saw the cigarette logos painted on the sides of the stock cars hundreds of times as they roared around the track. By sponsoring the races, R. J. Reynolds got its brand back on television—with a bonus. It could leave out the surgeon general's warning required on its cigarette packages and in its printed advertisements that said tobacco could kill.

At the racetrack, R. J. Reynolds also learned to confront fans directly. The tobacco company had forty of its "agents" roam the stands, looking for fans who smoked. The agents invited the smokers to the company's Winston tent, where they were given free cigarettes and NASCAR collectibles. The fans gave RJR their names and other personal information. The experience helped the tobacco company form "a relationship" with the smoker. RJR also erected driving simulators for kids to sit in, giving them a driver's-eye view of the race. Its marketing tactics proved potent. In 2000 the Winston brand had a 5 percent share of the national cigarette market but was favored by 20 percent of the NASCAR fans who smoked.

RJR ended its contract with NASCAR in 2003 as its marketing became more controversial. "With tobacco, you can't market to kids," Chip Williams, the former NASCAR public relations director, told *Auto Racing Digest* in 2003. "That might not sound like a big deal to some people, but it's becoming a larger and larger issue. Most of our clients—most of the companies involved in motorsports team sponsorship—are marketing to families. How can you market to families without marketing to kids, too?"

But NASCAR officials quickly found other major sponsors to fill the space left by Big Tobacco. In 2004 race fans saw the No. 6 Viagra Ford go up against the No. 18 Wellbutrin Chevrolet. In other words, it was prescription-enhanced sex competing against prescription-enhanced happiness.

Parents could now clothe their children in No. 6 Viagra leather jackets. They could give them toy race cars, in either the Viagra or Wellbutrin models. There were Viagra beach towels and posters and even a fuzzy Viagra teddy bear.

The drug companies also copied some of RJR's direct marketing techniques. GlaxoSmithKline, the maker of Wellbutrin, had "Racing for Life" trailers at the track where fans were screened for depression and other diseases. An added attraction at the trailer was a visit from Bobby Labonte, the driver of the No. 18 Wellbutrin car, and his crew chief, Michael "Fatback" McSwain.

NASCAR lovers are among the most dedicated of sports fans. They are known to show their loyalty by buying the products sponsoring their favorite drivers. Mark Martin and his No. 6 Viagra car had fanatical fans all over the country, including Iowa.

"I cried last week when he won the race," wrote Kathy Richey, of Osage, Iowa, on a guestbook that Mark Martin maintained on his website in 2005, along with photos of his Viagra mobile. "I think the world of him."

Annette Vozenilek, of Oxford Junction, Iowa, wrote in the guestbook, "I am a big fan and want you to know that I have a shrine of your collectibles and purchase more monthly."

Mitch Doherty, of Fort Madison, was a bit more blunt, writing a message that would have delighted any marketer at Pfizer. "Good luck and go get em!" he wrote to Martin. "From way up in Iowa we're watching and pullin HARD! for you."

EVEN GOD WAS not off-limits to the pharmaceutical marketers.

Pfizer had begun to market both its corporate image and its products inside churches around the country. In July 2004 it offered to pay for coffee and refreshments in the parlor of any church that allowed its public relations staff to promote its low-cost medicine program to the congregation. In another program, it paid to screen members of urban African American churches for glaucoma. There was a good chance that any churchgoer found to have signs of the eye disease would be prescribed Xalatan, Pfizer's high-priced prescription eyedrops.

The pharmaceutical companies had also become among the biggest advertisers in the spiritual magazine called *Guideposts*, which was founded in 1945 by Dr. Norman Vincent Peale. The magazine attracted millions of readers with stories of hope and divine guidance like one entitled "What Prayer Can Do." The magazine's publisher aggressively courted the drug companies and their advertising dollars, saying its faithful readers represented "a virtually untapped audience for healthcare marketers." In 2000 the publisher performed surveys that showed its readers were 78 percent more likely than the average American to have seen their doctors six times or more in the past year. "Our readers look to the magazine as a source of inspiration and a touchstone for balance and fulfillment," Janine Scolpino, the publisher of *Guideposts*, explained. "It is a totally positive environment for advertisers."

The promotion of prescription drugs in churches and in spiritual publications gave the pills a kind of holy endorsement from above. One of my mother's friends gave me a copy of *Guideposts* published in the summer of 2005. Tucked among stories about "finding hope in tough times" and "a young girl's moment of truth" was a four-page spread advertising the heartburn drug called Nexium, including an offer for a free seven-day supply. "The healing purple pill," the ad proclaimed, "has some very healing news."

One of the most powerful drug marketing campaigns aimed at Christians was performed not directly by the industry but by a theologian named Dr. Paul Meier, a popular radio talk show host and the owner of a chain of mental health clinics. His book *Blue Genes* was published in 2005 with help from Focus on the Family, a national group popular with many Christian conservatives in Iowa and across the country. The book was a kind of spiritual guide for those dealing with depression or anxiety. It described the new psychiatric medicines as offering "opportunities for healing that truly reflect God's care and love." In one of the book's stories, Dr. Meier compared taking a quick-dissolving wafer of Klonopin, a prescription tranquilizer, with taking Holy Communion. "If Edward felt panicky, he should peel out the wafer, suck on it like a communion wafer, dissolving it in about two seconds, and within four minutes his panic attack would be completely gone."

Dr. Meier wrote that he had personally come to depend on the meds he took for attention deficit disorder. "I write about two or three books every year while on medications and could write only one book every two or three years without them," he explained. "So if I were too prideful to admit that I had any mental dysfunction, and I refused to take psychiatric medications, I would hinder God."

Dr. Meier and his coauthors acknowledged that they had spoken to representatives from the drug companies, who had provided them inside information.

A BASIC GOAL of the pharmaceutical marketers was to create an enthusiasm among the public for lifelong medication use, which they called compliance. A two-day conference for industry executives in November 2005 was devoted solely to techniques used to keep people complying with their prescription schedules. Consultants estimated the drugmakers could add billions of dollars to their annual sales if they could keep people taking their meds.

A step in the process of gaining compliance was the collection of personal and medical information on every American they hoped to convince to be a longtime customer. For decades, the drug companies had been building giant databases of detailed information on physicians—from their artistic tastes to their outlook on life and their best friends—which sales reps used to gain access to the doctors and become like a friend. More recently the industry had begun collecting and analyzing intimate details on other Americans.

Some pharmaceutical companies paid physicians or pharmacies to let their sales representatives review their patient files. It was easier, however, to purchase the information from consulting firms that specialized in collecting patient data. A firm called PharMetrics said in 2005 that it had the complete set of pharmacy and medical claims of more than fifty-five million Americans, more than one-sixth of the population. PharMetrics said its database of personal medical histories, including prescriptions, diagnoses, hospitalizations, and lab tests, had been obtained from insurance companies, pharmacies, and other medical providers. The firm said its data did not include names and addresses, but such information was easy to obtain.

The drug companies had also begun collecting the private data directly from Americans through what some executives called one-on-one relationship marketing. To do this, the marketers created websites to attract people looking for health information. The websites offered gifts to those willing to fill out surveys and provide personal information. The companies added each new piece of data to their in-house databases, which allowed them to create profiles of individuals and better understand what motivated them. One marketing executive explained that this transformed customers from "anonymous and unengaged" to "profiled and active."

The data collection began with toddlers watching Big Bird and Ernie on *Sesame Street*. Iowa parents watching the show with their children on public television in 2006 were apt to see a promotional spot for a website called everydaykidz.com. AstraZeneca, the maker of the asthma drug Pulmicort, had paid the creators of *Sesame Street* to promote everydaykidz.com during its television episodes and in *Sesame Street* magazine. The Everydaykidz website was designed for children ages one to eight. It offered a host of games, stories, and art activities, as well as Pulmi, a froglike animated creature adept at cartwheels, that the company called a "thing-a-ma-jiggie." To access the games, parents were required to provide the drug company with their children's names, addresses, birth dates, and details on their health conditions. In fine print, AstraZeneca said it was storing the information in a corporate database for its marketing purposes.

Similarly, Serono, a Swiss company, was operating a website in 2005 with games and animated stories for American kids and teens. The site promoted the firm's growth hormone product, Saizen, and collected names and e-mail addresses. The children could sign up for the "cool.club" and win free songs for their MP3 players by providing their personal data and watching promotional cartoons, like one in which Chaz, the cool tenth grader, reveals to his gang that he takes Saizen.

The companies used the data they collected to become closer to the person or, as one marketer described, to be like a dinner "date" by "striking up conversation, piquing their interest, and leaving them wanting for more." For example, the drug company Roche created a program for overweight patients who were prescribed Xenical, its weight loss drug. The company asked doctors in Iowa and throughout the country to give their patients starter kits for its Xenicare program. Roche asked these patients thirty personal questions, logged the information into its sophisticated database, and then used it to act like a coach or well-wisher to the person. The company sent holiday cards and congratulatory notes as the weeks passed and the patient continued taking the pills. Marketers wrote the notes and letters with "the cool tone of a doctor or nurse speaking to you while looking over your chart," explained Micromass Communications, the firm that helped design Xenicare. The marketers even used special printers that gave the letters "a homespun feel." It was all, however, little more than a marketing ploy aimed at keeping people on their meds.

EVEN THE MOST compelling consumer marketing campaign will not be successful, however, if physicians refuse to prescribe the medicines their patients request. That is why the companies were spending most of their marketing budgets on physicians. Each doctor would write prescriptions worth millions of dollars during their careers. The drugmakers ranked the physicians according to their lifetime prescribing potential.

"Segment physicians according to their value," instructed Dr. David Lefkowitz, a consultant to the industry, in an article in 2003, "and focus resources on those with the greatest worth."

Those "resources" included offers of cash, travel, and entertainment. A frequent prize for high-prescribing Iowa physicians in 2005 was an expensive night on the town, and many of the state's finest restaurants were benefiting as a result.

"On behalf of Salix Pharmaceuticals, you and your colleagues are cordially invited to attend an educational program," said one invitation, embossed in silver ink and mailed in June 2005. Paula Gray, the territory sales manager for Salix, had invited Iowa physicians to attend a presentation and dinner at the Linn Street Café in Iowa City, where the Moroccan rubbed rack of lamb with saffron-yogurt cream sauce goes for twenty-eight dollars and the wine list includes a three-hundred-dollar bottle of 1994 cabernet sauvignon.

These soirees fostered a feeling of entitlement among the physicians. Some doctors demanded even more. A study in 2003 found that the industry got 82 percent of the physicians they invited to an event to go when they also offered cash. The companies described these payments as "consulting" fees. Critics saw them more as a bribe.

Iowa's physicians were not shy about asking for gifts. In 2005 two sales reps from Schering-Plough paid to take an Iowa physician to a strip club in Cedar Rapids called Woody's at his request. The drug company later fired the sales reps, saying their trip to see nude dancers had gone too far. One of the salespeople explained why she had agreed to the doctor's request during a hearing at which she successfully pleaded for unemployment benefits. "He was a target that I had to actually, physically, track for the company," she testified at the hearing. "He had the potential to be a big prescriber and to increase my market share.

"He is entertained four nights per week by pharmaceutical representatives," she added. "And he is known far and wide for prescribing not on a clinical . . ." She had stopped in midsentence. "It's on who he likes," she continued. "He rewards people. He rewards people personally."

To protect the public, the nation has rules and laws regulating the giving of gifts by stockbrokers and the receiving of gifts by federal judges. Radio broadcasters cannot legally take cash or any other gift in exchange for playing specific songs because it could be viewed as a bribe. But in the medical world, doctors depended on the industry's largesse. The gifts were part of the culture, part of a physician's daily practice. Doctors had continued taking the loot despite studies showing that even gifts as small as a pen could imbue them with the sense that they owed the pharmaceutical company a favor, a quandary that could be swiftly solved by writing more prescriptions.

———

THE PHARMACEUTICAL COMPANIES had another way of marketing their products to physicians, one that was growing in importance every year. The drug companies had seized control of a part of American medicine that was considered so critical to the health of patients that many states, including Iowa, required every licensed physician to take part. That activity was the continuing education of doctors after they graduated from medical school. By 2005 the drug industry and other medical companies were paying hundreds of millions of dollars to the organizers of the nation's accredited medical education courses, enough to cover between 65 percent and 80 percent of the cost. As a result, most of these events had become little more than pharmaceutical sales bazaars.

By paying for doctors' continuing education, the drug companies made sure physicians learned what was best for the corporate bottom line. Doctors learned how to diagnose their patients with the marketers' hottest diseases of the moment, which in 2005 were maladies like irritable bowel, restless leg syndrome, and attention deficit disorder (in adults). They also learned about the benefits of the industry's newest and most expensive medicines. There were few refresher courses on older and cheaper medicines that had been proven to help patients but were no longer promoted. There were few discussions on how to get patients to exercise or lose weight. Doctors did not learn all the dangers of the new drugs or how to recognize when these products were making their patients worse. And patients who were truly sick, but not with a disease considered to be profitable, were often forgotten.

At the annual educational conference for the Iowa Academy of Family Physicians in the summer of 2005, pharmaceutical sales representatives seemed almost as numerous as doctors. At a time when many Iowans struggled to pay medical bills and families wondered how they would afford the fast-rising tuitions at public universities, the state's doctors were enjoying low-cost, corporate-subsidized education in four-star accommodations. At the Marriott Hotel in downtown Des Moines, the physicians sat in ballrooms with crystal chandeliers, where the tables were covered with white tablecloths, and attendants kept them supplied with coffee and hard candy. They took breaks for pastries, yogurt, and soft drinks in a large hall, half the size of a football field, which was filled with sales booths erected by pharmaceutical companies. To pay for the event, the academy had charged the drug companies a thousand dollars for each eight-by-ten-foot booth. Tables in the booths were piled high with gifts for any physician wandering by. There were Zoloft wall clocks, bottles of Paxil hand cream, and enough pens, staplers, notepads, clipboards—all emblazoned with pharmaceutical brand names—to supply a nearby office building. I watched as a white-haired physician wandered through the hall, stopping at each booth and picking up one or two items from each table. He carried three large shopping bags, each brimming with swag.

In 1900 the influential physician Dr. William Osler said in a speech that doctors could not just end their education after medical school. Physicians, he said, must be lifelong students to maintain their competence. Dr. Osler, a Canadian who became physician in chief at Johns Hopkins in Baltimore, said this education was best done in hospitals where doctors learned by observing patients and talking about the best way to treat them. For decades, American hospitals educated physicians using Osler's methods in what they called grand rounds. Physicians would gather in a room in the hospital where a medical professor or senior physician would present the case of an actual patient, who often was also in attendance, lying on a gurney or sitting in a chair.

As the years passed, it became clear that this continual education of physicians was necessary to keep them up-to-date with treatment standards, and many states passed laws requiring doctors to attend annual educational courses. The typical course in 2005, however, had few similarities to that advocated by Dr. Osler. Rather than a lively debate on how best to care for an actual ailing patient, the courses were slide presentations by corporate-paid physicians on how to prescribe the latest in industrial medicines. Many of the lecturers had even been trained to speak by marketing firms working for the drug company that sponsored the event.

Joe Torre, chief executive of the global advertising firm Interpublic, explained how this process worked in an interview in 2002. His ad firm had organized continuing education events for dozens of drug companies over the years. The divisions inside the ad firms that did this work were called medical education companies.

"Very often doctors are more influenced by what other doctors say than what pharmaceutical companies say," Torre said. "So companies work through medical education companies to have doctors who support their products talk about their products in a favorable way. That's called medical education."

The drug industry's practice of hiring local physicians to lecture their peers about prescription products was almost entirely unregulated. In 2005, a physician could make $750 to $2,000 for a thirty-minute speech, while some doctors demanded far more. Pharmaceutical reps complained in private that some physicians could not get enough of these corporate handouts. A sales rep in New Jersey told me in 2003 that a physician on his rounds was giving talks on ten different prescription products and demanding $1,500 a speech. "Doctors are corrupt," he grumbled. "They say, 'If you hire me as a speaker, I'll prescribe.'"

The drug companies also warmed the doctors' hearts at these educational events by providing extra cash for fun and entertainment. After the lectures the doctors often enjoyed beach parties, banquets, and barbecues, courtesy of the corporate sponsors. In 2001 the Iowa Academy of Family Physicians held its summer educational event at The Inn on Lake Okoboji, a popular resort in northwestern Iowa. Seventeen drug companies helped pay for the conference, which included a golf tournament with prizes of gift certificates and sports merchandise. The available recreation changed with the seasons. In March 2005 ear, nose, and throat specialists from Omaha held an educational conference in Silverthorne, Colorado, and physicians were told to bring their whole families to ski at Vail, Breckenridge, or Keystone. Nine pharmaceutical and medical device companies helped pay for the five-day event.

Organizers of some of these seminars attracted hundreds of physicians by hosting them in exotic locales and including plenty of amusements, where cost was not an issue. Dermatologists from around the country were invited to a continuing education symposium at a beachfront luxury hotel in Miami's South Beach in 2004 that included lectures by physicians like Dr. Roger Ceilley, a prominent Iowa dermatologist, as well as nightly social affairs. The biggest bash was on the final night, when DUSA Pharmaceuticals, a company based in Massachusetts, was footing the bill for a party on the lawn overlooking the Atlantic. The agenda promised the physicians a night to remember:

> The evening begins with the opportunity to have your photo taken with several amazing parrots. During the reception, a magician will be strolling throughout the crowd performing magic that will astound you and an aerial acrobatic team will take your breath away with a show that you will have to see to believe! We will also have traditional island foods and featured island cocktails. All the while, a traditional beach band will be playing the sounds of the beach. Of course, dancing is optional . . .

The drug industry did not stop its efforts in medical education with physicians. As I paged through postings of these events in Iowa, I found that Pfizer had paid in 2004 for occupational health nurses to lunch and attend a class at a sparkling new conference hall overlooking the Mississippi. A few months later, Pfizer treated Iowa pharmacists to dinner and "education" at the CR Chop House, a pricey establishment in Cedar Rapids with steaks and other expense account fare.

The Iowa Physician Assistant Society had worked hard to improve its "pharmaceutical relations," according to the group's board minutes in 2002. At each educational event the society asked the companies to pay for speakers, refreshments, and door prizes. In 2004 one of the society's board members worried openly that the group was too slow in accepting the companies' offers. She had heard from four different drug companies that wanted to help pay for the society's fall conference. "We need to be more responsive to this type of interest," she explained. "Companies need to have information early so they can get speakers lined up." Her advice was heeded. By the time of the society's fall conference in 2005, twenty companies had agreed to help pay the bill.

No INSTITUTION IN the state had been more transformed by the pharmaceutical marketers than the University of Iowa's medical school. The university, its hospital, and its professors courted the drug companies and their cash.

The university's physicians and scientists applied for $65,000 grants to become the Pfizer fellow of pediatric health, the Pfizer fellow of biological psychiatry, or the Pfizer fellow of just about any medical specialty one could think of. Pfizer wrote checks to pay for the department of internal medicine's annual Research Day, an event where the company handed out financial grants to medical students and residents for travel. Pfizer helped buy the medical school a mobile clinic. Even the director of the university's hospital had sat on a Pfizer advisory board. The global pharmaceutical giant had paid to become an influential player inside the state's most important hospital, but so too had dozens of other firms manufacturing drugs and medical devices.

To solicit the industrial money, the university created an "office of corporate partnerships." It also set aside land for "a research park" on campus, where companies could rent office space and laboratories and easily interact with the faculty.

"It used to be the case that if you were involved in business, you were considered a bad academic," Bruce Wheaton, the director of the research park, explained in 2003. "It was considered really cheesy. Now it's almost considered a badge of honor."

While other state employees were banned by law from accepting gifts valued at more than three dollars from any industry, the state-employed physicians were accepting tens of thousands of dollars from companies making drugs and medical devices. The drugmakers paid the academic physicians to give speeches about their products, to sit on their advisory boards, and to work for them as "consultants." In 2006 some Iowa professors were working for a half dozen or more companies at a time. One of the few requirements was that some professors had to report any annual payment of ten thousand dollars or more from a single company to university officials. The university kept these reports secret even though they were of tremendous importance to the public. These industry-paid physicians made decisions every day that could mean the difference between life and death.

It was clear, however, that the public's health was no longer the only thing on the minds of the academic physicians in Iowa or at other teaching hospitals across the country. Dr. Jean E. Robillard, the dean of the

University of Iowa's college of medicine, explained this change of thinking in a speech to the faculty on a March night in 2003. In his talk, Dean
Robillard called for new rewards for faculty who won industrial contracts, which the university referred to as technology transfers. According to the notes to his presentation, Dean Robillard said that in addition
to the school's duty of taking care of Iowans' health, "we have also a responsibility in creating wealth."

Some of the most lucrative industrial deals went to those university
physicians who recruited Iowans for clinical trials in which medicines
were tested in humans. In recent years, Iowa researchers had tested
dozens of experimental products for the industry, from Strattera, a drug
for children with attention deficit disorder, to LibiGel, a testosterone
cream for women with lapsing libidos.

In the promotional materials used to attract the drug companies, university officials offered up their fellow Iowans as research subjects. They
explained that among the university's "resources" for the industry was its
sprawling academic hospital, which attracted "a large population of potential research participants."

Indeed, Iowans were becoming known to the drug industry as people
who made good study subjects because of their willingness to follow directions and stick with experiments they volunteered for. In other words,
they made good guinea pigs.

In 2004 the university boasted it had 136 scientists managing clinical trials for the industry. It was involved in so many drug trials that it had
negotiated standard written contracts with more than a dozen companies to save time.

But there were problems. Drug companies were asking for waivers
from the university's requirement that the results be published soon after
the trial was completed. Without this rule, there was a risk the public
would never learn about a study that found a medicine had dangerous
side effects or did not work as expected.

The university also tried to get the companies to agree to pay the
medical bills of any volunteer injured in an experiment. If a company refused, the university made sure it did not promise to pay for the treatment of the volunteers' injuries either.

But the thorniest problem lay in the tangle of financial ties between the industry and the academics leading these trials, a web that grew more complex every year. How could the university ensure that a professor, who had a lucrative consulting and speaking contract with a pharmaceutical firm, would keep an independent frame of mind as he performed a trial of that company's product? Could an industry-paid researcher keep the safety of human volunteers a priority and honestly report the results of the study, even if his corporate backer was not happy with what he found? Could patients at the hospital be kept safe when their physicians were earning thousands of dollars from the manufacturers of drugs they prescribed? Would safety be kept a priority when even some of the university's surgeons were high-paid consultants to the manufacturers of the pacemakers, the hip replacements, the metal spinal disks, and other devices they implanted in their patients?

The university had plenty of rules for professors who worked for the industry. But the bottom line of each of these policies, based on my review of them in 2006, was that in many cases the conflict could be "managed" or explained away. Or the physician could get what university officials called a waiver. The "management plan" could include nothing more than disclosing the industrial work to university officials, who assured the professor that they would not disclose the information to the public. Even the Iowans signing up for the experiments managed by these industry-paid professors might not learn about the money deals. The university's policy said only that it "may" disclose these financial conflicts to patients in clinical trials. All this was discussed in internal meetings among professors to which the public was not invited.

A small amount of information about these financial deals leaked out. At times, the professors had to disclose their industrial relationships at events where they spoke or in articles they wrote. The few facts that became public were enough to see how deep the conflicts had become among Iowa's faculty.

For example, this was how Dr. Jennifer Robinson, an associate professor in the College of Public Health, listed her financial ties on an educational website for medical professionals in 2006: "Jennifer G. Robinson, MD MPH has openly disclosed that s/he: has grant/research support from

Pfizer, Merck/Schering Plough, Hoffman La Roche, Astra Zeneca, Wyeth Ayerst, Bristol Myers Squibb, Atherogenics, Proctor and Gamble, Glaxo-SmithKline, Sankyo and Abbott [sic]; and has resolved all relevant conflicts of interest." She did not explain how she had "resolved" all these conflicts.

In 2005 Dr. Robinson also disclosed that Pfizer was paying her not only to do research but also as a speaker and a consultant. She made this disclosure in a letter to *The New England Journal of Medicine* in which she argued that a group of German researchers had been wrong to conclude in their clinical trial that Pfizer's medicine Lipitor did not help diabetic patients who were on dialysis. In the German study, fewer diabetic patients taking Lipitor had heart attacks or died from heart disease, but more of them died from stroke than those who had taken sugar pills. Dr. Robinson argued that the researchers should have looked only at the heart disease data and ignored the slightly higher death rate from stroke. The German scientists were blunt in their reply to Dr. Robinson's suggestion that they selectively report their data so that Pfizer's product, also known as atorvastatin, looked beneficial. "The fact that we cannot explain the higher rate of ischemic stroke in the atorvastatin group," they wrote, "does not mean that strokes did not occur."

It was telling that Dr. Robinson worked in the College of Public Health. The practice of public health had long been defined as that of protecting and improving the health of a community through such preventive measures as education, vaccines, sanitation, and monitoring environmental hazards. Public health scientists, funded by government grants, have also looked more broadly at the long-term risks and benefits of prescription medicines. But in Iowa the College of Public Health had become a magnet for industrial drug trials, some of which did not end up serving the public's health.

For instance, in 2000 the Bayer Corporation paid the university's public health scientists to make Iowa one of the research sites that recruited patients to take a very high dose of a cholesterol pill called Baycol. The results of that study, published in the spring of 2000, concluded that the 0.8 milligram tablet of Baycol was safe and effective. Just over a year later, federal officials pressed Bayer to take Baycol off the market. More than one hundred patients had died while taking the drug. The number of deaths had surged when patients began taking the 0.8 milligram dose.

With no limit on the amount of money faculty could receive from the industry, some professors were receiving annual fees from a single company that could buy a classy Mercedes or pay to send a child to Harvard. For example, I found the name of Dr. Vincent Traynelis, one of the university's spine surgeons, on the list of physicians that Medtronic had paid as consultants in 2002. A former Medtronic sales representative gave me the list, which said Dr. Traynelis would receive $65,000 that year. He may have felt underpaid. Medtronic, a maker of spinal disks and screws, was paying a surgeon at the University of Wisconsin $400,000 that year.

Some Iowa professors blatantly promoted the products sold by the companies who paid them fees. In 2004 Novartis quoted the university's Dr. Satish Rao in a press release sent to journalists to promote a pill called Zelnorm, which it sold to treat irritable bowel syndrome. In the press release, Dr. Rao said that Zelnorm was the "first drug" to show improvement in treating "the multiple symptoms" of constipation.

In 2004 Dr. Rao, a professor of gastroenterology, participated in an Internet seminar for physicians, which Novartis paid for. As part of that event, Dr. Rao disclosed that he worked as a consultant and speaker for Novartis and sat on the company's advisory board. He said he also worked as a speaker for AstraZeneca, Janssen, and Tap Pharmaceuticals. He had received "educational grants," he said, from AstraZeneca, Janssen, Novartis, Solvay Pharmaceuticals, and Tap Pharmaceuticals. He also sat on the advisory boards of GlaxoSmithKline, Sanofi-Synthelabo, and Solvay.

Many Iowa physicians learned about Zelnorm from Dr. Rao, even before the drug was approved in 2002. Dr. Dean Abramson, a gastroenterologist with a private practice in Cedar Rapids, said that after listening to a talk by Dr. Rao, he came to believe that Zelnorm would be some kind of wonder drug. But when the drug finally gained federal approval, he was deeply disappointed in how it worked for his patients.

In fact, Zelnorm had shown so little benefit and had so many side effects that by 2006 the European Union had twice turned down the request of Novartis, a Swiss company, to sell the drug there.

"He is Dr. Zelnorm," Dr. Abramson said of Professor Rao.

Many months after I spoke to Dr. Abramson, the FDA demanded in July 2007 that Novartis sharply limit the use of Zelnorm to women who met strict requirements. The agency said that patients taking the drug had a small but increased risk of having a heart attack or stroke.

Dr. Abramson said he was troubled by all the money that flowed from the pharmaceutical industry to the professors at the University of Iowa and to medical schools across the country. He said he had lost trust in the studies paid for by the industry that he saw published under the names of academics.

"Years ago people who went into medical research were content not to earn a lot of money," he said. "They were content to help mankind."

These days the academic-industrial partnerships are proliferating, he said, because they benefit all parties involved. Professors boost their salaries by tens of thousands of dollars or more. The university earns money from the clinical trials and does not have to pay its academics as much because of the fees they earn on the side. The drug companies get a potent form of promotion that generates vast sales. Everyone wins, he said, except patients.

"It's pervasive," Dr. Abramson said of the drug companies and their influence. "They're out there everywhere."

THE WOMEN WERE sipping glasses of sauvignon blanc while watching the salesgirls from the Aveda salon demonstrate how to brighten their appearance with lipstick and blush that came in warm summer colors. One of the Aveda girls introduced herself as Kelly. She had dark hair cut in a short, punky style. She wore a black T-shirt inscribed with a line written by Emily Dickinson: "Beauty is not caused. It is."

"I do hair," Kelly said. "I do waxing. If I'm not having a good hair day, my day is shot."

About sixty Iowa women had come to the Celebrate You club, a monthly event held at the Jordan Creek Town Center, a newly built shopping mall in West Des Moines. Its developers had turned cornfields into what resembled, with its pastel-colored painting scheme and an artificial

lake, a megashopping complex in Southern California. With stores like
J. Jill, Godiva, and Barnes & Noble and restaurants like the Cheesecake
Factory, the Jordan Creek Town Center could be Any Mall, U.S.A. The
promoters of the shopping center had joined with Mercy Medical Center, one of the largest hospitals in Iowa, to create the Celebrate You club.
At monthly events, medical professionals taught women about health,
while the stores promoted their products. I went to a club gathering on
a June evening because I was curious about what one might learn about
medicine at a free seminar at the mall.

For half an hour, Kelly and the other Aveda girls demonstrated their
company's cosmetics, lotions, and shampoos. At one point Kelly massaged
the scalp of a volunteer with the company's "energizer" oil. Her volunteer
fell into a relaxed, compliant stupor under Kelly's expert hands. But then
the Aveda girls were told their time was up. Another woman named Kelly,
Dr. Kelly Reed, took the floor. Her presentation was entitled "Migraine
Thoughts in 2005."

Dr. Reed looked as if she had just walked out of the Ann Taylor store
that was downstairs. She had pulled her blond hair back into a knot. She
wore a striking lime green herringbone jacket with black pants and green
sandals to match. She strolled back and forth in front of the crowd, holding the microphone, with the easy style of a talk show host.

She talked about how more women suffer from migraines than men
and how many migraine cases are never diagnosed. She said many women
believe they are suffering from sinus headaches or allergies when their
real problem is migraines. "It hits us in the prime of life," she said as the
scent of the Aveda oils wafted by on the breeze from the air conditioner.

Dr. Reed devoted part of her speech to telling the women about the
new migraine medicines called triptans. "We have some fabulous medicines now to treat migraines," she said as a group of shoppers on their way
to the Younkers department store paused to listen. She said the drugs,
which include brands such as Imitrex and Relpax, "can work beautifully."
They can provide "pain relief in twenty minutes," she said.

After speaking for just short of a half hour, Dr. Reed asked if the
women had questions. One woman told Dr. Reed that she had taken one
of the triptans and the pill made her head hurt the next day. She asked if

she should change medicines. Dr. Reed told the woman that the next-day pain could not have been caused by the drug and was instead part of the migraine's cycle. "It is not because your medicine has not helped you," she said.

There were no other questions, and the women gave Dr. Reed a warm round of applause. The pharmaceutical companies had been nowhere in sight that June night, but they had profited greatly. Dr. Reed had described the triptan drugs in ways that a pharmaceutical sales representative could not do without generating complaints. The triptans did not offer all patients the twenty-minute fix that she had described. Only a little more than half the patients taking Imitrex, a triptan sold by GlaxoSmithKline, felt relief from their pain after two hours, according to trials the company performed to get the drug approved. Even the sugar pills worked well in these studies. About a quarter of the people getting the placebo were also relieved of their pain after two hours.

Dr. Reed also did not talk about the triptans' possible side effects, which include rare heart attacks and strokes. If the risks were listed on one of her slides, she did not point them out, and they passed without notice. The twenty-three pages of prescribing instructions for Imitrex warn doctors not to prescribe it to people with heart disease or high blood pressure. The instructions say that some patients have suffered "serious cardiac adverse events" and died within a few hours of taking the drug. Some of those who died had no histories of heart disease. Even a fourteen-year-old boy had a heart attack within a day of taking the drug.

Moreover, all headache medicines, including the triptans, can cause pain the next day or rebound headaches, the problem the woman seemed to be asking Dr. Reed about. A study by German scientists in 2001 found that people who overused triptan medications like Imitrex could suffer from withdrawal headaches lasting four days.

Later I learned that Dr. Reed, like hundreds of physicians in Iowa and tens of thousands of physicians in the United States, had previously given speeches at events paid for by pharmaceutical companies. For example, in 2004 she gave a talk paid for by GlaxoSmithKline. Her migraine presentation that night at the mall was similar to one that GlaxoSmith-Kline had paid for that summer that involved a physician assistant from

Dr. Reed's office. One of the other doctors practicing in her office had received payments from GlaxoSmithKline and three other drug companies. There was nothing unusual about this. It was simply an example of a tiny strand of the ubiquitous web of doctors that the drug companies had created to promote their products even when they were not around.

I rummaged through my files to find the brochure Dr. Reed had handed out to the women at the mall. Called the *Headache Impact Test*, it included six brief questions to use to rate the severity of headaches. Even a person who was "rarely" bothered by headaches but "sometimes" felt too tired to work because of the pain was urged to talk to his or her doctor. At the bottom of the questionnaire, in very small letters, the brochure said it had been copyrighted by GlaxoSmithKline.

THREE

Chemical Imbalance

IN AN OFFICE above Sally's Beauty Supply, Patrick Hurley is talking fast, telling me how Ritalin and Prozac changed his life.

The hands on the clock on his wall are ticking backward, a novelty timepiece that he says only he and his clients really understand. Hanging above his desk is a black frame holding the silver badge from his days as a Johnson County sheriff's deputy. Dangling from a string placed over that frame is a bright blue name tag, a memento from a conference he recently attended. The name tag is imprinted with the careful script of Eli Lilly's corporate logo.

Hurley is a big, friendly man in his early fifties, with thinning blond hair and a round face. He is grinning and waving his arms as he recounts a time, nine years ago, when as a father of four children, he cheated on his wife. His marriage broke up, he said, and he became depressed and lost his self-esteem. At the urging of his brother-in-law, he went to a psychologist in Iowa City, who diagnosed him, at age forty-two, with attention deficit/hyperactivity disorder. The doctor gave him a sample of Ritalin, he said, and suddenly just about every troubling experience from his past made sense in his mind, including why he had had that "stupid" affair.

"It was the ADHD," he said, beaming. "I was impulsive. I didn't think through the consequences."

He said that after his diagnosis, he understood why he had been the class clown as a child and struggled in school. "I'd remember every jingle from television but couldn't get my work done. The nuns said, 'He just doesn't apply himself.'"

He also now knew why he had five cans of WD-40 and five hammers in his house and still couldn't find them when he needed them.

Hurley told me he knows many people who say their diagnosis with attention deficit disorder "was the best news they ever got." That is why, he said, he decided a few years back to rent the office in a strip mall in Cedar Rapids and begin promoting himself as a coach for those with the disorder. That is also why he is now constantly searching for others with lives as messy as his once was. He believes he can help turn these people around by getting them to a doctor for a simple diagnosis and a prescription for daily meds.

He has sent forty-seven people to the Iowa City clinic of Dr. Frank Gersh, he said, and forty-six have come back with a diagnosis. "Dr. Gersh tells me I have a knack for finding them."

Dr. Gersh also probably appreciates the business.

One of the people Hurley sent to the psychologist's clinic was his second wife, who works as a principal in an elementary school. When he started dating her, he said, he noticed her office was cluttered with piles of papers, one of those "classic ADHD things." But it was not until he helped her move, he said, that he knew she had the disorder. "I opened a box marked 'Kitchen,'" he said, "but there wasn't anything for the kitchen in it."

His son went to Dr. Gersh two years after he did. He was diagnosed when he was a junior at Iowa State. His daughter got her diagnosis in seventh grade. Of twenty-three nieces and nephews, he says, six have been diagnosed with a form of attention deficit disorder.

Hurley told me he believes many people with the disorder are really geniuses who have been held back because they are not taking meds. His son now works as a mechanical engineer. His daughter got a doctorate in psychology. His clients, whom he coaches through the disorder, include a lawyer, a nurse with a Ph.D., and three engineers from Rockwell Collins, a large military contractor that has its headquarters in Cedar Rapids.

"They think some of the greatest minds had ADHD," he said, going on to mention Leonardo da Vinci, Benjamin Franklin, and Bill Clinton. "Thomas Edison and Einstein," he noted, "were both kicked out of school."

This theory—that a pill will unmask the latent genius within you—seemed to come straight out of the ads for drugs that treat the disorder. "Does living up to your potential feel like a game that never goes your way?" asked an ad on the website where Eli Lilly was promoting Strattera, a drug for attention deficit disorder, in the summer of 2005. The ad featured a bespectacled man, somewhere between ages twenty and thirty, who vaguely resembled Bill Gates. "Focus on the possible."

Hurley said he keeps his Ritalin bottle next to his alarm clock on the table beside his bed. When the alarm rings in the morning, he takes his pill and hits the snooze. In fifteen minutes, when the alarm buzzes again, his pill has kicked in, and he jumps out of bed. "Boom," he said. "I know it works."

He said he once worried all the time what people thought of him. But Ritalin took those thoughts away, he said. "Now I don't need input from people saying I'm a wonderful guy. I know I'm a wonderful guy. I know it was the medications."

I asked him about side effects. "I haven't had any, except I sweat more than I should," he said, raising his arms to show me the dark spots on his olive green T-shirt. I asked him about the increased blood pressure and heart problems I had read about in the warning labels printed by Novartis, the maker of Ritalin, and he raised his brows as if to say, "Now, that is a new one." He said he knows that some people believe the stimulant has stunted their children's growth. But as far as he knows, "Ritalin is the most tested medication that is on the market.

"My wife will tell me she sees kids who are zombies after taking their meds," he said. "I say, 'Well, they're taking the wrong ones.'"

Hurley said he likes to tell the people he meets, "Hi. I'm Pat Hurley, and I have ADHD." But he almost didn't get his diagnosis. According to Hurley, Dr. Gersh told him on his first visit that he believed he had had

ADHD as a child but had grown out of it. Hurley begged the doctor to screen him anyway. So the tests began.

In the first test, the doctor showed him some simple stick figure drawings of a house with a window and door, took them away, and asked him to draw them. He passed without a problem. Next was a computer test in which he had to hit a key every time he saw what looked like an orange seed appear on the screen. Again Hurley passed. Then the doctor asked him questions like "What color is the sky?" The answers were written in inks of varied colors, including the correct answer to the sky question, blue, which was written in yellow ink. Once again he succeeded. But the tests were only getting started. The doctor next read him a story for thirty seconds and asked him to repeat it. Hurley did well. In the test that followed, he listened to a tape-recorded voice recite a long list of numerals in a monotone. He was asked to count how many times he heard a certain number like 8. This was easy for him. Then, still listening to the tape, he was asked how many times he heard a certain numerical sequence, like 8 followed by 2. Again he passed.

The doctor continued to make it more complicated. The series of recited numbers had sequences such as 2 8 8 2 8 2 8 thrown in. "I was just lost," Hurley said. He agreed with me, however, that many people would not be able to get this right. The doctor then read twelve words slowly and asked him to repeat them back. It took him a dozen times, he said, to get them all right. The doctor had found his diagnosis. Hurley remembers the doctor exclaiming, "Oh, my God, we have these two bad scores."

The doctor then gave Hurley a tablet of Ritalin and prepared to give him the tests again. "Five minutes before the test this calmness came over me like nothing I ever felt before," Hurley says. "It was unbelievable."

Medicated on Ritalin, he passed all the tests. Hurley remembered how before his visit to Dr. Gersh, he had been "sort of a nonbeliever" in ADHD and daily medications. "Now I plan to be on them for the rest of my life."

IT WASN'T JUST Ritalin and Prozac that had become as socially acceptable as once-a-day vitamins. For many Iowans, their lives now revolved around their prescriptions.

Daily they swallowed their proton pump inhibitors and COX-2 inhibitors, tricyclics and analgesics, benzodiazepines and amphetamines, anticoagulants and antihypertensives, as well as their lipid reducers, serotonin escalators, and mood stabilizers.

On average, each Iowan now picked up fourteen prescriptions a year from the pharmacy. Some of the highest users needed that many medicines every day. Local newspapers were the first to document the predicaments of those prescribed ever more pills. Colleen Keith told the *Iowa City Press-Citizen* that she had taken nothing more than aspirin when she retired fourteen years earlier. Now, at seventy-four, she used a dozen medicines and had struggled recently to pay a four-hundred-dollar medicine bill.

"I don't know what to do," she said. "Truly."

Between 2000 and 2005 the average number of prescriptions used annually by each Iowan increased by 28 percent, a rise similar to that found across most of the nation. The number of prescriptions had continued to multiply even as the government decided that some heavily used drugs like Claritin and Prilosec could be purchased without prescriptions. This surge in the use of medications could not be tied to any outbreak of disease. Instead, the steady promotional buzz of the medicine merchants had made more Iowans believe they were sick, while fewer felt healthy and normal.

Health-minded people took pills with a host of side effects, believing they were a ticket to feeling better and more alive. On college campuses the prescription amphetamine stimulant called Adderall had become a study aid. "If I have an important test coming up, especially during finals, I can't get enough," Kelly Mikan, a sophomore at the University of Iowa, complained to the campus newspaper in 2005. Ms. Mikan said she often got her Adderall tablets from a friend who had been prescribed the drug after being diagnosed with an attention disorder.

"It's like asking a friend for a Tylenol when you're hung over," another student, Yvonne Lyngaas, explained.

Some elderly Iowans took so many meds prescribed by so many different physicians that they risked life-threatening interactions. A few drugstores like Lutz Pharmacy in Altoona, a suburb of Des Moines, began offering to sort through their customers' pills. Gene Lutz, a pharmacist and the store's owner, suggested his customers gather up their pill bottles, place them in a brown paper bag, and bring them in.

Lutz said there was "no question" that some of his customers were taking too many drugs or were taking heavily advertised ones when other older and far cheaper pills would be better. "The way medications get used or managed in this country," he said, "is broken."

It had gotten to the point where Iowans didn't even need a prescription. Viagra and diet pills were for sale, according to a classified ad in the *Forest City Summit*, a local newspaper in northern Iowa. "No prev. prescription or DR visit req'd," the ad promised. All a person required was a phone and a valid credit card.

Iowans of every age were on regimens of medications. Some toddlers were growing up in a permanently medicated state. Two-thirds of the day care centers surveyed in eastern Iowa reported that they were distributing doses of medicines for attention deficit disorder to some of their young attendees, according to a 2003 study by researchers at the University of Iowa. On a typical day almost 6 percent of the infants, toddlers, and children in those day care centers were given some kind of medicine, which ranged from antibiotics to insulin. That number did not include the children who took prescription drugs at home before their parents dropped them off.

In elementary school, children had grown accustomed to a daily medication break, just the way students before them had counted on milk time. When researchers from Iowa State University arrived at an elementary school in the 1990s, they found youngsters standing in a long line outside the office of the nurse, who was handing them their medication. The group found that 25 percent of the school's students were taking Ritalin or another stimulant for attention deficit disorder.

"Putting children on Ritalin became an easy solution," said Dr. Susan Hegland, an associate professor of human development and family studies, who organized the study. Dr. Hegland said that officials at the elementary school were even giving pills to one child who had not been diagnosed with the disorder. She later learned that the school had formed a partnership with a local mental health group, which had placed a staff person inside the school with a folder of blank prescriptions. She remembered how the principal of the school had commented, "Wow! These kids are active."

In 2005 some Iowa schools still had employees prescribing medicines to children. The schools employed nurse practitioners who can prescribe drugs just like physicians.

Even a few drivers of the eighteen-wheeled semitrucks speeding across Iowa on Interstate 80 fretted that their employers would find out they used prescription stimulants like Ritalin, Adderall, or Provigil to stay awake on their cross-country hauls. The truck drivers talked openly about their worries on an Internet blog that let them keep their identities hidden.

"Hey dude. I'm in the same boat," wrote a driver who identified himself only as birddog4334. "I take Ritalin and I've got to get my first medical this week . . . People like you and I function much better on Ritalin and the roads are much safer if we are taking the medication. So just don't tell them and give your system a few days to flush it out."

Another driver, meanbone79, said the drivers didn't need to fret. "DOT only checks for opiates, thc, barbituates [sic] and cocaine based drugs," he wrote. "Anything else goes unnoticed on a drug screening for truckers unless someone is killed then they do a blood test and check for everything. Hell I know drivers that take Lorcet, xanax, soma and other prescriptions and pass with no problem."

THE RISING POPULARITY of prescriptions was even changing the midwestern landscape. All over the city of Des Moines and its suburbs, the Walgreens pharmacies were rising. Workers had recently constructed more than a half dozen red-brick Walgreens drugstores, most of them on the high-priced prime corner lots that had long been home to gas stations. Someone driving across Des Moines on University Avenue in 2005 would spot three or more of these sprawling new pharmacies. The Walgreens stores sold everything from liquor to laundry soap, but 64 percent of their total sales came from the pills dispensed at the counter in the back.

In 2005 Walgreens opened drugstores in America at the rate of one every day. It now had more drugstores than Domino's had pizza kitchens.

And it had not stopped its expansion with Des Moines. It was staking out property for new stores in Iowa's more rural areas, anyplace where residents took enough prescriptions to meet its corporate goals. Walgreens' aggressive expansion plan in Iowa and the rest of the country was very much in line with its corporate credo, which reads in part, "We believe that we can get what we go after."

Walgreens was not the only company in Iowa to find increasing profits in the practice of filling prescriptions. Building pharmacies had become such a big business that one company bragged in 2004 that it could construct one in just three days.

Dozens of supermarkets in Iowa had recently added a pharmacist and a prescription counter. Hy-Vee, one of the largest supermarket chains in Iowa, was offering discounted groceries to anyone who transferred a prescription. Pharmacies had also been built inside the megastores like Wal-Mart, Costco, Target, and Kmart.

On Civic Mills Parkway in the booming suburban city of West Des Moines, the newly built pharmacies came one after another. In the last four-mile stretch of the parkway, which ended just as it became gravel and turned into cornfields, pharmacies outnumbered gas stations and fast-food joints. There were four pharmacies, including three built within the last year or so, as well as one Hy-Vee supermarket with pharmacy "coming soon," according to a white and red sign posted in a large lot.

The neighborhood, which just a few years before had been farmland, was a prosperous one with developments of gray-roofed homes, golf courses, and a new multimillion-dollar football stadium at the public high school. While I had to wait to pump my gas, a pharmacist was waiting and eager to help at each of the four pharmacy counters. I asked each pharmacist the price of a thirty-day prescription of twenty-milligram Lipitor tablets. With all those pharmacies, I had believed residents would benefit from lower prices as the stores competed against one another. But all of them charged more for Lipitor than the $96.99 price I found on the Internet site drugstore.com. The new Walgreens pharmacy was charging the most at $116.69. The most helpful pharmacist, the one behind the counter at Drug Town, suggested I ask the doctor to write a prescription for forty-milligram pills and then cut the tablet in two, allowing an order of fifteen pills, costing $59.09, to last the month through.

With construction rampant on Civic Mills, there was a good chance more fast-food restaurants and gas stations would soon be built. But it was clear from my visit in the summer of 2005 which businesses had the money to be the first in the neighborhood as the city of West Des Moines pushed west into the cornfields. It was the drugstores, as well as four or five banks.

One of the pharmacies on Civic Mills was inside the newly constructed Super Target, a store the size of an aircraft hangar that sold everything from furniture and clothing to choice-cut steaks. I walked through the doors, around the twenty checkout stands, past the Starbucks, to the pharmacy, where a large sign hanging over the counter said, LIVE FULLY. FEEL YOUR BEST. Of all the drugstores I visited in Iowa, Super Target was working the hardest to make medicines appear hip. The store had introduced its own scarlet red pill bottle, which it bragged would soon be on display in Manhattan's Museum of Modern Art. The bottle, which Target called "a revolution in pharmacy," came with a cap that could be color-coded for each family member so that parents didn't mistake their pills for those of their six-year-old twins.

Target was promoting its red pill bottle in 2005 as if it were a new line of clothing. It was even running advertisements to promote the bottle, which featured good-looking young adults and playful children. There were no grandmothers, no one who looked older than sixty, and no one who looked ill. In one ad, beautiful women read books that were magically transformed into red bottles. In another, three young children played in brightly colored inner tubes, each toy representing the color-coded cap on their prescription bottle. The implied message in the ads: taking meds can be as trendy as wearing a pair of Manolo Blahnik stiletto heels or as much fun as splashing in the pool.

Iowa pharmacies were also taking cues from the likes of Burger King and Jiffy Lube, serving up prescriptions fast and conveniently, any time of the day or night. If someone in Iowa City remembered at midnight he was out of tablets of Paxil or Provigil, he did not have to wait for morning. He could drive down to the Walgreens at the busy corner of Highway 6 and First Avenue in Coralville, which was staffed with a pharmacist twenty-four hours a day. Iowans needing to refill prescriptions did not even need to park their cars. Drugstores had drive-through windows, where one could pick up a bottle of pills just like a Big Mac.

Many people got their pills without ever leaving their homes. They simply pressed a few keys on the Internet or called a toll-free number and had their pills delivered just like a mail-order purchase from Sears or L.L.Bean. These orders went to giant prescription-filling factories like Medco or Express Scripts, where robots filled the bottles at a rate of five thousand per hour, before sending them down a conveyor belt to be wrapped, addressed, and dropped in the mail.

This was medicine in a minute. People wanted their fix, and they wanted it quick. Health care was becoming just another part of the economy that was run like a fast-food restaurant, a trend that the sociologist George Ritzer has called the McDonaldization of society.

At many pharmacies in Iowa, a mother needing a medicine for her child could pick from forty-two flavors, as if she were selecting a milk shake in strawberry, chocolate, or vanilla. This medicine-flavoring service, offered by a fast-growing company called FLAVORx, was advertised prominently in most of the pharmacies I visited. At the Kmart pharmacy in Marshalltown, Iowa, FLAVORx had erected a five-foot cardboard cutout of a smiling pink spoon. Written in crayon and in the block letters that a child would use was the line "We make medicine a lot less yucky." In an ad on the company's website, a freckle-faced boy exclaimed, "FLAVORx is so yummy . . . I wish they filled donuts with it." The staff at FLAVORx had even performed research to find the best flavors for specific medicines. Prozac, the antidepressant, tasted best when flavored in raspberry, grape, or banana, according to the company's analysis, while Tylenol with codeine went down smoothly when mixed with the artificial essence of citrus punch.

At the same time, pharmacies were now selling many drugs that had once been available only by prescription as freely as they sold snacks or cosmetics. In recent years, pharmaceutical companies had successfully lobbied the federal government to remove the "by prescription only" status from many medicines, including big sellers such as Zantac, Tagamet, and Prilosec. No longer did the consumer need a physician. It was becoming easier to self-medicate.

The drug companies promoted some of these over-the-counter medicines as sugary confections. In 2006 Johnson & Johnson, for example, sold Tylenol in chewy melt-aways flavored in Grape Punch, Wacky Watermelon, or Bubblegum Burst. "Kids prefer it," said the company's ads. For the more discerning consumer, the company sold Tylenol Cool Caplets, a sort of breath enhancer and pain reliever in one. The company covered the medicine caplets with a strong mint-flavored coating, which it described in its ads as "super cooling." The Cool Caplets and Tylenol melt-aways were what Madison Avenue called brand extensions. The result was a potentially deadly pain reliever that looked and tasted like the sweet treats offered in a candy store.

Some of these heavily promoted over-the-counter drugs could be especially dangerous for the elderly, according to studies, but their easy availability made them appear as safe as soda or salad dressing. The heartburn drug Tagamet, for instance, was included on a well-known list of drugs that the elderly should avoid because it can cause dizziness, confusion, and memory problems. This information was not included on the Tagamet boxes I found being sold off the drugstore shelf.

In 1951 Congress had tried to protect Americans from dangerous drugs they did not need by amending the law to require patients to get prescriptions from physicians for most medications. Before that, pharmacists could give consumers whatever drugs they desired. This protection, however, was fast disappearing in the land of McMedicine.

A few supermarkets and pharmacies had even begun to add their own in-store medical clinics, allowing a customer to see a health professional for a prescription and then finish her shopping while it was filled. The stores often built these new exam rooms just steps from their pharmacies, which could count on increased business. In 2006 a Hy-Vee supermarket in Davenport, Iowa, opened an in-store clinic. The NOW OPEN sign promised "really, really, fast health care right here in your neighborhood."

Wal-Mart had also begun adding medical clinics to its superstores. In Minneapolis a company called MinuteClinic was building exam rooms inside Cub Foods, Target stores, and CVS pharmacies. "You're sick. We're quick" was the motto of the company run by the former chief executive of Arby's, the fast-food chain. For a reasonable fee of forty-five or fifty dollars, a nurse practitioner would examine a customer and write a prescription in just fifteen minutes.

While the operating principles of a fast-food restaurant may work when you sell grande lattes or change oil in automobiles, there are dangers in reorganizing medicine for speedy and easy mass consumption. Medicine is a complex art that cannot easily be reduced to a cookbooklike checklist that can be applied to every patient. Such standardization may help a teenager assemble a bacon double cheeseburger, but it leaves room for potentially deadly mistakes when used to diagnose and treat an ailing human being.

The close business relationship between these in-store clinics and pharmacies also created a conflict of interest. The more meds prescribed in the clinic, the more money made at the pharmacy counter. There was a danger that patients would get drugs they did not need or whatever medicine happened to make the most money for the pharmacy, whether it was the best one for them or not.

IT HAD COME to a point where almost any bodily function or any feeling could be tweaked with the help of a pill. Some of the most popular medicines in Iowa were those that brightened, calmed, or otherwise altered the public's moods. A deep melancholy seemed to have crept across the farmland and prairie, or so it seemed on the basis of the rising prescriptions for antidepressants and other mood-altering drugs.

In 2003 Wellmark, the state's largest health insurer, announced that the number of antidepressant prescriptions written for those it insured in Iowa and South Dakota had risen by more than 90 percent in just four years. Almost 14 percent of the Iowans covered by its plan were taking Paxil, Zoloft, Effexor, or a similar drug, Wellmark said. This was higher than the national rate of antidepressant use, which the insurer said was 10.7 percent. Almost three-quarters of the Iowans who took the pills were women.

The rate of antidepressant use varied from town to town with the residents of Ames, the home of Iowa State University, taking the most. In Ames almost 18 percent of the adult population was on an antidepressant.

Wellmark, the insurer, had helped spur the rise in antidepressants by asking physicians in its network to have patients—whether visiting the doctor for asthma, an annual physical, or a broken leg—answer nine written questions about their mood. Wellmark said doctors should give the quiz to patients who appeared tired, complained of unexplained symptoms, had many worries, could not get enough sleep, were having problems at work or home, or had already visited a physician several times that year. This would cover a substantial number of the patients in any physician's waiting room. The questionnaire allowed primary care doctors to swiftly diagnose depression and prescribe an antidepressant as just one part of the fifteen-minute office visit. Pfizer, the manufacturer of Zoloft, had paid to create the questionnaire, known as Prime-MD, for use across the country. Pfizer also paid to have the checklist distributed and promoted to Iowa doctors.

The drug company's marketers were so successful in promoting Prime-MD that by 2005 family physicians around the world were using the questionnaire. Pfizer's consultants had even refined the screening method to the point where doctors were said to be able to find depressed patients through a two-question test that took just a minute. Medical journals were jammed with articles about the need for family physicians to screen patients for mental illness whether they complained of depression or not. Proponents of the screening ignored studies that had found as many as a quarter of patients diagnosed with depression by their family physician—a doctor not trained in the intricacies of psychiatric disorders—did not meet the symptoms of depression.

In Iowa, a group of researchers announced in the fall of 2005 that the use of Pfizer's questionnaire in two rural clinics had done little to help patients. "We found that the same thing that has been reported so many times in the past," explained Dr. George Bergus, an associate professor of family medicine at the University of Iowa, who led the study. The questionnaire increased the number of people diagnosed with depression, he said, "but the outcome that we were really after, that of improving depression, is not achieved."

Yet it was not just adults who were being screened and prescribed more antidepressants. Doctors were prescribing more of these same psychiatric medicines to children. The year 2003 marked the first time that Americans spent more to treat their children with Ritalin, Prozac, and other psychiatric drugs than they spent on children's antibiotics or asthma medications. That milestone was reported by analysts from Medco Health Solutions, who noted that there had been a startling 369 percent rise in just three years in spending on Ritalin and other drugs for attention disorders in children not yet old enough for kindergarten.

> "Since I went back to work, he started doing the baby thing," the mother of a young boy was telling the physician over the speakerphone.
>
> "It looked like he had untreated attention deficit, but now I'm not so sure," the doctor replied. "I want to try Lexapro."
>
> "I'm on Lexapro," the mother said. But she added that she was uncertain whether the antidepressant would be right for her son. "He doesn't swallow pills well."
>
> "It's teeny tiny," the doctor replied. "It's like a dot . . . The diagnosis I'll give him is generalized anxiety disorder."
>
> "Okay," the mother said.
>
> "I'd like to see him before he goes back to school," the doctor continued. "The biggest side effect of this is a little bit of an upset stomach."
>
> The doctor got the child back on the speakerphone.
>
> "I'm concerned about all the worrying you do," the doctor told the boy. "Would you be willing to try a medication to get rid of all those worries?"
>
> The child hesitated. He said he didn't like taking pills.
>
> "You can barely see it," the doctor said. "It's so tiny."

Dr. Sharon Collins was recalling the stories of her young patients, telling them quickly, one after another, as if for too long she had kept them locked up inside. She told me she had been almost afraid to speak.

"Our system is broken," she said in a gentle, measured voice. "I get fiery angry."

Dr. Collins is a slight woman with kind brown eyes. She was sitting in her small office near Mercy Medical Center in Cedar Rapids, where she is director of pediatrics. Her desk was the cluttered one of a busy pediatrician. Beside the piles of medical journals and papers were frames holding photos of her own three children.

Dr. Collins had moved to Iowa from a rural part of Kansas sixteen years before. At that time, she said, about one of every ten of her young patients was taking prescription stimulants like Ritalin for attention disorders.

"Now, if I have children just on Ritalin, I consider it a happy day," she said. "Now they're on four or five drugs."

Dr. Collins said she sees many children who are angry, scared, and depressed. What concerns her most, she said, is that the children who need help so desperately almost always receive it in a chemical form.

"People want the quick fix," she said. "People want something now—yesterday actually."

She hears from parents who have been told by school officials that their child needs medication to control his behavior. In other cases, parents have seen the calming effect a drug had on their friend's child and want the same thing for their son.

"I had one father who came in and said, 'This kid is a problem, and I want him on medication.' I said, 'I'm not comfortable with that. I need to know more.' He was livid with me."

She recounted how another doctor had prescribed Ritalin to one of her young patients who was just starting kindergarten. About a week later the boy began having seizures. Dr. Collins said she believed that the stimulant may have played a role in bringing on the seizures, and she asked the boy's family to stop giving him the pills. Novartis, the maker of Ritalin, had warned that some children have had seizures after taking the drug.

The boy's other physician disagreed with her theory, Dr. Collins said, and started his Ritalin prescription again. This time the boy's seizures were out of control, and doctors began talking about how he might need brain surgery to stop them. Dr. Collins said she again talked to the family and convinced them to stop the Ritalin for good. The boy's seizures stopped, she said, and haven't reappeared after four years.

"No one cared about his seizures," she said. "They wanted his behavior controlled."

And then there was the day the stepmother of one of her patients called to say she was worried because the girl was depressed. Dr. Collins referred the family to a counselor she knew, but the visit was brief. The counselor talked to the girl for twenty minutes, before sending her back to Dr. Collins. The counselor told Dr. Collins that she believed the girl had lost her joy for living and needed an antidepressant. When the girl arrived, Dr. Collins began asking her question after question, trying to find out just what it was that had saddened her. "I asked her one question, and the tears just started to flood," she said. "She was very angry her parents had divorced. She loved her stepmom but felt bad about her mom. I said, 'Oh, my gosh, I can understand. That would be hard.'"

Dr. Collins called the counselor to tell her that she needed to talk to the girl about her parents' divorce. A couple of weeks later the counselor called to say the girl had not returned. Worried, Dr. Collins called the girl's stepmother, who told her the girl's mood had brightened since she had talked to Dr. Collins. "She's great," the stepmom had said.

Dr. Collins's voice rose as she thought back to the child. "Nobody is talking to these kids," she said. "Nobody is pointing out where their struggles lie . . . You can't just keep medicating people and medicating people and not dealing with the underlying issue."

Physicians don't take the time to find out what is bothering the child, she said, because that is not what insurance companies pay them to do. "I don't get paid for forty minutes of talking," she said. "Instead, I get paid for a fifteen-minute examination, enough time to prescribe an antidepressant."

DR. COLLINS IS not the only physician in the state to be shaken by the rising number of psychiatric drugs taken by Iowa's children.

"We're seeing kids on three, four, five, six drugs," said Dr. Jeffrey Lobas, the director of fourteen clinics in Iowa that specialize in children's health. "It's what I see as a common practice."

I first met Dr. Lobas, who is also a professor at the University of Iowa, at a pediatrics conference in Washington in May 2005. We both were attending an early Sunday-morning session for physicians on how to treat attention deficit disorders in preschoolers. Five doctors spoke about how to diagnose these young children and treat them with prescription stimulants such as Ritalin, Concerta, Adderall, and others. Three of the speakers, all considered top experts in their field, disclosed that they had financial relationships with one or more pharmaceutical companies. One speaker, Dr. Laurence L. Greenhill, a professor at Columbia University, noted that he had a financial arrangement with seven drug companies, including the makers of the biggest-selling drugs for attention deficit disorder. Even the doctor who moderated the session worked as a consultant to two pharmaceutical firms.

Dozens of pediatricians from all over the country listened to the presentations. The doctors gave each speaker a round of applause. But when the presentations were over, it was clear that a few pediatricians in the audience had been unsettled by the talk of prescribing Ritalin to three-year-olds who were always on the go. When the panel asked for questions, Dr. Lobas had walked to the microphone and said he was seeing children in Iowa on multiple medications, a practice that doctors call polypharmacy. Dr. Lobas said it appeared that some doctors caring for these children were of the mind "Why use one drug when you can use three?"

One of the speakers, Dr. Christopher Varley, from the University of Washington, told Dr. Lobas he understood his concern. There were almost no studies that looked at what happened when children took more than one pill, Dr. Varley explained, and there was not a single study that followed kids who took four or more drugs at a time. In essence, treating children with more than one drug was an experimental venture.

The clinics that Dr. Lobas directs in Iowa see more than five thousand children each year. Twenty years ago, he said, most kids going to the doctor had physical problems. Today most children visiting the clinics, he said, are being treated for mental, emotional, or behavioral problems.

Ritalin, or a similar drug like Adderall or Concerta, is often the first medicine these children are prescribed. The fast growth in the use of these drugs began in the early 1990s, as the pharmaceutical companies increased their promotion and after federal lawmakers made attention deficit disorder a protected disability under the Individuals with Disabilities Education Act. Lawmakers also agreed that families could collect federal disability payments known as supplemental security income (SSI), in cases in which children were impaired by the disorder.

Doctors wrote almost five times as many prescriptions for Ritalin and similar drugs in 1996 as they had just six years before. Most of these were written for children. By 2004 2.5 million American children were taking these drugs, including almost 10 percent of all ten-year-old boys.

Researchers have found that the prescription rate for stimulants such as Ritalin can vary radically between cities, with the highest use in relatively white, suburban, and affluent areas. In 2004 Dr. Farasat Bokhari, an assistant professor of economics at Florida State University, and his colleagues published a study that showed that the counties with the highest rates of psychostimulant use had higher income levels, less unemployment, and more children in private schools.

The communities of Iowa City and Cedar Rapids in eastern Iowa have some of the highest rates of Ritalin use in the whole country, as does Iowa as a whole. Other states with high numbers of medicated children include New Hampshire, Vermont, Michigan, and Delaware, according to the Drug Enforcement Administration, which closely tracks the flow of the drugs because of their potential for addiction and abuse.

These statistics tend to feed on themselves. When numbers are released from an area of the country where prescriptions are high, officials at schools with lower numbers can be quick to believe that they have children suffering from the disorder who have not yet been diagnosed. For example, a 2002 newsletter for Iowa's school nurses detailed a new study that found that 15 percent of white boys in the fourth and fifth grades in Johnston County, North Carolina, had been diagnosed with ADHD. The headline in the Iowa newsletter: IMPACT OF ATTENTION DEFICIT-HYPERACTIVITY MAY BE UNDERESTIMATED.

But Ritalin is often just the beginning of what becomes a long history of medications for the child. The stories that Dr. Lobas and Dr. Collins tell of the increasing number of children on multiple meds have been confirmed in studies from around the country. For example, one research team used national data to look at office visits at which the doctor had prescribed Ritalin or a similar drug to a child diagnosed with ADHD. They found the doctor had prescribed Ritalin *and at least one other psychotropic drug* in 25 percent of those office visits in 1997 and 1998. This was a fivefold increase from just four years earlier, when only 5 percent of such office visits resulted in prescriptions for two or more medicines.

Experts have all sorts of theories on why American children are taking more psychiatric medicines every year. Some critics fault the tests used to diagnose children with attention disorders and other mental illnesses. They say these tests use criteria that are far too vague and that normal childhood behaviors are now considered symptoms of mental illness. There is no blood test or other way to test physically for attention deficit disorder or any other mental illness. Instead doctors use the *Diagnostic and Statistical Manual of Mental Disorders*, a nine-hundred-page guide written by psychiatrists and published by the American Psychiatric Association, which has gained enormous power in America today. The *DSM*, as it is commonly called, states that a child has an attention deficit disorder if he or she displays six of nine described behaviors. These behaviors include failing to pay close attention to details, not listening when spoken to, failing to finish schoolwork, forgetting things, or being easily distracted. The doctor may add hyperactivity to the attention deficit diagnosis if the child often fidgets or squirms in his or her seat, runs or climbs in situations where such activity is inappropriate, has difficulty playing quietly, or is often "on the go."

Ten years ago, most children diagnosed with a mental illness were said to have an attention deficit disorder. Today, doctors diagnose attention deficit disorder and then frequently tack on one or more of the dozens of other psychiatric diagnoses listed in the *DSM*, which might include depression, obsessive-compulsive disorder, conduct disorder, generalized anxiety disorder, or something called intermittent explosive disorder for children who show extreme anger at what others consider minor incidents. Many of the disorders described in the current edition of the *DSM* did not even exist thirty years ago. In 1952 the manual listed 106 mental illnesses. By 1994 the list had expanded to 357. Critics of the *DSM* have argued that its authors have been far too eager to add new disorders, even when the science supporting their existence is lacking.

At the same time, psychiatrists have changed the definition of depression and other mental illnesses that have long been recognized so that they include larger groups of people. When a scientist at the pharmaceutical company Ciba-Geigy came up with the first antidepressant, a drug called Tofranil, in the 1950s, the company had little interest in marketing it because so few people were thought to suffer from depression. As few as one in ten thousand people was then thought to be depressed. By 2005 some scientists estimated that as many as one thousand to two thousand of every ten thousand people suffered from depression, or as much as 20 percent of the public. This would mean there had been a thousandfold increase in the rate of depression over fifty years.

This expanding number of psychiatric diagnoses, as well as the growing number of people said to suffer from them, has led to a bitter national debate: Is life being redefined as a string of mental disorders, each requiring treatment with pills?

Dr. Stuart A. Kirk, a professor of social welfare at UCLA, has spent years studying the *DSM*, how it was created and how it is used. He says he has come to believe that the psychiatrists who wrote the *DSM* are "making us all crazy" by their continual expansion of behaviors they defined as psychiatric disorders. In an essay in 2005, Dr. Kirk wrote that psychiatrists now see signs of a mental disorder in children when they "are deceitful, break rules, can't sit still or wait in lines, have trouble with math, don't pay attention to details, don't listen, don't like to do homework or lose their school assignments or pencils, or speak out of turn." American psychiatrists and drug companies, he said, are eyeing the lengthening list of disorders in the *DSM* "like a lumber company lusting after a redwood forest."

Indeed, at times the drug companies have blazed ahead of even the psychiatrists writing the *DSM*. In 2001 Forest Laboratories paid for an experiment in which it hoped to show that Celexa, its antidepressant, was an effective treatment for something called compulsive shopping disorder. The drug company's study created a frenzy in the media. The newscaster Charles Gibson told viewers of *Good Morning America* on ABC that this new disorder could affect as many as twenty million Americans, 90 percent of them women. Appearing as an expert on the program was Dr. Jack Gorman, a professor of psychiatry at Columbia University. Dr. Gorman was also a consultant to Forest Laboratories and a dozen other drug companies, although his audience did not learn those facts. He told viewers that 80 percent of the compulsive shoppers in the study slowed their purchases after taking Celexa. The flurry of publicity caused the American Psychiatric Association to put out a statement saying it had no intention of adding such a disorder to its next revision of the *DSM*.

Other experts have blamed societal changes for the rising number of psychiatric prescriptions for children, including the high divorce rate in America, the increase in the number of mothers who work, and parents who increasingly find themselves too busy to give their children all the attention they desire. In Iowa about 70 percent of children under the age of six have parents who both work.

Some scientists have pointed a finger at television. A study in 2004 found that the more television children watched between the ages of one and three, the more likely it was that they would be diagnosed with an attention disorder by age seven.

Other studies have theorized that children with attention disorders are not getting enough exercise or eating nutritious foods. Some researchers blame the large classroom sizes in many public schools, which may make some teachers push for their unruly students to be medicated. Or perhaps in some cases, high-achieving parents have desired high-performing children and believed they could boost their potential by getting them prescriptions.

Dr. Lobas lays some of the blame for the rising use of psychiatric medicines by Iowa children on the lack of counseling and other nonmedical help available for parents who are overwhelmed. Society should aim to improve children's behavior through families and the community, he said, rather than use the medical system to hand out pills. Parenting is a skill that can be taught, he said, and the state could help by having more social workers visit troubled families at home. While psychiatric medications might be okay for some adults, Dr. Lobas said, most children need help in ways that don't involve pills. "Kids are not small adults," he said. "Kids need to be supported and loved and they'll turn out okay."

IN RECENT YEARS, the administrators of Iowa's schools had been bombarded with claims that their students were suffering from mental illnesses that had not yet been diagnosed. In 2005 many Iowa school boards heard presentations about a program called TeenScreen, a program started by Dr. David Shaffer, a professor of psychiatry at Columbia University, who has worked as a consultant to some of the leading makers of psychiatric drugs. Dr. Shaffer was the leader of a team that reported in 1996 that nearly 21 percent of American children suffered from a mental disorder, a study that started a flurry of discussions across the nation about "a crisis" in children's mental health. The team's estimate meant that in every classroom of thirty students, six were mentally ill.

The staff of the TeenScreen program, which had its offices in Manhattan, offered to test schoolchildren regularly for a variety of mental illnesses. Their mission—to reduce teenage suicides—was a noble one. The problem was that scientific studies had not been able to prove that the benefits of such screening outweighed the possible harm, which includes the danger of diagnosing and prescribing medications to students who are not mentally ill.

The pharmaceutical industry had long been involved in promoting Dr. Shaffer's work. For example, at the press conference in 2000 at which Dr. Shaffer announced that he had shown that screening adolescents at school could find those at risk of suicide, Solvay Pharmaceuticals, the maker of the antidepressant Luvox, presented two checks, each for $250,000, to the Foundation for Suicide Prevention, where Dr. Shaffer served as president. The checks were part of Solvay's pledge to pay $1 million to the foundation, which has helped spread the word about TeenScreen. In 2005 the foundation's chairman was David A. Dodd, the former chief executive of Solvay. Other directors of the foundation included executives from Pfizer and Johnson & Johnson.

By the end of 2005 at least seven school districts in Iowa were using

TeenScreen, and not all parents were happy about it. Pam Wheeler, a Des Moines mother of three, said she worried the screening would identify children who were not actually ill but simply coping with some of the rough times that are typical in the life of an American teenager. "If you ask a sixteen-year-old girl whether she has had a hard time getting out of bed, there is a good chance she will say yes," Mrs. Wheeler said. "She could have just broken up with her boyfriend or had a fight with her mom. My concern is that this is a way to squeeze in more diagnoses for mental illness that may not exist."

The TeenScreen program focused on teenagers, but some of the antidepressant manufacturers had also pushed in recent years to screen Iowa children who were much younger. For example, Pfizer, GlaxoSmithKline, and Eli Lilly paid in 2001 to promote mental health screenings for all kids during what organizers called Child Health Month. The event's main message was that one out of every five Iowa children had a mental illness that could be diagnosed and treated. The organizers said that those children who were not treated were more likely to end up unemployed, abusing drugs, physically ill, or serving time in prison. Iowa governor Tom Vilsack, the University of Iowa, and the state's pediatricians urged parents to have their children tested.

At least one pharmaceutical company had even been able to place a storybook it published in a library used by Iowa's public schools. Solvay Pharmaceuticals had distributed the book *Kids Like Me* across the country to promote its antidepressant Luvox.

The book featured Marc Summers, the host of *Double Dare*, a children's game show on Nickelodeon. Summers wrote about how he had been diagnosed with obsessive-compulsive disorder, a mental illness he described as a "brain with hiccups" or as a "chemical imbalance."

The book then told the stories of children it said also suffered from the disorder, which is often referred to by its initials, OCD. In one story, eight-year-old Alicia can't stop saying her prayers until she believes she has said the words just right. Alicia's lengthy prayers prompt Father Joseph to tell her she may be suffering from the disorder. The priest gets Alicia an appointment with a doctor and promises she will soon feel better.

Another story in the book features Joey Martinez, a young boy who declares he has to bounce the basketball exactly nine times before taking a shot. This worries his father, who takes Joey to see Dr. Reese. The doctor quickly has a solution for the child.

> "Joey," continued Dr. Reese, "I'm going to give you a medicine that should help you with your OCD."
>
> But before Joey could answer him, his dad quickly spoke up. "Why does he need medicine? Why can't he just make himself stop thinking all of these bad thoughts?"
>
> "Mr. Martinez, Joey doesn't think about these horrible things because he wants to. People with OCD have a brain chemical that isn't working correctly. Sometimes the medicine can help correct that. If your son had an eye problem and needed to wear glasses to see better, would you tell him not to use them?"
>
> "Of course not!" Mr. Martinez laughed.

Solvay was not the only antidepressant manufacturer trying to convince Americans of all ages that they could eliminate their anxiety or sadness by swallowing a pill that restored the chemicals in their heads.

"Life is too precious to let another day go by feeling not quite 'yourself,'" declared a magazine ad for Paxil CR in 2002. "If you've experienced some of these symptoms of depression nearly every day, for at least two weeks, a chemical imbalance could be to blame."

Pfizer made similar claims in advertisement after advertisement as it built its product Zoloft into a billion-dollar drug. "Zoloft may help correct the chemical imbalance of serotonin in the brain," stated Pfizer's guide for patients taking Zoloft. "This helps relieve your symptoms."

Pfizer even promoted the idea of a chemical imbalance in an elaborate museum exhibit about the brain that it created and then sent to travel the circuit of the nation's science centers, beginning with a six-month stay at the Smithsonian in Washington in 2001. By 2005 the exhibition had not yet come to Iowa, but the state's science teachers were recommending the company's virtual tour of the museum display to classrooms across the state. Kids could navigate through the virtual tour of the exhibit by hitting icons resembling oval-shaped prescription tablets. The site included the *Neuron Run* video game as well as "fun facts" for kids. The exhibit claimed that "half of all the people in the United States experience some degree of brain dysfunction at some time in their lives." It also explained the cause of this dysfunction. For example, this was its explanation for anxiety: "Chemical imbalances in the brain—often involving the neurotransmitter serotonin—are almost certainly involved."

Pfizer then told visitors to the museum exhibit what they could do about these chemical imbalances. "More medications than ever before are available," it explained.

The manufacturers of drugs for children with attention deficit disorder had waged similar campaigns. In 2005, for example, Johnson & Johnson discussed brain chemicals on a website promoting its drug Concerta. Under the heading "Science Made Simple," the company claimed its drug worked this way: "The Cerebellum, Basal Ganglia, and the Prefrontal Cortex are rich in brain chemicals (norepinephrine and dopamine) that impact emotion, behavior, thinking, and attention skills, which are related to ADHD. Medications like Concerta help restore brain chemical communications to more normal levels."

And in 1997 Novartis, the maker of Ritalin, distributed a booklet to teachers across America, urging them to explain the drugs to parents in this way: "These medicines do not 'drug' or 'alter' the brain of the child. They make the child 'normal' by correcting for a neurochemical imbalance."

Doctors and hospitals in Iowa helped the drug companies spread the word that many people suffered from chemical imbalances that were easily treatable with prescription pills. At an event for children at the Jordan Creek mall in West Des Moines in 2005, a clown was painting youngsters' faces and the staff of Mercy Hospital was offering its services in diagnosing children with attention deficit disorders. The hospital employees were handing out brochures that said drugs like Ritalin "medicate parts of the brain which aren't working as well as they should."

The idea of a "chemical imbalance"—that mental suffering was caused by nothing more than a lack of certain brain chemicals—was a concept that Iowans could readily embrace. It was an alluring theory that anyone coping with severe stress or unhappiness could be tempted to believe. It freed the person from blame for anything that might have caused the unhappiness. It also made any kind of mental anguish something that could be easily and swiftly remedied by taking a pill. By getting the public to believe that sadness could be corrected with an antidepressant just as diabetes could be managed with insulin, the companies sold billions of dollars' worth of medicines. By 2001 drugs for the brain and central nervous system were accounting for almost a quarter of the prescriptions written in the United States, and sales were growing at a pace of 20 percent a year.

The problem with the notion that mental illness is caused by a chemical imbalance is that it is little more than that. It's a theory—oversimplified by drug marketers—that scientists have not been able to prove despite decades of work.

Some psychiatric experts have tried to set the record straight. They point out that the brain is immensely complex and that scientists understand very little about how it works.

"I spent the first several years of my career doing full-time research on brain serotonin metabolism, but I never saw any convincing evidence that any psychiatric disorder, including depression, results from a deficiency of brain serotonin," said Dr. David Burns, an adjunct clinical professor of psychiatry and behavioral sciences at Stanford University, when he was asked about the serotonin imbalance theory in 2003. "In fact, we cannot measure brain serotonin levels in living human beings so there is no way to test this theory. Some neuroscientists would question whether the theory is even viable, since the brain does not function in this way, as a hydraulic system."

Wrote Dr. Elliot S. Valenstein, professor emeritus of psychology and neuroscience at the University of Michigan, in his 1998 book *Blaming the Brain*: "It may surprise you to learn that there is no convincing evidence that most mental patients have any chemical imbalance . . . The theories have changed very little over the years despite much evidence that they cannot possibly be correct."

In 2005 Dr. Kenneth S. Kendler, professor of human genetics and psychiatry at Virginia Commonwealth University, wrote, "We have hunted for big, simple neurochemical explanations for psychiatric disorders and have not found them."

Scientists have also failed to tie attention deficit disorders in children to an imbalance of brain chemicals. At a 1998 meeting organized by the federal government, a group of top scientists in the field concluded that there were "no data to indicate that ADHD is due to a brain malfunction."

Similarly, Dr. William B. Carey, professor of pediatrics at the University of Pennsylvania, wrote in 2002, "The assumption that the ADHD symptoms arise from cerebral malfunction has not been supported even after extensive investigations."

GRANDMA WAS THE first to notice. She was sliding the new school picture of her ten-year-old grandson into a frame, covering up the photo that had marked the year before.

"Look at Peter's eyes," she told her daughter, Sandy Koppen. "They look dead."

One hot afternoon in the summer of 2005, Sandy pulled her son's school photos from a drawer, and we lined them up, from kindergarten to high school graduation, on her dining room table. It was then that the story of a young boy prescribed one drug, only to have doctors add two more, began to fall into place.

In the third-grade photo, before his first prescription of Ritalin, Peter is grinning; his eyes are bright. By the fifth grade the smile has disappeared. His eyes are vacant. His mood appears as sullen and gray as the color of his sweater. In the photo taken the following year, he has a funky crew cut at the age of eleven and a half, but the same blank stare.

"That's what really woke me up," Sandy said, recalling the discussion with her mother about Peter's empty gaze. "I thought, where is he? He's all locked up inside because of all these meds."

Sandy said she once believed in the medicines. But that was before she saw what they did to Peter and her younger son, Aaron, as they grew up in a farmhouse they called Windridge Acres. The house was built by her husband, John, on top of a hill about three miles outside Shellsburg, a town with a one-block-long downtown business district and just a few more than nine hundred souls. The WINDRIDGE ACRES sign still welcomes any visitor who turns off the gravel road and onto the lane leading up to the house. But the sign has faded with the years, and Sandy now says she would have done things differently if only she had known what she does now.

PETER'S TROUBLES BEGAN on a cold day in 1990, when his father, John, died. Peter was seven, just old enough to know what he had lost. Sandy took Peter to a grief counselor, but the talking didn't seem to help. His schoolteachers began to complain that he wouldn't pay attention and seemed to be lost in space. One day Peter crawled into the tunnel on the playground and refused to come out. "The counselor thought he hadn't gotten over his dad's death," Sandy recalled. "Everybody said, 'Put him on meds.'"

A psychiatrist diagnosed Peter with attention deficit disorder and scribbled a prescription for Ritalin. But the drug seemed to do more harm than good, and the doctor switched him to a pill called Dexedrine. The doctor told Peter to take the pills in the morning, at noon, and, if he had activities after school, at 4:00 p.m.

Dexedrine is approved to treat hyperactive and distractible children as young as age three. The medicine is a type of amphetamine that is strictly controlled by drug enforcement officials. They explain that Dexedrine, like Ritalin, can have an effect similar to cocaine. The drug's label warns that it can cause episodes of psychosis, restlessness, tremors, and tics. It can elevate blood pressure and cause the heart to race. No one really knows how it works.

In the 1950s and 1960s amphetamines such as Dexedrine were marketed as a remedy for exhausted long-haul truck drivers, overweight persons of every sort, and even bored housewives who troubled their husbands with too many complaints. The U.S. military has long given Dexedrine to pilots on long-range bombing missions. The pilots refer to the drug as their "go pills."

Young Peter hated taking the orange-colored tablets that had a triangular shape. "I found pills shoved into furniture and down into plants," Sandy recalled.

Drug manufacturers boast in their ads for stimulants like Ritalin and Dexedrine that the pills will boost children's grades. But they did nothing for Peter, who continued to get Cs and Ds. He also became angry sometimes. Anger is a known side effect of Dexedrine.

When told of his bad temper, the psychiatrist gave Peter an additional diagnosis of oppositional defiant disorder. Sandy believes that is why the doctor wrote yet another prescription for her son, this time for the antidepressant Paxil. Doctors diagnose children with oppositional defiant disorder if they often lose their temper, argue, or disobey, behaviors not uncommon in boys. Some studies have said that as many as 20 percent of schoolchildren meet the symptoms of the disorder as listed in the *DSM*.

The government has never approved the use of Paxil by children, but doctors can legally prescribe it to whomever they want. The antidepressant comes with its own long list of side effects. Some people taking it have become manic, impulsive, and ceaselessly restless.

Peter remembered how the mix of the powerful drugs made him feel "loopy."

"I was out of it all the time," he said. "I just needed someone to spend more time with me."

Neither Peter nor Sandy remembers exactly why the doctor then prescribed Depakote, a drug that its maker, Abbott Laboratories, markets for conditions ranging from migraines to seizures to mania. Peter believes the doctor told him it would help him fall asleep and escape the effect of his daily doses of stimulants, which are known to keep children wired and awake all night. Sandy thinks the doctor prescribed Depakote because Peter was spacey.

"The doctors would see the kids for just a couple of minutes," Sandy said. "Every time there was a side effect, they would add a new med."

But each new medicine meant even more adverse effects. Depakote has a warning on its label, printed in a box with black borders so doctors won't miss it, which states that people have died after the drug caused the pancreas to become inflamed or the liver to fail. Perhaps taking such a high-stakes risk would have been worth it if Peter had been helped by the drugs. But the brighter mood, better report card, and growing circle of friends promised in the advertisements for such psychiatric drugs never came to Peter.

When he was a junior in high school, he dropped out of school.

AARON, THE YOUNGER boy, got his first psychiatric diagnosis in the second grade. Sandy ties his diagnosis back to the day of a class trip and an unwritten note of appreciation. Aaron's teacher asked students each to write a thank-you note to the group that had hosted the outing. Aaron refused. For two hours he sat, refusing to write, until the teacher hauled him to the principal's office. The psychiatrist said that Aaron had attention deficit disorder, like Peter, but was also hyperactive, making the formal diagnosis attention deficit hyperactivity disorder. The doctor prescribed Ritalin for Aaron, but, when it did not work, switched the drug to the same one Peter was taking, Dexedrine.

As the months passed, doctors wrote prescriptions for more drugs for Aaron, just as they had for Peter. First came Paxil, which Sandy believes was written after a second diagnosis, just like Peter's, of oppositional defiant disorder. At some point the doctor switched the Paxil prescription to one for Wellbutrin, another antidepressant.

But the drugs made Aaron feel worse, just as they had Peter. His appetite disappeared, and he got so skinny that Sandy could see the sharp outlines of his bones in his back. "I'm sure it was the meds," Sandy said.

FOR YEARS LIFE in the farmhouse surrounded by pines and maples revolved around the pills. After her husband died, Sandy began taking Prozac. She had started tensing her muscles, she said, and having panic attacks. She had once been able to breeze through the speeches and presentations that were part of her job at the United Way in Cedar Rapids. But after John's death she froze. She learned her decision to get a prescription was not all that unusual. "I was shocked at the number of people at work who were taking Zoloft or Paxil because they were stressed."

She took the drug for about six months, about the time it took her to discover that talking to a counselor was providing much more relief.

It was when Peter dropped out of school that Sandy and her sons started talking about stopping the pills. Dr. Collins in Cedar Rapids, who had been the boys' pediatrician, recommended a counselor they could see. Sandy called the psychiatrist who had been prescribing the pills and told him they weren't coming back.

Dr. Collins helped reduce the doses of the drugs until the boys could stop taking them altogether. Peter went back to school to finish his junior and senior years. He joined the football team. In the photo taken for his high school graduation, he's sitting in the grass under a tree, wearing a white sweater and jeans. He's looking out toward the camera with the eyes of a young man who knows what he is doing. The long-lost smile of the third grader is back.

SANDY TOLD ME about the family's experience five years after they had stopped taking the meds. Peter is now twenty-two and in the Navy. He recently scored better than 93 percent of the sailors taking a written test and was promoted to the rank of petty officer, third class. Aaron is getting As and Bs in high school and playing the piano for his church group. At fifteen, he still has the energy that years ago the psychiatrist called hyperactive. In the summer he works in the cornfields on a crew that pulls the tassels from the top of the hybrid plants that will produce next year's seeds. Among the teenage crew of detasselers, some call him the Energizer Bunny because he always wants to do one more row.

Sandy said she blames herself for the troubles her boys had on meds. She remembers how she put in sixty-hour weeks at work when her boys needed her at home. "I was stressed out," she said. "I'm sure I got into the habit of criticizing and labeling. I was putting the kids down."

She was forced to quit working in 2000, when she became disabled from the rare disease she had been battling since childhood. The connective tissue disease called Ehlers-Danlos syndrome has crippled her with arthritis. She now needs a cane to walk. Her eyesight is almost gone. She loses the phone when she puts it down. But she hasn't lost her spirit.

When I admired the view of the wooded hills from her living room, she said, "I can't see it anymore, but I know it's beautiful."

She said it was when she was forced to stay home that things got better for her boys. "If I had it to do over again, when my husband died, I would have worked part-time and lived on a lower income and been around for the children. So many people think they can't do that, but by working, they're hurting the kids.

"We've gone to treating with drugs only," she said, "and not looking at the real cause."

Part II

THE RISE OF
THE MEDICINE MERCHANTS

FOUR

The Early Years

MARKETERS AND SALESMEN did not always rule the nation's pharmaceutical companies. For decades, scientists, physicians, or men who devoted their companies to science held top executive posts at some of the most prominent drug firms. Some of these executives spoke of how they knew if they used science to discover lifesaving medicines, the profits would come easily. There would be little need to promote.

Take the pharmaceutical giant Merck. In December 1950 the company's longtime president George W. Merck gave a speech at the Medical College of Virginia, describing a deep belief that drove his decisions. At the time, academic scientists working with Merck's company had just won the Nobel Prize for Medicine for their discovery of cortisone, a drug that allowed people crippled and bedridden with arthritis not only to walk, but to climb stairs and dance.

"We try never to forget that medicine is for the people," Merck said in the speech. "It is not for the profits. The profits follow, and if we have remembered that, they have never failed to appear."

His words were more than merely good public relations. George Merck had a history that illustrated his philosophy. He had become president of his father's company in 1925, a time when the American drug companies had little interest in science. The industry then was largely a group of chemical companies manufacturing millions of bottles of pills that did little to treat real disease. The nation's academic pharmacologists held these pill peddlers in such low esteem that they refused to allow any industrial scientist to become a member of the American Society for Pharmacology and Experimental Therapeutics, which had been founded by Dr. John Jacob Abel. Dr. Abel operated a laboratory at Johns Hopkins University and is widely regarded as the father of American pharmacology.

"It is well known that the advertisers of drugs and medicines have often failed to confine their statements to actual facts," Dr. Abel complained in a letter to a colleague in 1915, "and have yet to get the confidence of our profession."

In 1925, the same year that George Merck became president of Merck & Co., Sinclair Lewis published his novel *Arrowsmith*, which expressed the sentiments of the nation's scientists at the time. Among the novel's characters was Professor Max Gottlieb, an immunologist who criticizes the blatant commercialism of the pharmaceutical firms. Soon, however, Professor Gottlieb is forced for financial reasons to join the fictional drug company Dawson T. Hunziker and Co., Inc.

Other scientists lament the professor's defection. "How could old Max have gone over to that damned pill-peddler?" a group of researchers wail.

"Of all the people in the world!" remarks a young physician. "I wouldn't have believed it! Max Gottlieb falling for those crooks! . . . I wish *he* hadn't gone wrong!"

Once inside the walls of Hunziker and Co., Professor Gottlieb finds his new employer just as he expected. It was producing, for instance, "a new 'cancer remedy,' manufactured from the orchid, pontifically recommended and possessing all the value of mud."

That distrust of the pharmaceutical industry in the early twentieth century carried over to America's physicians. Many doctors warned their patients about the dubious medicines being sold. In 1915 a committee of the American Medical Association urged serious scientists to stay away from the industry. "It is only from laboratories free from any relations with manufacturers," the committee wrote, "that real advances can be expected."

George Merck vowed to change this widespread impression of the industry by creating a scientific laboratory that would be on par with that of any university. He promised that any scientists who worked for Merck & Co. would be free to disclose their discoveries at meetings and in scientific publications. The industry's secrecy and refusal to allow the sharing of scientific information had become a leading complaint of the academic scientists.

But Merck was not the only pharmaceutical executive to begin investing in science. Between 1920 and World War II, many of the nation's pharmaceutical manufacturers opened their first scientific laboratories and worked hard to gain the trust of academic scientists they hoped to hire. Some of the companies, including Merck and the drugmaker Squibb, promised to keep their new laboratories separate from their corporate interest of making money.

When the Indianapolis-based drugmaker Eli Lilly and Company dedicated its new laboratory at a ceremony in the 1930s, Dr. George Henry Alexander Clowes, the company's director of research, told the audience that the firm was dedicated to fundamental science. The company's leaders, Josiah K. Lilly and Eli Lilly, he said, "were not only willing, but eager and anxious, that we should conduct investigations in certain fields in which there could be no possible hope of any commercial return."

The executives did not always follow through on such promises. During World War II, American drug executives twice turned down requests by the government and Dr. Alfred Newton Richards of the University of Pennsylvania that they help manufacture the antibiotic penicillin for the troops. The amazing new drug had been discovered quite by accident in Britain, and no one yet knew how to produce it in large quantities. The drug executives did not want to spend the time or money trying to devise a process to manufacture it, even though they understood its ability to save patients dying from infections and the impact it could have on the battlefield. On Dr. Richards's third attempt, George Merck changed his mind and helped convince three other pharmaceutical companies to join

Merck & Co. in the effort to manufacture the drug, which has proved to be one of the great medical discoveries of all time. By D-day there was enough penicillin to cover the needs of all the wounded at Normandy.

George Merck again showed his concern for the advancement of medicine over profit in 1946, when he gave the patents his company had obtained on the antibiotic streptomycin to a public trust.

Dr. Selman A. Waksman, the inventor of streptomycin and a scientist at Rutgers University, had worked with the company to produce the drug, the first antibiotic found to work against tuberculosis, the deadly lung infection. As part of the deal between Waksman and the company, Merck received the commercial patents on the medicine. In exchange, the company would pay a royalty to Waksman and the university. Dr. Waksman later won the Nobel Prize for his discovery and attributed part of his success to the help he received from Merck's laboratories. There, he said, he had found "a university-like atmosphere where basic research was understood and pursued."

Just as Merck was getting ready to sell streptomycin, however, Dr. Waksman began to fear a public outcry over the commercialization of such an important lifesaving drug. He convinced George Merck to relinquish the company's patents to a university trust fund, which then licensed the right to make the antibiotic to several companies. Merck was still the first company to sell streptomycin in 1946, but the price of the drug plunged as other manufacturers joined in.

Some writers and historians trace the pharmaceutical industry's interest in science to a 1938 law that was passed to protect the public from ineffective and dangerous medicines. As the writer Philip J. Hilts has explained, American drug regulations were so lax before 1938 that "anyone could concoct a medicine in his kitchen and sell it, with no testing required as long as it didn't contain narcotics or one of a few listed poisons."

The need for stronger drug regulations had become clear after the S. E. Massengill Company of Bristol, Tennessee, decided that the public, especially children, would be pleased if it offered a popular drug called sulfanilamide in the form of a sweet-tasting syrup. The company's chemist created a pink preparation consisting of the drug, a raspberry extract, and a solvent called diethylene glycol, an industrial chemical sometimes used in the manufacture of explosives. Just weeks after Massengill shipped bottles of Elixir Sulfanilamide to stores across the country, the president of the Tulsa County Medical Society in Oklahoma sent an urgent telegram to the American Medical Association. He said that six patients had died immediately upon swallowing it. The message from Oklahoma was the first of many reports of deaths from the drug. The company and the government tracked down the bottles of the elixir and destroyed them, but not until more than one hundred Americans had died. By one calculation, the drug killed as many as 30 percent of those who took it. Dozens of the victims were children, including some who had taken it for nothing more than a sore throat. Another death was that of the company's chemist, who killed himself.

"The most amazing thing about the company was the total lack of testing facilities," explained a federal agent who was investigating the tragedy in 1937. "Apparently they just throw drugs together, and if they don't explode they are placed on sale."

The deaths compelled Congress to pass the Food, Drug, and Cosmetic Act, which President Roosevelt signed into law on June 15, 1938. The law required the companies to test the safety of medicines before they were sold.

The testing requirements of the 1938 law added a new urgency to the drug industry's search for academic scientists it could hire. As the companies invested even more money in research and laboratories, the American pharmaceutical industry was transformed from a group of chemical manufacturers that had disdained science to an industry that saw science as crucial to its survival. By the 1940s some fifty-eight thousand scientists, up from only a few thousand in the 1920s, worked in the industry's research laboratories.

The results of this push into scientific research were a revolution that James Harvey Young, an authority on the history of drug regulation, called "one of the major events in medical history."

More truly effective drugs were invented between 1935 and 1955 than in all previous human history. Penicillin was followed by other antibiotics, new vaccines, synthetic vitamins, antihistamines, tranquilizers, and steroid drugs like cortisone. Some of these new medicines set new standards because they didn't just soothe symptoms of illness. They actually cured or prevented life-threatening diseases. Children and young adults especially benefited. A child cured of tuberculosis by streptomycin could credit the antibiotic for decades of living. In 1951 two scientists at Burroughs Wellcome Company in Tuckahoe, New York, synthesized one of the drugs that would help children suffering from leukemia survive their disease. In 1955 Dr. Jonas Salk announced the effectiveness of his polio vaccine, which prevented a disease that was killing and crippling thousands of American children.

By investing in science aimed at ameliorating real disease, the industry reaped great financial rewards. Between World War II and 1957 the pharmaceutical industry more than doubled its sales. In December 1957 the 214 corporate members of the American Pharmaceutical Manufacturers Association gathered in Manhattan to celebrate their success. "This has been the best year in history for the pharmaceutical industry," proclaimed Francis C. Brown, the president of Schering Corporation, during the meeting, "and we have no intention of stopping there."

This great scientific success in the 1940s and early 1950s, which has not been repeated since, changed forever the way Americans think about their prescriptions. The new lifesaving medicines, especially penicillin and Salk's polio vaccine, heralded the age of the "miracle drug." The public began imagining a world without disease.

Reports in newspapers and magazines and on radio and television hailed each new medicine that was introduced as another therapeutic wonder produced by modern medicine. Almost always these reports were exaggerated, but the media knew what their audience wanted to hear. *The Saturday Evening Post*, for instance, did not mention a drug in its editorial columns during 1936. Twenty years later, in 1956, the magazine's stories referred to seventy-two different medicines a total of 330 times. "Readers are not just more medically conscious," a drug trade journal stated at the time, "but more drug conscious too."

It took years before doctors began to understand the dark side of these miracle drugs. The pharmaceutical companies were not required then to provide the government with reports of the injuries and deaths blamed on their products. Even the greatest discoveries were later found to have deadly risks. For example, long after Merck had begun selling cortisone to widespread acclaim, doctors determined that it was causing severe osteoporosis of the spine and life-threatening stomach ulcers. It became clear that cortisone was not the "cure" for rheumatoid arthritis that doctors and the public had believed. Patients could tolerate the drug for only a short time before suffering severe side effects.

As for streptomycin, doctors found it cured many patients of tuberculosis but left some deaf. The antibiotic proved to be especially toxic in children, and eventually doctors began using other antibiotics to treat the deadly lung infection.

These early reports of the deaths and disabilities caused by the miracle cures showed just how powerful this new technology could be. The new medicines could save lives, but they could also kill. The injuries that were coming to light showed how critical it was for doctors to give a medicine to patients only when its potential benefits outweighed the risks.

The American public continued to believe, however, that the world had entered an age when science would deliver marvel after marvel. There was an impression that scientists and pharmaceutical companies would continue to invent cures if only people paid them enough money. The pharmaceutical companies took credit for the new drugs, even though the best of them were largely serendipitous discoveries made by academic researchers. The public's belief that each new prescription drug introduced was yet another magic bullet like penicillin made the industry wealthy and powerful. It also greatly eased the job of the pharmaceutical marketers.

"Americans have come to believe, that science is capable of almost everything," said Dr. Louis M. Orr, the president of the American Medical Association, in 1958. "Any glib salesman who has a white coat and calls himself a doctor can take a black box, a powder, a pill, or a liquid and set out to capitalize on it."

THE INDUSTRY'S GOLDEN age of medical invention soon came to an end. The rate of discovery of beneficial medicines slowed. Why this happened is not clear, although there are theories.

Many of the blueprints for the new drugs had come from the universities, where scientists had been working for decades to advance their
understanding of disease. Once the industry convinced academic scientists to become its partners, the companies swiftly mined the best ideas.
At the same time, infectious diseases, like tuberculosis and polio, have a
single, identifiable cause. As scientists began to understand how bacteria
and viruses caused disease, they made great strides in wiping them out.
Other diseases have proven harder to solve.

The writer Dr. James Le Fanu has pointed out that the postwar therapeutic revolution came about even though scientists did not understand the basic processes of most diseases caused by something other
than bacteria or another infectious agent. They did not understand, for
example, what caused airways to constrict during an asthma attack or
how neurotransmitters worked in the brains of those suffering from
schizophrenia. Lacking that knowledge, the industry instead resorted to a
rather crude method of discovery. The corporate scientists synthesized
millions of chemicals and then tested them to see whether they were
lucky enough to have some kind of therapeutic effect.

Whatever its cause, the fall in the number of significant new medicines marked the beginning of another shift in the pharmaceutical industry. The companies began looking for the easy money.

A system developed whereby one company would introduce a medicine and other firms would quickly begin selling similar products, each
just different enough to get its own patent and secure its own monopoly.
These copycat medicines eventually became known derisively as the me-
too drugs.

In the marketplace, consumers benefit when more companies begin
selling a product because competition drives down prices. But in the American drug market of the 1950s, prices stayed the same or even increased
as more companies sold medicines that were barely distinguishable from
one another. Normal economics no longer applied.

To help create this system, the companies lobbied successfully in
Washington for changes to laws that made it easier for them to patent a
medicine and hold control of it for years. They also succeeded in chang-

ing laws so that it became illegal to advertise the price of drugs, and soon no one really knew how much medicines cost.

More important, the industry learned a simple lesson: it could sell high volumes of most any medicine by spending more on promotion. Flashy advertisements, which were aimed in the 1950s only at physicians reading medical journals, could make up quickly for whatever a medicine lacked. Advertisements could even sell medicines that did not work. There was no requirement at that time for companies to prove their medicines were actually effective and treated disease as the company claimed.

Dr. A. Dale Console, a former executive at E. R. Squibb & Sons, described the industry's practices at a hearing in Congress held by Senator Estes Kefauver. The senator, a Democrat from Tennessee, had shown he was not afraid to take on a group as powerful as the pharmaceutical industry. As the chairman of the Senate's Antitrust and Monopoly Subcommittee he had already taken on the steel and railroad industries. A few years earlier he had made the cover of *Time* magazine for his investigation of organized crime. In December 1959 Senator Kefauver turned his attention to the pharmaceutical industry and began what would be a long series of hearings probing its practices. Stories had begun to appear of patients searching for a cheaper antibiotic and finding them all priced the same, sometimes to the penny. At the same time, doctors were complaining that the industry was introducing hundreds of medicines that were ineffective and not needed and that the companies were promoting these products like the snake-oil nostrums sold at the nineteenth-century medicine shows.

At one of the hearings, Senator Kefauver asked Dr. Console just how much of the industry's research was aimed at producing drugs that the public did not need—that is, those that were useless or worse.

"I think more than half is in that category," the former Squibb executive testified. "And I should point out that with many of these products, it is clear while they are on the drawing board that they promise no utility. They promise sales."

Dr. Console said the pharmaceutical companies had become adept at creating myths, including one that claimed their advertising was a kind of postgraduate education for physicians. The industry, the former executive said, was "unique in that it can make exploitation appear a noble purpose."

Senator Kefauver's hearings, which lasted for months, exposed the modern pharmaceutical industry's marketing and pricing practices to the public for the first time. The hearings made headlines that turned the marketing of prescription drugs into a national issue. The public also got to listen to pharmaceutical executives tell their side of the story.

In his opening statement to the committee, Francis C. Brown, the president of Schering Corporation, explained his theory on why the public was complaining about high medicine prices. It was not that companies were charging too much, he said. The American people simply did not earn enough money.

"It seems to me that this problem must be viewed in its true light," Brown said. "It is a matter of inadequate income rather than excessive prices."

But Kefauver was not about to let the executives get away with such answers. His staff soon presented a chart showing that Schering and three other drug companies were each selling the steroids prednisone and prednisolone at exactly the same price of $35.80 for a bottle of two hundred tablets. In fact, the price of those two hundred pills had not changed since 1956, when they were introduced. The senator asked Brown why the prices had remained high despite such intense competition.

"I have never understood this kind of a competitive system," Kefauver said. "How is it, if you want to be really competitive, you don't lower your price to get more of the business?"

"Senator," Brown replied, "we can't put two sick people in every bed where there is only one person sick."

As the testimony continued, Kefauver unearthed eye-opening financial details of the drug companies' expanding marketing operations. Dr. E. Gifford Upjohn, the president of the Upjohn Company, testified that to keep up with competitors in the marketing race, his company was spending 28.6 percent of its budget on promotion, including a force of a thousand salesmen. Upjohn's research costs, on the other hand, amounted to just 9 percent of the corporate budget. Despite their expensive marketing and overhead costs, the drug companies were producing record profits. Kefauver's staff presented tables showing that the industry's average profit was 21.4 percent of its net worth, almost double the 11 percent profit for all American industries combined.

It also became clear during the hearings why the industry needed to spend so much on marketing. Too many of the drugs being introduced, according to testimony by Dr. Louis Lasagna, the head of clinical pharmacology at Johns Hopkins, were "not as good as what they replace."

Dr. Walter Modell, a pharmacologist from Cornell, expanded on this fact in an article that appeared in *Clinical Pharmacology and Therapeutics* in 1961. The companies, he wrote, were playing a game of "structural roulette" by having their chemists make minor changes to the molecular makeup of a competitor's drug to get around patent restrictions. He said this "molecule manipulation" was done to "horn in on a market which has been created by someone else's discovery."

There was a bewildering array of some 150,000 drug preparations in use, Dr. Modell wrote, of which 90 percent had not existed twenty-five years before. About 15,000 new mixtures and dosages were hitting the market each year, he said, while about 12,000 of these drugs died out.

"At the moment," Dr. Modell said, "the most helpful contribution is the new drug to counteract the untoward effects of other new drugs. We now have several of these."

Despite the mounting evidence that the industry was manipulating its prices and aggressively promoting medicines that were dangerous and ineffective, Senator Kefauver could not find enough votes for the legislation he proposed to restrain some of the egregious practices. It took another tragedy to prompt Congress to act.

As the Senate hearings began, a drug manufacturer in Cincinnati named the William S. Merrell Company was in the midst of distributing tens of thousands of tablets of an experimental drug called thalidomide to thousands of American doctors for "testing" in patients.

The Merrell firm was a subsidiary of the Vick Chemical Company, the maker of Vicks VapoRub. In 1959 Merrell had agreed to license thalidomide from a German company called Chemie Grünenthal, which had already gained approval to sell it in many countries around the world. Grünenthal was promoting the drug as a strong sedative that did not have the dangerous side effects of barbiturates. In promotional materials, Grünenthal said that thalidomide was "completely safe." With these promises, millions of people outside America had begun taking the drug to help them sleep. Foreign doctors were also giving the medicine to pregnant women to alleviate the nausea and vomiting of morning sickness. The German company proclaimed in its advertisements that the drug was "especially well-suited for calming down anxious, nervous and restless children . . . Excellent for babies."

Merrell, the American company, had not yet finished testing thalidomide in animals when it armed its sales representatives with samples and told them to have doctors try it on their patients. Merrell had explained that the doctors would be part of "a trial" of thalidomide. Actually, the "trial" was later revealed to be more about promoting the sleeping pill than about gathering scientific information. For one thing, the company's marketing department was in charge of it. And according to internal documents later obtained by *The Sunday Times* of London, Merrell told its sales reps that the "objective" of signing up doctors to participate in the trial was "for the purpose of selling them on Kevadon," the company's brand name for the drug.

Court documents and depositions later explained more on how this was done. Dr. Ray O. Nulsen, an obstetrician, was one of the physicians who agreed to try the sedative on his pregnant patients. Dr. Nulsen, who practiced in Cincinnati, near Merrell's headquarters, was a friend of some of the company's top executives. The physician later testified that he had not kept track of how many tablets he dispensed or to whom. He said that "the girls in the office" had filled out questionnaires on how the patients fared.

At one point Merrell asked Dr. Nulsen to write for a medical journal an article on his success in treating pregnant women with the drug. The company then gave this article to the FDA as part of the package of evidence that it said proved the experimental drug was safe for broad use. The article, however, was not written by Dr. Nulsen, although his name appeared as its author. It was actually written by an executive at Merrell, Dr. Raymond C. Pogge, one of Dr. Nulsen's golfing partners.

Unknown to Americans at the time, a disaster was unfolding in countries that had already approved the drug. Some women who had taken the sedative during their pregnancies were giving birth to babies who were grotesquely deformed. The infants suffered from what is called phocomelia, which comes from the Greek words *phōkē*, meaning "seal," and *melos,* meaning "limb." The bones in the infants' arms or legs were so grossly short that their hands or feet appeared to sprout directly from their torsos like the flippers of a seal. Some of the babies also lacked openings for their ears or bowels.

It later came to light that the first thalidomide baby had been born in Germany in 1957, the same year that country had approved the drug. The public did not learn of the cases, however, until November 1961, when a German newspaper gave the disturbing account of Dr. Widukind Lenz of Hamburg. Dr. Lenz had found eight infants in the German city who were born deformed after their mothers had taken thalidomide. He estimated that at least forty more cases had occurred in Hamburg in the last two years. Before thalidomide was introduced, phocomelia had been so rare in Germany that most doctors did not see a case in their lifetime.

After the newspaper revealed the horrors that Dr. Lenz had found, Grünenthal removed thalidomide from the market in Germany. Other countries also quickly halted its sales.

Thousands more Americans would have taken the sedative if it had not been for a doctor at the FDA named Frances O. Kelsey. She had been reviewing the application that Merrell submitted to gain approval to sell thalidomide in the United States. Dr. Kelsey had become concerned, however, about the poor quality of the company's scientific data. She had also found a report in the *British Medical Journal* in December 1960 that said the sedative appeared to damage the nerves of some patients. Merrell executives had become furious with Dr. Kelsey for delaying the sale of their product as she asked them for more data to prove it was safe.

It is now estimated that thalidomide caused deformities in some eight thousand infants around the world. Thousands of other babies were so malformed that they died before they were born. Only about forty of those cases were in the United States, although there has never been an accurate count. Some of the worst cases in America were reported in patients in Cincinnati who had been treated by Dr. Nulsen. He testified he did not deliver any thalidomide babies, but it was shown that he had given the drug to dozens of pregnant women and had delivered three deformed babies without recognizing the problem. Two other babies of women treated by Dr. Nulsen died of their deformities before birth.

Public outrage about the thalidomide tragedy stirred Congress to reconsider Senator Kefauver's proposal. On October 10, 1962, members of both the House and the Senate unanimously passed the Kefauver-Harris amendments. None of Kefauver's proposals aimed at reducing drug prices was left in the bill, but the new law greatly strengthened the FDA's control over the marketing and promotion of prescription drugs. It also required the companies once again to focus on good science.

Under the new law, the companies were required to perform careful clinical trials that proved not only that a medicine was safe but that it was effective for its intended use. At the same time, doctors and scientists performing the trials had to show they were qualified to do the work. The companies could no longer distribute samples of an unapproved drug to doctors for experimental purposes as Merrell had done with thalidomide.

The law also required drug companies to tell regulators about the injuries and deaths that had been blamed on their products. It became illegal to keep these reports hidden in corporate file drawers. In addition, the law forced the companies to change their promotional tactics. No longer could they only describe the expected benefits of a drug in their advertisements, which were then directed only at physicians. They had to describe the risks as well.

Many pharmaceutical executives complained bitterly about the new law. More regulation meant more paperwork and more costs, they said, which would hurt profits and force them to spend less on research aimed at finding new medicines. Some companies, the executives said, would be forced out of business.

Few of these worries materialized. The companies that were hurt by the new requirements were those that had not spent money for good science in the first place. They were the molecule manipulators that had made money by copying their competitors' medicines.

Later some executives at the big drug companies agreed that the additional scientific requirements had benefited the industry. In a paper presented at an industry conference sponsored by the American Enterprise Institute in 1974, Harold A. Clymer, the vice president for planning and business development at the SmithKline Corporation, said the amendments to the law in 1962 changed the industry's direction.

"They wrenched some of us out of old ways and headed us toward more thorough work and better science," Clymer wrote. "They made research and development expenditures aimed at anything less than superior therapy a waste of stockholders' money."

But this way of thinking was not to last.

ASK ANY NUMBER of drug executives why medicines cost so much, and they'll give you the same answer that corporate medicine men have repeated for decades: companies need money to pay for the expensive science required to find new drugs. Discovering a new medicine can take more than a decade, the executives say, and run up a bill that by 2006 was approaching one billion dollars.

This estimate of the cost of discovering a drug comes from a group of professors at Tufts University's Center for the Study of Drug Development. The center was started in 1976 by the influential pharmacologist Dr. Louis Lasagna. Today it is funded mostly by the pharmaceutical industry and its other corporate partners. Since its founding, the Tufts professors have surveyed the drug companies and used the information to calculate how much must be spent to find and develop a new drug. The center's estimate, which has been widely quoted by the industry and media, has climbed rapidly. In 1979 the center said each new drug cost the industry an average of $54 million to discover. By 1991 the cost had climbed to $231 million. Ten years later the Tufts researchers said the industry spent $802 million to develop a new drug.

A wide-ranging group of critics have attacked these estimates. They have pointed out that nearly half the estimate consists not of actual expenses but of what the Tufts professors call "the cost of capital," or the money the companies could have earned if they had invested their research money in stocks or other moneymaking ventures. The critics have also shown how the Tufts researchers have failed to adjust their estimate downward for the billions of dollars in federal tax benefits that the pharmaceutical companies receive each year by spending money on research.

Others have pointed out that the industry likes to take credit for discovering all the medicines that Americans count on, even though most of the nation's critical lifesaving drugs, like those that treat cancer and AIDS, would not be sold today if taxpayers had not paid for the science that led to their discovery. Pharmaceutical executives admit that they count on taxpayer-funded research. They explain that the job of the federal government is to pay for basic science that advances the understanding of medicine, which the companies then "apply" to create new products. But the industry's reliance on money from federal taxpayers goes beyond even this for many of the nation's most significant medicines. For example, Bristol-Myers Squibb's bestselling cancer drug Taxol was discovered by scientists funded through government grants. The federal government then paid to manufacture the drug and to test it in patients, before granting a license to Bristol-Myers to sell it.

In fact, of the nation's twenty-one most important drugs introduced between 1965 and 1992, fifteen were developed using knowledge from federal-funded research, according to a report in 2000 by the Joint Economic Committee of Congress, then headed by Republican senator Connie Mack. Among the drugs mentioned by that report was the cancer drug cisplatin. It was discovered by researchers at Michigan State University and tested in patients with testicular cancer with the help of millions of dollars from taxpayers. The university then licensed the drug to Bristol-Myers, which for years promoted itself as a leading cancer research company through a partnership with the cycling champion Lance Armstrong. The cyclist beat back advanced testicular cancer at the age of twenty-five and went on to win the Tour de France, cycling's most prestigious race, seven times. Bristol-Myers paid money to Armstrong's cancer charity for a campaign in which he credited the company with saving his life. After one of Armstrong's Tour de France victories, the company paid for advertisements proclaiming, "This miracle is brought to you by Bristol-Myers Squibb." However, the truth behind the discovery of the medicines that saved Armstrong got lost in the frenzy of international publicity as he appeared for Bristol-Myers on television shows like ABC's *Good Morning America* and *Live with Regis and Kathie Lee*. Bristol-Myers did indeed *sell* three of the drugs that helped the cyclist defeat his cancer, including cisplatin, and it made tens of millions of dollars in profit from them, but it did not *discover* them. Instead, Bristol-Myers was their licensed seller and marketer.

The most troublesome problem with the Tufts estimate of the cost of discovering a drug, however, is that there is no way to verify it. The pharmaceutical companies' actual research costs are one of the world's most closely guarded industrial secrets. In the 1970s and 1980s the companies waged a decade-long legal battle to keep even government auditors from reviewing the costs of their research laboratories.

While it appears the estimate by Tufts has been greatly inflated, no one can dispute that inventing a lifesaving medicine is an expensive task. At the same time, it's also unquestionable that it's far less costly simply to follow in your competitors' footsteps, copying their work before adding your own twist.

These facts were strikingly evident in a hard-fought marketing battle between two drugmakers in the 1980s that ushered in the age of the pharmaceutical blockbuster in America and transformed the industry yet again. One of these companies spent heavily on research, funding a team of corporate scientists for more than a decade until they discovered a drug so original and beneficial that it changed the practice of medicine.

Unfortunately, it was the story of the second company that became the essence of the industry's playbook that is still used today. That company learned that to reap great profits in the modern-day pharmaceutical business, one did not need a lifesaving drug or, for that matter, a medicine all that different from the one sold by the competition. All that was needed was a copycat pill that could be sold as an enhancement of the American lifestyle and a masterful marketing campaign for which expense was not an issue.

FIVE

An Awakening:
The Age of the Blockbuster

DR. JAMES W. BLACK arrived at the British laboratory of Smith Kline & French in 1964 with a passion for the scientific method, boundless curiosity, and a theory he could not get out of his head.

The bespectacled Scotsman was driven by his belief that he could invent a new medicine to help the millions of people suffering from stomach ulcers, an excruciating condition that in its most severe form can lead to death.

Already Dr. Black had achieved extraordinary success for a scientist, even though when it came to experimentation, he was largely self-taught. His achievement seemed to emanate from the fact that he was an independent sort. He was not always at ease traveling the well-worn path of his scientific peers.

Born the fourth of five boys in a staunch Baptist family, he admitted he had been a bit of a daydreamer growing up. The family lived in the coalfields of Fife, an eastern region of Scotland, where his father worked as a mining engineer. At the age of fourteen, he had discovered that he loved mathematics. One day he proved to his teacher that the answers printed in his calculus textbook were wrong, an event he later described as an epiphany. If his textbook was wrong, he realized, there were probably many other things that should be challenged or questioned. There was a real need in the world for someone who looked at things with a skeptical eye and was not always willing to accept what others said to be true.

With the help of a scholarship, he studied medicine but realized he didn't want to be a physician. He said he wasn't comfortable with how many doctors at that time in the 1940s seemed to treat patients. He thought they had a way of dehumanizing their patients, treating them as livers or hearts or whatever organ was aching rather than as the individuals they were. Instead of doctoring, he turned to academia and research. As he learned more about pharmacology and the intricacies of experimentation, ideas began to bubble in his mind. One was the blueprint for a drug that he believed could help patients with angina, the chest pain caused when the heart does not get enough blood.

In 1958 the thirty-four-year-old scientist took this idea to ICI, the giant British chemical company. Over the next six years, as an employee of ICI, he laid the groundwork for the discovery of a new type of lifesaving heart medicine called the beta-blocker. The drug would transform the treatment of angina and much more. It became one of the first effective treatments for high blood pressure, and eventually doctors recognized its potential to help patients suffering from congestive heart failure.

Yet Dr. Black wasn't about to sit back and enjoy his success. He soon decided to leave ICI, he later recounted, because he did not wish to get caught up in the final development and marketing of the new drug. It was also clear that he did not crave the limelight. He was happiest when at work on questions still unanswered.

He vowed to take the science further, using the same idea that had led him to the heart medicine—that is, that he could develop a chemical that blocked the action of another chemical in the body—to find a drug that healed stomach ulcers. Dr. Black's past triumph, however, did not make his new idea any less risky or controversial. He had not been able to get ICI interested in the project. Executives at Smith Kline, a drug company based in Philadelphia, decided to give him a chance.

DR. BLACK MOVED his work into Smith Kline's laboratory in Welwyn Garden City, a town about twenty miles north of central London, in 1964. Doctors treating patients with serious ulcers at that time had little more to offer than their surgical knives. A hot topic of discussion among surgeons that year was just how much of the stomach could safely be cut out to get rid of the ulcers and keep them from coming back. Some surgeons were advocating the removal of as much as 40 percent of a patient's stomach, while others worried there was no way of telling which patients might die during such operations or shortly afterward.

Smith Kline's new scientist was imagining an entirely new approach. Dr. Black's goal was to stop the stomach from producing acid, which was believed then to be the cause of most ulcers. To do this, he hoped to synthesize a chemical drug that blocked a substance in the body called histamine. That substance had long been suspected of prompting the stomach to produce acid.

Dr. Black hoped his new project would take a few years, but as it is with science, he and his team suffered hundreds of failures. By 1970 the team had tested more than seven hundred chemical compounds for their ability to reduce the flow of acid. To their dismay, they found the compounds that actually worked that way were so potent that they poisoned other parts of the body. And scientists around the world remained skeptical. At a symposium at Johns Hopkins University in 1973, a leading gastroenterologist announced that it appeared that any chemical that blocked the acid-stimulating effects of histamine was "inherently toxic," a poison far worse than the disease. This lack of scientific support for Dr. Black's idea intensified the pressure on Smith Kline to drop the project, which seemed to be going nowhere.

In a way, the team was trying to crack a safe, tediously dialing in new combinations, hoping to hear a click that would let them at the gold inside. They kept tweaking the chemical structure of drug compounds, searching for the one that reduced stomach acid without the poisonous effects. One promising compound worked in animals but then failed in human tests. They were gleeful when another drug worked when swallowed by humans, only later to be let down when they found it dangerously depressed the infection-fighting white cells in the bone marrow.

Then, seven years after Dr. Black had walked through the doors of the company's laboratory, the team scored a breakthrough. They discovered that one of the chemicals they had synthesized—a drug they called cimetidine—worked to stop stomach acid without the terrible adverse effects. By 1977 the pale green tablets were on sale in the United States under the brand name Tagamet. Dr. Black had become the inventor of a second lifesaving medicine, a feat that later earned him a Nobel Prize, as well as an appointment by Queen Elizabeth II to the Order of Merit, one of the highest honors the British monarch can bestow.

Tagamet proved so effective at healing holes in the stomach that doctors began to attribute the steep decline in the number of ulcer surgeries to its healing effects. The new ulcer medicine also richly rewarded Smith Kline for its financial investment in a risky scientific project. By 1981 some fifteen million people in the world had taken Tagamet.

Executives at other pharmaceutical companies had been watching. They had been quietly performing their competitive intelligence and gathering data on the activities at Smith Kline. In London, executives working in the head office of Glaxo were especially intrigued with the progress of Dr. Black and his team, who were making their discoveries just a short train ride away.

The Glaxo executives were fortunate that Dr. Black was a former academic, who believed science benefited from the free flow of ideas. He viewed science as a collaborative venture. He attributed his discovery of the beta-blocking heart drug to work done earlier by Dr. Raymond Ahlquist, a pharmacology professor at the Medical College of Georgia. He said he had a revelation after reading a paper by Dr. Ahlquist, which was published in 1948 but had largely been ignored.

To generate discussion among his peers, Dr. Black gave lectures on his work, including one in the early 1970s about his quest to find a remedy for ulcers. Sitting among the students and scientists in the audience was Dr. David Jack, the head of pharmaceutical research at Glaxo. The speech was an eye-opener for Dr. Jack and other Glaxo executives. They swiftly shifted the work assignments of the company's scientists, ordering them to follow along behind Dr. Black and the rest of his team at Smith Kline. Their decision would be momentous.

At the time Glaxo was best known in Britain as the company that "builds bonnie babies," a reference to its longtime marketing of a dried milk formula for infants. It also had a successful medicine business but had no operations in the United States, where sales of prescription drugs were booming.

An unabashedly self-assured accountant named Paul Girolami was determined that Glaxo would discover America. Girolami had joined Glaxo as financial controller and worked his way up the ranks to become chief executive in 1980. Three years later Glaxo and Girolami introduced Americans to a new ulcer medicine called Zantac. The drug was not in fact "new." It was nothing more than a revision of the drug that Dr. Black had invented.

Dr. Jack later explained that the discovery of Zantac required little more than solving a problem of chemistry because all the original work had been done by Jim Black. Zantac worked in the same way as Tagamet but was just different enough not to infringe the patent that Smith Kline had obtained to protect its drug from competition.

Because Zantac was nothing more than a copycat pill, financial analysts on Wall Street were not impressed. They estimated that at most Glaxo's drug would get 5 to 15 percent of the market for ulcer drugs, just a fraction of Tagamet's sales.

Girolami, however, had something else in mind. In a move that changed the pharmaceutical industry forever, he upset the market with his pricing strategy. Rather than set Zantac's price at a discount to win more sales, the Glaxo chief decided to charge a premium over Tagamet of as much as 50 percent. The message of Glaxo's higher price was like that of an underweight boxer trying to fool the prizefighter with his swagger. The high price implied that Zantac was far better than Tagamet. That was not the case. It did not have to be taken as frequently as Tagamet, but it was essentially the same drug.

To cement Zantac's image of superiority, Glaxo used the extra money that came from its premium price to pay for studies aimed at showing that it worked better and was safer than Tagamet. Girolami also began one of the most expensive and aggressive promotional campaigns the industry had ever seen, one that even today is talked about by the nation's drug marketers. To start, he greatly expanded Glaxo's fledgling sales force in America by contracting to use hundreds of sales representatives who were already visiting physician offices for Hoffmann–La Roche, a Swiss company that had been aggressively promoting the tranquilizer Valium.

More important, Girolami decided he was not satisfied with selling Zantac only as a remedy for stomach ulcers. There was a far larger market in selling it to America's overeaters of pizza, French fries, and other heartburn-inducing foods. Glaxo's marketers, however, faced a conundrum. Few Americans believed heartburn was a malady that required a trip to the doctor. Instead, most people soothed their acidy stomachs with cheap rolls of Tums or Rolaids and tried to avoid foods like greasy fried chicken. Girolami saw this problem as a marketing opportunity. He and his marketing staff set out to make heartburn into an acute and chronic "disorder" that came with serious consequences if not treated twice daily with the company's two-dollar pill.

In marketing brochures and press releases, Glaxo marketers began referring to heartburn as the more worrisome-sounding gastroesophageal reflux disease, which they reduced simply to GERD. The four-letter acronym was easily promoted to consumers in advertisements and became like a password between patients and physicians.

Girolami then worked to convince America that nearly half the country was needlessly suffering from heartburn when an effective treatment was available. In 1988 Glaxo paid the Gallup Organization to survey Americans about their heartburn. The corporate-paid survey found that 44 percent of Americans suffered heartburn each month, a number that the company promoted in a grand public relations campaign called Heartburn Across America.

That same year Glaxo recruited the actress Nancy Walker, whom Americans knew better as the mother of Rhoda Morgenstern on *The Mary Tyler Moore Show*, to tell the public about her longtime personal struggle with GERD. In interviews with journalists, Ms. Walker recounted how she had helped solve her acid reflux by visiting her doctor for a prescription of Zantac.

Even after paying to have a Hollywood star add life to the campaign, Glaxo's marketers had money to spend. They decided to devise an appeal that appeared scholarly and scientific and had the feel of independent medical education. The marketers created what they called the Glaxo Institute for Digestive Health, which said its mission was to give financial grants to physicians around the country for "research" and to raise "public awareness" about stomach problems. One of the doctors Glaxo paid was Dr. Donald O. Castell, the chief of gastroenterology at the Bowman Gray School of Medicine in Winston-Salem, North Carolina, which was not far from Glaxo's American headquarters in the Research Triangle Park. Dr. Castell told *The New York Times* in 1989 that Glaxo gave him fifteen thousand dollars for a study in which he gathered a dozen members of a Winston-Salem running club, fed them a light meal of orange juice, cornflakes, low-fat milk, and banana, and sent them on a run. He then monitored them for heartburn, which he called runner's reflux. Dr. Castell said he had relieved the runners' heartburn by giving them Zantac before they exercised. Glaxo then hired a public relations agency, Ketchum Communications, to spread the word across the country about this newly discovered problem among the nation's runners and the medicine that brought them relief.

Girolami's promotional plan worked so well that Zantac was soon minting money for Glaxo. In 1986 Zantac passed Tagamet to become the biggest-selling drug on earth. And the once-sleepy Glaxo became Britain's largest company. Queen Elizabeth knighted Girolami as "Sir Paul," and the company hired a sculptor to immortalize him in the form of a bronze bust to be placed in its headquarters.

The company's transformation was unsettling to some of its scientists. Dr. Jack left the company in 1987, and he later told the British writer Matthew Lynn that Glaxo had become an uncomfortable place to work under the command of Girolami.

"I can tell you quite frankly, he doesn't have any great regard for scientists, or for science as a way of living," Dr. Jack said. "His whole purpose is to make money. I don't think there is much folly in his mind about doing good."

Girolami had set a new standard for all pharmaceutical companies to follow. The industry learned that Americans would pay almost anything for a new pharmaceutical product, even if it wasn't really new. The executives also realized that every dollar spent on marketing a drug that enhanced the American lifestyle would be quickly rewarded with a dozen times that in sales. The same could not be said for money spent on risky ventures in laboratories looking for highly elusive new drugs that actually saved lives.

"There was an awakening that the amount of marketing money you could spend on a high-margin drug for chronic illness was vast," explained Marc Mayer, an analyst at Sanford C. Bernstein & Co., an investment house in New York, to a reporter for *Fortune* magazine in 1991.

Added Paul Brooke, an analyst at Morgan Stanley: "The $50-million-a-year drug of the 1970s became the $500-million-a-year drug of the 1980s."

Glaxo had shown its competitors the way to the future.

IN THE FOLLOWING years, driven by investors hungry for profits, every major pharmaceutical company strove to outdo Glaxo's success. Gradually a set of selling tactics emerged that came to be known among industry insiders as the blockbuster model. The recipe goes something like this: Focus your money and marketing efforts on drugs for chronic illnesses or problems like heartburn, cholesterol, and depression. The most profitable of these medicines are taken every day and don't cure illness. They only treat symptoms. Each patient on these once-a-day pills, like a smoker hooked on cigarettes or a coffee lover addicted to espresso, becomes an annuity, paying the company handsomely for years.

Under the blockbuster model, it helped to have discovered an innovative new medicine, but that was not required. The key ingredient was promotion—to the American masses.

The pharmaceutical companies now spend twice as much on marketing as most other industries. Executives at AstraZeneca explained in 2000 that companies must spend as much as $1 billion to promote a drug if they wanted it to become one of the coveted blockbuster sellers that brought in sales of more than $1 billion a year. About 25 percent of that money—or $250 million—must be spent, they said, even before the new drug is shipped to pharmacies for its first sales.

Because a blockbuster demanded salesmanship more than science, at the turn of the twenty-first century, many large drug companies, including the one once led by George W. Merck, were run by marketers or businessmen who had little or no training in scientific medicine. In 2001 Peter Dolan, a young executive who had made his early mark promoting Jell-O for General Foods, became the chief executive of Bristol-Myers Squibb. The drug company Novartis hired the Pepsi marketer Thomas Ebeling and by 2000 had given him responsibility for running its global pharmaceutical business. When Randall Tobias took over as the head of Eli Lilly in 1993, he had spent most of his career as an executive for the phone company AT&T. And Bill Steere, who turned Pfizer into the world's largest pharmaceutical company and a marketing powerhouse that others tried to imitate, was one of the industry's many top executives who began their careers as drug sales reps.

The industry's own hiring statistics show its shift from research to marketing. Between 1995 and 2000 the number of marketing personnel at the large pharmaceutical companies in America increased by 59 percent to 87,810, according to surveys of the companies by the industry's trade group. Over those same years, the number of staff devoted to research and development fell by 2 percent to 48,527.

The industry's move away from science was first noticed in the late 1970s, about the time that Glaxo was devising its marketing plans for Zantac. Dr. Steven N. Wiggins, a professor of economics at Texas A&M, had interviewed executives at the major pharmaceutical companies for a paper he delivered at an industry conference in 1979. Scientists had begun to lose their power inside the big companies in the late 1960s, Dr. Wiggins said. Before the power shift, he said, marketers could not offer advice on what medicines the company's scientists should work on. "The degree and exact timing of the change varied across companies," he wrote, "but in all companies there was a lessening of scientific power over research resources."

The basic instinct of a scientist is to discover and to expand on what is already known. The best scientists see little need in developing yet another me-too medicine. Businessmen see things differently. They are schooled in how to make money most efficiently in ever-rising amounts. Inside the drug companies these two ways of thinking often clashed.

"In the beginning, the pharmaceutical industry was run by chemists," said Pierre Simon, a scientist who had been in charge of research for Sanofi, a French drug company, in an interview with the medical historian David Healy in 2000. "Now most of them are run by people with MBAs or things like that, people who could be the chief executive of Renault, Volvo or anything."

Dr. Simon had been an academic pharmacologist before being hired by Sanofi in 1985. He said he had grown disenchanted with the industry's practice of developing copycat medicines. "When you have seen the quantity of money spent by the pharmaceutical industry for the research of me-too drugs, which sometimes have some minor benefits, it's in between 70 percent and even 90 percent of the research money," he said. "It's not for innovation. This is a terrible waste of money."

The federal government has made it easy for the drug companies to imitate the work of others by not requiring them to prove a new drug is better than those already on the market. The result of these lax requirements is reflected in the list of drugs that have been approved by the FDA. Between 1990 and 2004 the FDA's Center for Drug Evaluation and Research approved about 1,100 new drugs. Only about 400 of them were actually "new," or what the FDA called a new molecular entity. In addition, federal regulators found that most of these "new molecular entities" were not significant improvements over the medicines already being sold. Only 183 drugs approved during those fourteen years, or about 16 percent, were actually both new and significant. The rest were nothing more than me-toos or drugs for which there was no real need.

"We've seen the rise of the me-too world," Matthew Emmens, the chief executive of Shire Pharmaceuticals, told the trade magazine *Pharmaceutical Executive* in 2006. "One could argue that it's commoditization. I could never imagine this business becoming like the chemical business, but in some ways it is, with the products becoming more alike."

Or as Dr. Duncan Moore, a former scientist who became a health care analyst for Morgan Stanley, the investment bank, wrote in 2006: "It seems clear that discovery in the large pharmaceutical companies has become quite stale compared to the situation in the 1970s and 1980s. The influence of marketing on the discovery process, added to the enormity of the enterprises, has fostered a trend for funding the probable rather than the possible."

This same observation about America's big pharmaceutical companies was made at a symposium at the University of Michigan in 2002. In the keynote address, Dr. Erling Refsum, an analyst at Nomura International, a securities firm, said the large drug companies had become little more than cash-flow machines for investors.

"The large pharma companies—they're financial-engineering vehicles," Dr. Refsum said. "They are not science-research operations. Financial-engineering is all about making your EPS and your shareholders happy. It's not about finding drugs. They don't care what they're actually selling. They are only too interested in making the money."

The truth is, however, the pharmaceutical companies *did* care about what they were selling.

"We sometimes joke that when you're doing a clinical trial, there are two possible disasters," Alex Hittle, a stock analyst at A. G. Edwards, explained to a journalist in 2003. "The first disaster is if you kill people. The second disaster is if you cure them."

Indeed, if the companies eliminated disease, they would eliminate sales.

One need look no farther than Zantac, the first blockbuster, to see how the industry's laser beam focus on finding ways to medicate consumers on a daily basis can prevent patients from receiving short regimens of cheap medicines that actually cure disease. This part of the Zantac story could be called the Case of the Cure No One Was Told About. It begins in the early 1980s about the same time that Glaxo started aggressively selling Zantac to Americans. On the other side of the world, a young Australian physician named Barry Marshall had stirred up a noxious concoction of beef broth and bacteria in his laboratory, put it to his lips, and swallowed. Within days Dr. Marshall had come down with an acute case of gastritis. He was delighted.

At age thirty-two, Dr. Marshall had become fascinated by a strange spiral-shaped bacterium that his colleague Dr. J. Robin Warren had discovered in biopsies taken from the stomachs of patients suffering from gastritis. Dr. Marshall decided to take that work further. He began studying more patients who suffered from ulcers, gastritis, and other stomach ailments. In each case, he found the patient's stomach was infected by the same puzzling bacteria. Then, in a lucky break, a patient told him that his dyspepsia had improved following a short course of the antibiotic tetracycline, which he had taken for an unrelated chest infection. To Dr. Marshall, the implications of this patient's report were clear: a bacterium, which came to be known as *Helicobacter pylori*, was the cause of his patients' stomach ills, and a short course of antibiotics offered a simple cure.

Other scientists dismissed Dr. Marshall's findings, saying bacteria could not possibly survive the hydrochloric acid produced by the stomach. Doctors believed then, just as Dr. James Black had believed in the 1960s, that most ulcers were caused by an excess of this acid in the stomach. Also, physicians had become awed with the ability of Zantac and Tagamet to reduce the acid and heal their patients' ulcers. Most patients using the drugs, however, found their ulcers came back in a year or so, requiring them to take several dollars' worth of the acid-suppressing pills every day, perhaps for more than a decade.

Even after Dr. Marshall reported his own illness from swallowing the bacteria-infested beef broth, scientists remained skeptical. Some wrote it off as a stunt by a young scientist, not long out of school, who was taking his findings too far. He got little more than silence when he wrote to Glaxo and Smith Kline in the hope that they would support his work in what he believed was a cure. By then the two drug companies had created a market for ulcer medicines worth billions of dollars a year.

"If the drug companies were truly into discovery, they would have gone straight after the *Helicobacter*," Dr. Marshall told *The New York Times*, just days after he and Dr. Warren were awarded the Nobel Prize in 2005 for their discoveries. "Had these drugs not existed, the drug companies would have jumped on our findings."

America's medical-industrial complex became so wedded to the heavily marketed pills that it was not until 1994, ten years after Dr. Marshall had swallowed the noxious soup, that a government panel announced that ulcers should be treated with antibiotics. One year after that announcement only about 5 percent of ulcer patients were receiving antibiotics. And by 1997 the government had been forced to begin a public information campaign, urging doctors to change their practices. The government pointed out that curing an ulcer with a seventeen-day course of antibiotics cost less than a thousand dollars. This was less than a tenth of the expense of using years of the expensive acid-suppressing drugs.

Pharmaceutical marketing had caused vast sums of the nation's health care dollars to be wasted on unnecessary medicines. It had also kept patients from a potential cure.

IT WAS NOT long after Glaxo turned Zantac into the bestselling drug in the world that investigators in Congress noticed the new aggressiveness among the industry's marketers. In December 1990 Senator Edward M. Kennedy held a two-day hearing on the industry's promotional practices. Witnesses described one case after another in which the companies had lavished physicians with gifts and cash or manipulated the public's impression of their products through secretive public relations tactics.

The star witness at the hearing was David C. Jones, a former executive with Ciba Geigy and later at Abbott Laboratories. Mr. Jones had been a vice president at Abbott when he left the company in 1986 because of marketing practices he said he found "untenable."

"I left the industry because I got to a point where I began to learn what the truth was," he told the senators, "and I could no longer tolerate that truth."

Mr. Jones explained that "everything changed" in the industry after the marketing of Tagamet and Zantac. The companies had learned, he said, how to fuel demand for their products beyond the real medical need. They had discovered how to "disguise" promotion as "education" and promote medicines for uses that were dangerous, not approved by the government, and not supported by science. The companies were creating "bogus organizations," he said, that were "nothing but a file drawer in the public relations or marketing department." They did this, he explained, "to hide the company's sponsorship of communications that are often questionable and sometimes blatant attempts to break the law."

He described how Abbott had promoted its antianxiety drug Tranxene to psychiatrists attending a major medical conference in Manhattan by paying to entertain them at a special performance at the opera. The singers performed songs that included stories of psychosis and neurosis. The program also promoted Tranxene.

Senator Kennedy asked Mr. Jones where Abbott got the idea for a night at the opera.

"It was put together rather late," Mr. Jones explained, "because as I understand it, we learned that another company—I think it was Pfizer—had rented a naval aircraft carrier in New York harbor for a major reception for psychiatrists, and we wanted to do something to counter that."

Mr. Jones said the companies were providing far more to physicians than mere entertainment. Most of the leading physicians in the various medical specialties, he said, were now paid consultants to one or more pharmaceutical companies. "The reach goes very, very far," the former executive said. "These corporations are not paying these physicians or anybody else out of disinterested philanthropy. They expect something."

Mr. Jones's testimony that day raised questions about pharmaceutical executives' often repeated claims that they needed to charge high prices to cover the cost of scientists working to discover new drugs. Mr. Jones said it was common practice in the industry to overstate research costs by recording some of the spiraling marketing expenses as "research and development" on the accounting books. For example, he said, industry accountants often coded the cost of promotion as a research expense if the drug had not yet been approved by the FDA. These early marketing costs were not insignificant. These are the same type of promotional costs that an Astra-Zeneca executive was referring to when he said in 2000 that a company must spend as much as $250 million on promotion before doctors write the first prescription.

"It is simply a corporate decision made through a department called 'MIS,' Management Information Systems, to charge that expenditure to

Phase 3 research or another component of the R & D budget," Mr. Jones explained when asked about the practice by Senator Kennedy. The accountants have not yet transferred the drug project out of the research budget, he said, "so all of the communications associated with that product can easily be cross-charged into the R & D budget."

When setting a drug's price, executives consider many factors other than the cost of research, Mr. Jones said. "There is at least some assessment in terms of the options that the patient has available—the fewer the options, the higher the price; the greater the desperation, the greater the suffering, the higher the price. These are routine conversations that occur with virtually every drug that is introduced."

Mr. Jones said that over the years he had grown disturbed by the rising number of unethical practices he observed. "As the industry learned how effective it could be in stretching demand, it began to drift away from its ethical moorings," he testified. As an example, he described how Abbott had decided to market a drug to patients suffering from Lou Gehrig's disease, even though the company's scientists had little reason to believe it would help them. The disease, also known as amyotrophic lateral sclerosis or ALS, is a cruel and fatal one; patients rapidly lose control of their muscles until they are paralyzed.

Abbott's executives, he said, saw the plan to market the drug to ALS patients as "a solution to a short-term revenue problem." One of their analyses, he said, estimated that it would take about six months for doctors to see the drug was not working for their patients. The executives estimated the plan would be worth millions of dollars to the company even though ALS is rare. That is because Abbott was charging each patient about ten thousand dollars for the drug, which was known as thyrotropin-releasing hormone or simply TRH. There had originally been a reason for that high price, Mr. Jones explained. At first, employees had made the hormone by hand. But in 1985 the company's chemists had found a way to manufacture the drug more cheaply, so the price could be dropped sharply to two thousand dollars for each patient.

"The task force working on TRH was called together for a meeting," Mr. Jones testified. "Company doctors and scientists gathered around the table with enthusiasm at finally being able to lower the price . . . But marketing executives asked why we would want to do that. Someone even said that we should not worry about the price because neighbors would hold garage sales to raise money for those with ALS. The people in the room were stunned."

Mr. Jones said he later met with the executive in charge of marketing of the drug and asked that the company lower the price and stop using publicity to recruit ALS patients to a clinical trial. The patients in the trial had to pay for the medicine even though they were helping the company test a product. "My recommendations were met with a blank stare," he said. "They were not acknowledged or discussed."

Soon afterward Mr. Jones answered a call to his office. On the line was a social worker in a small town in Arkansas who pleaded for the company to provide TRH to a family that could not afford it. The father of the family had just died of cancer, the social worker explained, and now a son had been diagnosed with ALS.

"I ended up repeating eventually the party line—that it was just so expensive to make," Mr. Jones testified. "It was not true. Not long afterwards, I left the company and the industry.

"These practices are commonplace in the industry," he continued, "and the industry works hard to hide what it is doing. Drug companies have institutionalized deception."

EVIDENCE PRESENTED BY other witnesses at that two-day hearing of the Senate's Committee on Labor and Human Resources showed that the cases Mr. Jones described were neither isolated nor exaggerated. Documents showed, for example, that American Home Products, the New Jersey–based drugmaker, had created a program whereby physicians could earn frequent flier miles by writing prescriptions for the company's recently approved blood pressure drug, Inderal LA. This medicine was not actually new. It was a long-acting version of the beta-blocking pill invented more than two decades earlier by Dr. James Black. The medicine had, however, a new and effective marketing campaign. A doctor writing fifty prescriptions for Inderal LA and filling out a short form on each patient prescribed the drug could earn a free seat on American Airlines to anywhere in the United States.

At the same time, Roche Laboratories had offered physicians twelve hundred dollars for prescribing the antibiotic Rocephin to twenty patients, according to a letter written on corporate letterhead. And the drugmaker Sandoz was sending checks for a hundred dollars to physicians who agreed to read a two-page article on how its organ transplant drug Sandimmune could treat psoriasis, a skin disease. Sandimmune had not been approved to treat psoriasis. In fact, it was so toxic that almost half the psoriasis patients taking it experimentally in one trial dropped out after it harmed their kidneys or caused their blood pressure to rise.

Witnesses also detailed how local television stations were regularly broadcasting during their news programs videos that had been created by pharmaceutical companies to promote their products secretly without scrutiny from the FDA. The companies made the videos look like the work of broadcast journalists, while concealing their own involvement. The film segments often featured articulate physicians, grateful patients, and elaborate computer-generated graphics. The written scripts distributed with the videos suggested introductions, questions, and closings that could be used by the stations' anchors to make the videos appear like real news.

At the hearing, the senators listened to one of these fake news videos that promoted an asthma drug called theophylline. The video included footage of a young girl named Lacy and her mother.

"Lacy, do you think it helped?" the anchor was prompted to ask about the drug. The station then could cut to the film of the child as if the anchor were doing a live interview. "Yes," Lacy said. "I think the Theophylline has helped a lot because before, the medicine didn't help me, and I couldn't run very fast in sports. But now, I can run fast and do very well."

Senator Kennedy invited the companies' executives to speak at the hearing to explain these videos and their other marketing techniques, but they declined. Instead, the industry sent Gerald Mossinghoff, the president of the Pharmaceutical Manufacturers Association.

Mr. Mossinghoff argued, as the pharmaceutical companies had argued hundreds of times before, that the companies should be left free to market their products in a "responsible" way in order to generate sales and money needed to discover new medicines. It was a warning to Congress that if it didn't keep its hands off the industry, Americans would not get the new medicines they needed.

And to show that the industry was capable of overseeing its own affairs, Mr. Mossinghoff testified that in fact, the industry had just that month adopted a Code of Pharmaceutical Marketing Practices, prohibiting many of the activities that were generating complaints. For example, the code declared that the companies could no longer pay to fly doctors to meetings and cover other travel costs. The American Medical Association had adopted a similar code, limiting what physicians could accept from the drug industry.

Senator Kennedy asked Mr. Mossinghoff whether the industry had any way of enforcing its new ethical code.

"Mr. Chairman, we do not," Mr. Mossinghoff answered. "These are voluntary guidelines."

Later Senator Kennedy told Mr. Mossinghoff that he had learned that even as the committee was meeting that chilly December day in Washington, a drug company was making plans to fly a group of physicians to a hotel in the sunny Southwest.

"We understand that one company has an all-expenses-paid trip for 100 doctors and their spouses scheduled for tomorrow in Phoenix for the treatment of gallstones," Kennedy said. "Do you know if that symposium will go forward?"

Replied Mr. Mossinghoff: "I don't know the answer to that."

DESPITE THEIR PROMISES, the companies continued their zealous marketing campaigns. In 1994 Dr. David A. Kessler, the commissioner of the FDA, joined four of his colleagues to detail the companies' dangerous practices in an article in *The New England Journal of Medicine*. The frenzy of corporate promotion was driven, the regulators said, by the fact that the drugs being introduced were "virtually indistinguishable" from one another. Only a minority of the 127 new drugs approved between 1989 and 1993, the FDA officials wrote, had offered any clear clinical advantage over drugs already being sold. The companies used promotion, they said, to show the new drugs were somehow different and necessary.

"Victory in these therapeutic-class wars can mean millions of dollars for a drug company," Dr. Kessler and his colleagues wrote. "But for patients and providers it can mean misleading promotions, conflicts of interest, increased costs for health care, and ultimately, inappropriate prescribing." The regulators said they were particularly concerned about the companies' practice of paying pharmacists to get doctors to switch patients to their products, even when such a switch could harm the person.

More troubling was some companies' practice of paying doctors to prescribe medications in what the companies called clinical trials but were really campaigns run by marketers. These "trials" served little or no scientific purpose, Dr. Kessler explained, and instead were "thinly veiled attempts to entice doctors to prescribe a new drug."

The regulators had obtained a memo written by an executive inside one of the companies that described one of these marketing campaigns that had been disguised as a scientific study. It read, in part:

> Make no mistake about it: The [name of drug] study is the single most important sales initiative for 1993. Phase I provides 2,500 physicians with the opportunity to observe in their patients . . . blood pressure control . . . provided by [name of drug] . . . If at least 20,000 of the 25,000 patients involved in the study remain on [name of drug], it could mean up to a $10,000,000 boost in sales. In Phase II, this figure could double.

There was a mounting pile of evidence that patients were being endangered by the industry's aggressive marketing. In the past, when government watchdogs discovered such perilous practices, they eventually acted to stop them. In 1906, with the boom in quack medicines like Swaim's Panacea and the Grand Restorative, Congress had passed a law that allowed regulators to police the industry. In the late 1930s, after more than a hundred Americans died from the sweet-tasting Elixir Sulfanilamide, lawmakers had passed a measure requiring manufacturers to test their products before selling them. And in 1962, after thalidomide proved disastrous when given to pregnant women, Congress had strengthened the FDA's control over drug promotion. In this modern-day medicine show the watchdogs acted differently.

Just six months after Dr. Kessler stepped down from running the FDA, the acting commissioner, Dr. Michael J. Friedman, announced that the agency had decided to loosen its drug-advertising restrictions and pave the way for a massive shift in the marketing of drugs from print advertising to the more powerful medium of television. What had held the drug companies back from television ads was the requirement that they provide consumers with detailed information regarding a medicine's possible risks. For most drugs, that information requires several typewritten pages. Instead, under the FDA's new rules, the companies were now free to provide simply a few of the drug's more common risks, along with a toll-free phone number where the curious could find out more.

Dr. Friedman, a bespectacled and bearded oncologist with a penchant for bow ties, did not explain in his announcement that consumers could plan on being bombarded with television ads that vastly understated the risks of medicines. Instead, he said the action would "help promote greater consumer awareness about prescription drugs." He said he wanted to "end the uncertainty" that had "plagued both consumers and industry" about the use of television ads.

The pharmaceutical industry, the ad agencies on Madison Avenue, and the owners of television stations across the country welcomed a new heyday. And Dr. Friedman soon left the agency. In 1998, President Clinton nominated Dr. Jane Henney to be the next commissioner of the FDA, and Dr. Friedman resigned the next year to become a senior vice president at Searle, a subsidiary of Monsanto, which had just introduced a new pain pill called Celebrex. The pain reliever quickly became one of the most heavily advertised drugs in America and a blockbuster seller that dazzled Wall Street investors and made the company's executives wealthy.

THE INDUSTRY'S NEW television advertisements transported consumers to a Kool-Aid–colored fantasyland where ruddy actors played the roles of the afflicted who had found relief and enough energy to celebrate by taking a daily pill. The television ads could make even ineffective pills like Claritin, the allergy medicine that studies had shown worked little better than nothing, look like panaceas.

Schering-Plough, the maker of Claritin, spent $136 million on consumer ads in 1998, the first year after the government relaxed the rules. That sum was far more than had ever been spent to advertise a prescription drug and more than was spent that year to advertise Coca-Cola Classic, Coors Light, or American Express. Schering's ads featured smiling people romping in green fields to the tune of "Blue Skies" by Irving Berlin. Other ads featured Joan Lunden, the former host of ABC's *Good Morning America*, hiking through a field of flowers and telling viewers that Claritin had cleared her head. The marketing worked beautifully. Led by Claritin, sales of antihistamines soared by 612 percent between 1993 and 1998. The cover story in *Medical Marketing & Media*, an industry magazine, in May 1999 praised Schering for creating memorable ads that were like the "edutainment" created by Disney.

Quickly, another new drug, introduced in 1998, took the game to a whole new level.

"Viagra changed pharmaceuticals as a business," J. Patrick Kelly, a top marketing executive at Pfizer, the drug's maker, told a reporter from *Advertising Age* in 2001. The company's sex pill became part of American pop culture almost as soon as Pfizer introduced it. Not even Prozac, the antidepressant first sold in 1988, had been the topic of so many discussions around the water cooler, at the dinner table, or on late-night talk shows.

With Viagra, Pfizer marketers showed they were experts at creating a style or personality for a pill. They gave the pill a masculine blue hue and a unique diamond shape, as well as an unforgettable name that evoked energy and vigor. It didn't hurt that Viagra rhymed with "Niagara," giving the suggestion of a forceful flow.

Pfizer's marketing team even changed the name of the disease that Viagra was said to treat. Impotence, they believed, was an embarrassing term that men did not want to talk about. Instead, the company promoted Viagra as treating "erectile dysfunction" or simply ED. Pfizer then spent millions of dollars hiring celebrities to promote its new pill, beginning with the aging Bob Dole, who admitted to having sexual problems after prostate cancer surgery. To expand the market to younger and healthier men, Pfizer later hired thirty-seven-year-old Rafael Palmeiro, the first baseman for the Texas Rangers. With the hiring of Palmeiro in 2002, the theme of the Viagra campaign became one about enhancing performance, whether on the baseball field or in bed. It had little to do with treating a medical condition.

Viagra soon joined McDonald's and Coca-Cola on the list of the world's most recognizable brand names. And lifestyle drugs, those treating the problems and irritations that come with age, such as hair loss, wrinkles, and reduced sex drive, became the industry's new rage.

Pfizer was perhaps the first in the industry to transform itself so clearly into a consumer-marketing machine. Since its founding in 1849 by Charles Pfizer and his cousin Charles Erhart, the drug company had shown a knack for getting people to take more medicine. The cousins had their first breakthrough when they took a bitter treatment for parasitic worms, blended it with a sugar-cream confection and shaped it into a candy cone.

From those early days on, Pfizer proved willing to break the norm. Soon after the antibiotic Terramycin was approved in 1950, Pfizer's chemists tried mixing it with chocolate syrup to make it tastier; they gave up when the bottles started to explode. The chemists had better luck with a different tactic: they mixed the antibiotic with animal feed to create "a growth enhancer" for hogs, chickens, and cattle. To promote this agricultural use, Pfizer organized a hog-judging contest at the Conrad Hilton Hotel in Chicago, which ended with two-hundred-pound squealing pigs running through the lobby as newsmen caught the mayhem on film. Delighted with the publicity, Pfizer hauled a steer into the lobby of the Waldorf-Astoria Hotel in Manhattan, where a waiter in a white jacket served the bovine hay on a silver tray. Later, at a sales convention, Pfizer salespeople attracted attention by showing off a tiger in a cage.

The more aggressively it marketed a drug, Pfizer learned, the greater the profits and success. In 1947 Pfizer spent just 6 percent of its revenues on selling and administrative expenses. Fifty years later it was spending 40 percent of its revenues on those costs.

In a brochure given to job candidates hoping to join its marketing force, Pfizer boasted that it had taken its promotional messages "everywhere from the *Today* show to *Sesame Street* to the NASCAR circuit." The writers of the 2002 brochure could have added Major League Baseball, a concert tour by Earth, Wind & Fire, and the San Francisco Zoo.

By 2005 Pfizer was spending $2.28 on marketing and administrative costs for every $1 it said it spent on scientific research. But even those numbers, taken from its financial statements, may understate the company's true marketing costs. That's because at Pfizer, promotion began in the lab.

Pfizer's marketers worked side by side with scientists in what the company began calling in the 1990s Central Research Assists Marketing or simply CRAM. The name made it clear who was in charge. When I visited Pfizer's sprawling research headquarters in Groton, Connecticut, in the summer of 2000, two scientists who had worked on an antibiotic called Zithromax provided an example of how this worked. They said the company's marketing executives had sent them around the world to give talks about the drug at medical conferences years before it was approved. The main message in these talks, the scientists said, was that animal studies had shown that Zithromax was a powerful drug that stayed in the body's tissues longer than other antibiotics. The marketers suggested the scientists talk about the drug using snappy, memorable phrases like "the tissue is the issue," which doctors would remember once the experimental drug was approved for sale.

But the influence that marketers had in Pfizer's laboratories went far beyond having white-coated scientists use zippy slogans to speak about experimental medicines in the pipeline. Marketing infused every aspect of a drug's development at Pfizer, according to the company's executives. Marketers decided what projects the scientists would continue to work on. Once the medicines were approved, marketers directed scientists to perform additional studies that could be used for new promotional claims and slogans. For example, Pfizer's marketers expanded sales of Zoloft, its antidepressant, by having scientists perform studies aimed at showing that it not only eased depression but also relieved fear in people who were extremely shy and suffering from what had become known as social anxiety disorder. These clinical trials performed *after* a drug is approved by the FDA are known in the industry as Phase IV research studies. The most controversial of these trials have no apparent scientific purpose and have been used by some industry marketers, as the FDA commissioner David Kessler said in 1994, to pay doctors to prescribe a drug.

"We'll spend as much on Phase IV as we do on getting a product approved," Bill Steere, Pfizer's chief executive, explained in 2000. Pfizer executives said then that about 25 percent of Pfizer's research budget paid for studies of drugs already being sold. This money was being used for promotion and to expand sales of existing products. It had nothing to do with discovering new drugs.

Pfizer's emphasis on marketing rather than science was reflected in the fact that it had not actually discovered many of the drugs it sold. Instead, it had licensed them from other companies or from the universities that had invented them. In 2004 seven of the eight experimental drugs that Pfizer was readying for sale and that Wall Street was tracking because of their financial significance had been discovered somewhere other than in the company's labs. The eighth drug was nothing more than a combination of two drugs Pfizer had been selling for years.

The company was such a powerful promoter that investors often quickly bought up the stock of any other firm that began a marketing partnership with Pfizer. For instance, the market value of the company Serono soared by two billion dollars the day it announced that Pfizer would help it sell Rebif, a drug for multiple sclerosis. Investors were betting that Rebif's sales would now skyrocket with the help of Pfizer's marketing might.

In 2000 Pfizer bullied its way into becoming the world's largest pharmaceutical company through a hostile takeover of Warner-Lambert, a firm that had been its partner in the marketing of Lipitor, the cholesterol drug. Warner-Lambert scientists had discovered Lipitor, but Pfizer wanted to sell it.

The takeover also made Pfizer the most profitable drug company in the world. In 2001 Pfizer rang up sales at a rate of almost $4 million an hour and, by the end of the year, had turned $7.8 billion of those sales into profit.

Bill Steere, the mastermind behind Pfizer's rise to power, announced in August 2000, a month after the details of the Warner-Lambert deal were finalized, that he would retire as the company's chief executive.

"It's the perfect time to leave," he told me during an interview in his office, high above Forty-second Street on Manhattan's East Side. "I've done my part. We're number one."

Mr. Steere is an intense man, who can seem more reflective than talkative. He had spent more than forty years at Pfizer, joining the company as a salesman after graduating from Stanford with a degree in marine biology. He was leaving with a pension that would pay him more than six million dollars a year for the rest of his life, stock and options worth more than a hundred million dollars, and such perks as lifetime use of a car and driver as well as the use of the company's aircraft, if he desired. When I asked him what he would do now that he was letting Hank McKinnell, the Canadian businessman who had been his close aide, take over, he smiled. He explained he had a home in New York and another in Florida. He planned to continue lobbying for Pfizer in Washington, he said, but hoped to spend more time scuba diving and spearfishing.

"I recently bought a boat but had nowhere to put it," he said, "so I bought a marina."

As THE TWENTY-FIRST century began, it was Pfizer that set the industry's pace. The other companies imitated its marketing techniques and came up with some of their own.

A key part of the blockbuster strategy was to have marketers work quietly behind the scenes to mold the public's opinions and impressions in ways that could boost sales. A brochure I picked up at a pharmaceutical marketing conference in 2002 laid out these recommended promotional steps in an easy-to-read matrix. The brochure was written by Ethical Strategies Limited, a consulting firm that promised to "add value" to any pharmaceutical marketing campaign.

The brochure said the marketing of a drug should begin years before it was approved, even before it was tested in human subjects. During this time, known as the preclinical stage, the company should identify and recruit doctors who would be paid to speak on the drug's behalf, the consultants said. The drug company should also begin looking for non-profit health groups, like the American Heart Association, that it could partner with to promote the product. It was also a good idea, the firm said, to start at this early stage to identify the "key journalists" who could be counted on to get out the drug's story.

When the experimental drug moved from being tested in animals to its first trials in humans, which are known as Phase I studies, the company should start paying for meetings at which the experimental drug can be promoted to certain physicians. At this time, even though the drug is still years away from approval, the company should begin paying as well to have articles written and published in medical journals that supported the drug's use. Ethical Strategies also suggested the company prepare its media strategy during this period to "seed market with pre-clinical information."

As the months and years passed and the drug continued to move through human studies, the company should train and ready its re-cruited doctors for their "lecture tours," the brochure said. It should also develop written "therapeutic guidelines" that doctors would use to diag-nose and treat patients with the company's product once it was on the market. As the drug got closer to approval, the company should "launch key messages and story platforms" by providing information to journal-ists. And "where gaps exist," the company should "establish" new patient groups to help promote the new drug. Ethical Strategies said that these steps were "a look at a typical program."

The brochure was not so significant for the promotional techniques it described. I had already observed companies using the tactics that

Ethical Strategies suggested, including planting stories in the news media and creating patient advocacy groups. What was fascinating, however, was how early the marketers were expected to begin work on creating a desire for their product and how the recommended tactics were laid out as distinct steps on a timeline. To create a blockbuster, the marketing had to begin when the drug was still in the test tube, and it had to be timed to perfection.

The industry's recipe for its blockbuster sellers was so effective that Wall Street quickly became addicted to the resulting high profits. By the late 1990s it was no longer enough for a drug manufacturer to show a respectable increase in sales and profits every year. Investors came to expect the major pharmaceutical companies to increase their sales and profits each year by 15 percent or far more. They swiftly punished any drug-maker who dared to disappoint them by announcing earnings that were growing fast but were a fraction below what Wall Street expected. If a drug company earned more than expected, its stock price soared, along with the value of its executives' stock options. The system made the drug companies and their executives bound not to patients but to the demands and desires of the stock market.

And soon even a drug that could bring in a billion dollars in sales in a single year was not big enough.

ON THE AFTERNOON of September 28, 2000, executives at Bristol-Myers Squibb invited scores of Wall Street analysts and investors to a ballroom in a grand hotel on the East Side of Manhattan.

On a stage with a multicolored backdrop, the company's top two executives, Charles Heimbold and Peter Dolan, stepped up to announce that Bristol-Myers was embarking on what they called the MegaDouble plan. The company would now focus its efforts, the executives said, on marketing only those drugs with the potential to bring in several billion dollars a year. They called these products megablockbusters.

Dolan, the company's president, laid out more details of the Mega-Double plan in an article in a magazine published internally for employees. "Everyone in the industry knows that Rx companies need blockbuster products for growth," Dolan explained. "We need them, too—but we need much more than that. We know that to substantially accelerate our growth rates over time, and to keep high-quality expansion going, will require mega-blockbuster products, mega-blockbuster ideas and a strategy that can make mega-growth happen."

Added Rick Lane, the executive in charge of Bristol-Myers's international medicines business: "We have one fundamental objective, and that's to grow faster than the other guys."

The executives made it clear they had little interest in drugs or other products that did not fit their aggressive plan for growth. A drug that could achieve $200 million in sales a year was no longer big enough.

A few months before, Bristol-Myers executives had started a central part of their plan in the company's research laboratories through an initiative they dubbed Opportunity Seeking Blockbusters or OSB. In internal documents, the executives had first referred to this initiative as O$B but later shied away from using that acronym, fearing it could be taken as a sign of corporate greed.

Dr. Peter Ringrose, the scientist in charge of the company's laboratories, said that OSB meant that Bristol-Myers would put its research money behind the scientific projects that had the greatest potential to reap massive sales. That meant that experimental compounds that may have proved to be lifesaving for patients but could never bring in the sales of a megablockbuster would be licensed to other companies or set aside to gather dust on a laboratory shelf.

Explained Rick Lane: "If you look at the companies in this industry that have performed truly exceptionally over the last 10 years, they've been driven by blockbusters or, increasingly, by mega-blockbusters. Drugs like Prilosec for AstraZeneca, Viagra and Lipitor for Pfizer, Zocor for Merck. We need drugs in that range."

FOR THE PUBLIC, the implications of such a business strategy can be devastating. People with rare diseases are ignored. So are the poor, who cannot afford the high prices that must be charged for a drug to become a megablockbuster. Instead, under this game plan, the drug company focused its resources solely on drugs with the potential to be sold on a massive scale to rich Americans.

And it was not just Bristol-Myers that had devised such a strategy. Its executives were only following in the footsteps of their competitors, the other masters of the medicine trade.

Third World countries, where most real disease exists, had long suffered because the industry's business plans did not include them. Of the 1,223 new drugs that reached the market between 1975 and 1997, only thirteen of them, or just 1 percent, treated the deadly or debilitating diseases found in the tropics, where most people are poor. And of those thirteen medicines, only four came from research done by the pharmaceutical industry to discover human drugs. The others were updates of some drugs already available, were discovered as corporate scientists looked for medicines to treat livestock or pets, or were invented through scientific work paid for by the military.

But the economics of the pharmaceutical business had changed to the point where it was not just the world's poor who were not getting drugs they desperately needed. As the drug companies concentrated on selling daily medications to treat chronic conditions and on lifestyle pills like Viagra, some abandoned efforts to discover products like antibiotics and vaccines that actually saved lives but were taken just once or for brief periods. In 2002, for example, Bristol-Myers, Abbott Laboratories, and Eli Lilly halted or substantially reduced their efforts to discover antibiotics. These decisions affected all the world's populations, including Americans who had so overused the available antibiotics that doctors were finding more and more cases where the drugs no longer worked against lethal infections. Tens of thousands of Americans die every year from infections that were once easily remedied with an antibiotic.

Howard Solomon, the chairman of Forest Laboratories, a drug company smaller than giants like Pfizer and Bristol-Myers, described how he viewed the strategy of his larger rivals in his annual letter to shareholders in 2002. "The very size of the pharmaceutical leviathans require blockbuster blockbusters to make a perceptible difference in their profit and loss, and there are only so many targets that affect so many people so often that a successful drug can have the requisite billions of dollars of potential sales," he wrote. "As the leviathan becomes more bloated it has to feed on whales and it ignores the minnows, and there are far fewer whales."

THERE WAS AN even deeper flaw in the industry's strategy of aggressively marketing medicines. It was killing thousands of people as doctors prescribed new drugs on the advice of the corporate marketers before all the risks were known.

In case after case, drug companies eager to "launch" new medicines succeeded in getting American physicians to write millions of prescriptions for a drug, only then to find the medicine was so dangerous that it had to be pulled from pharmacy shelves. Between 1975 and 2005 at least twenty prescription drugs, including big sellers like Rezulin, for diabetes, and the diet pill Redux, were removed from the market. In 2002 a group of researchers studied the deaths and serious injuries caused by the newest medicines. They found that of the hundreds of drugs approved between 1975 and 1999, more than 10 percent were either taken off the market or given the government's most serious warning, one that is outlined in a boldfaced black box on the label and meant to send an alarm to doctors that the product can kill. The researchers concluded that the serious risks of a medicine could not be known for many years. Patients taking the new, heavily advertised drugs they saw on television had little idea of what they were getting themselves into.

The danger lay in the fact that most new drugs are tested in only *a few thousand* patients in experiments that may last just a few weeks. The companies carefully choose patients for those experiments, frequently leaving out the elderly, women, and patients who are very weak or ill. Once the government approves the drug, marketers and salespeople work feverishly to get doctors to prescribe it to *millions* of patients.

A single class of new medicines promoted to treat irregular heartbeats is estimated to have killed fifty thousand Americans in just a few years. That tragedy in the late 1980s showed that heavily marketed medicines could kill the equivalent of an entire city the size of Biloxi, Mississippi, with almost no public outcry if the drugs caused a type of death that was common in the population, like cardiac arrest.

At the same time, the industry's method of selling blockbusters had a way of tempting executives to keep a dangerous medicine on the market long after its deadly risks had become clear. Sales of a new drug could rise so fast that an executive's decision to remove it from the market would mean the loss of hundreds of millions of dollars in annual revenues and a large percentage of the company's total sales. Thousands of sales reps and other employees assigned to the drug would be left without their main reason for employment. And the company would lose the hundreds of millions of dollars it had invested in the product's research and promotion.

The pressure was intense for executives to look the other way.

AMERICA DID NOT need another cholesterol-lowering drug when executives at Bayer introduced Baycol in 1997. Other companies were already selling five of these drugs known as statins, including Lipitor, Zocor, and Pravachol. But that did not stop the plans of the executives at the German chemical giant. They needed a new bestseller and were excited by the fast-rising use of statins by Americans, who were reminded every day to watch the levels of cholesterol in their blood. Thanks to the marketers of the first statin pills, "Know your numbers" had become a mantra of the fifty-and-older set.

There was something about Baycol, however, that made it stand out from the others. Clues to its distinction began to appear almost as soon as Bayer began selling it. Within a hundred days of the first Baycol prescription in the United States, the company received disturbing reports of seven patients who had taken it. The patients had developed a potentially fatal condition known as rhabdomyolysis or had tested positive for an enzyme that was a sign of the condition.

Rhabdomyolysis is the rapid breakdown of the body's muscles. As the muscle cells disintegrate, their contents flow into the bloodstream. Mild cases can cause severe pain and muscle weakness. In serious cases, the condition can cause paralysis and death as the kidneys shut down. All statins had been found to cause rhabdomyolysis in rare cases. But some Bayer executives began to worry that the risk for patients taking Baycol was higher than for those taking the other drugs.

The company's drug safety office was soon deluged with injury reports. On December 30, 1999, employees wrote that they had received sixty reports of patients hit by rhabdomyolysis in the United States in the last two months. "The steadily increasing numbers of spontaneous reports of rhabdomyolysis associated with Baycol, along with the additional telephone activity, has overwhelmed the available safety assurance resources," they wrote in an internal memo.

The next month a group of Bayer's scientific relations staff met to talk about Baycol and a database the company had created to track the injuries. An unidentified executive scribbled notes of what transpired at that meeting on a copy of the typed agenda. The person wrote that some Bayer executives were reluctant to probe too deeply into the increasing number of injury reports. Some executives were "scared to uncover such data (bad data)," the person wrote, because the company was anticipating higher sales as it launched a new version of Baycol containing a higher dose.

"If FDA asks for bad news, we have to give," the executive wrote, "but if we don't have it, then we can't give it to them."

The next month Patricia Stenger, a manager in Bayer's scientific affairs division, e-mailed Dr. Richard Goodstein, the vice president for scientific relations at Bayer. Ms. Stenger said she was concerned that there was "widespread knowledge" among the company's sales reps "that there have been some deaths related to Baycol."

"So much for keeping this quiet," she wrote.

Despite the hesitation of some executives to probe too deeply into the drug's safety, Bayer employees did perform an internal analysis of the injury reports at about that time. In March 2000 Steve Niemcryk, an epidemiologist at Bayer, and Paul Cislo, a database analyst, reported to Bayer executives that Baycol "substantially elevates" the risk of rhabdomyolysis compared with similar drugs. But the two analysts said the magnitude of the problem could not be determined from Bayer's data.

They wrote that the company was working to gather data from other organizations that would provide a more accurate analysis of the drug's injury rate. Their report remained a corporate secret that was not shared with the public.

About that same time, Dr. Goodstein sent an e-mail to two dozen Bayer executives working on marketing Baycol in the United States. Dr. Goodstein said that reports of "alleged cases" of rhabdomyolysis caused by Baycol were coming into his office at a rate of about one a day. "Many of the cases are ugly," he wrote, "involving paralysis, dialysis, long hospitalization, disability and two potentially related deaths."

As the number of injuries continued to rise, Bayer executives did what other pharmaceutical companies do when they receive reports of people who have been hurt by their products. They added language to Baycol's written label explaining that such injuries had been reported. The label, which is also known as the prescribing instructions, is the official guide to a drug and is carefully monitored by the FDA. The language added by Bayer about the rhabdomyolysis cases served as a warning to physicians. It also served to protect Bayer from lawsuits brought by patients. The company could now point out that it was not hiding the danger. The problem was that studies had shown that many doctors ignored these labels. They greatly aided the company's defense lawyers but often failed to safeguard those they were meant to help.

Despite the increasing reports of injuries, Bayer did not slow its aggressive marketing of the drug. In July 2000 executives on the Baycol Project Team said their goal was to capture 15 percent of the statin market. Reaching that goal would require a big promotional push. At the time of the meeting, according to its written minutes, Baycol had only 5 percent of the market. Dr. Wolfgang Plischke, the president of Bayer's North American pharmaceutical division, attended the meeting and declared his optimism for higher sales. Dr. Plischke "reiterated the need to drive future sales," the minutes said, "and his belief that we can achieve blockbuster status."

When both corporate executives and government regulators agree that a prescription drug comes with a small but real risk of death, how many deaths does it take before there is one too many? It was not until late July 2001 that the staff at the FDA pressed Bayer about the deaths and injuries. The regulators told the company's executives that they had serious concerns about the drug's safety, especially when it was nothing more than a me-too drug. There were plenty of safer drugs available. Bayer executives reluctantly removed Baycol from the market. By that day in August 2001 the drug had been linked to more than a hundred deaths.

There were bigger disasters ahead.

IT WAS TWO weeks before the opening ceremonies of the 2000 Olympic Games in Sydney, and the former gold medalists Dorothy Hamill and Bruce Jenner were on *Larry King Live*. The Olympians were not talking about the upcoming athletic competition. They were complaining about their arthritis.

"I just—I felt old, I felt depressed, tired all the time," explained Ms. Hamill, winner of the Olympic gold for figure skating in 1976. "I mean, having chronic pain is exhausting. And I got to the point this year, I was on tour and I couldn't skate. And so, I went to a doctor, and we finally got to the bottom of it, and my doctor prescribed Vioxx for me, and it's as if I've been given a new life. It's just—it's been amazing. I feel twenty years younger."

Jenner, who won the Olympic decathlon in 1976, told the television audience that he had just turned fifty and found that his knee needed two weeks to recover after a game of tennis. "I'm dealing with a lot of pain here, you know, what are my options?" Jenner said. "And for me it was great—Vioxx."

That night's television talk show on CNN was part of what had become the most expensive and aggressive pharmaceutical marketing battle at the turn of the century. And this time the company once led by George W. Merck was at the heart of it.

Merck & Co. had grown to become the world's largest pharmaceutical company in the late 1980s, largely through the power of its science. At that time Ray Vagelos, a doctor who was fascinated with research, had been in charge. Dr. Vagelos gave the company's scientists a fair degree of freedom to pursue promising ideas. The strategy appeared to work as the company turned out a string of breakthrough drugs, including Mevacor, the first cholesterol-lowering statin to be approved by the FDA. Employees proudly pointed out that Merck, unlike many of its competitors, had never removed a drug from the market for safety reasons. This was a sign, they said, of the company's strong scientific practices and ethics. Executives and workers alike were often known to recite the words of George Merck from the speech he gave in 1950 that "medicine is for the people."

Now, in late 2000, Raymond Gilmartin, an electrical engineer with an M.B.A. from Harvard, was in charge. And it was the introduction of the pain reliever Vioxx that showed just how much power the marketers had gained inside Merck, as it struggled to keep up with promotional powerhouses like Pfizer and GlaxoSmithKline.

Merck had paid both Dorothy Hamill and Bruce Jenner to promote Vioxx to the American public in a campaign called Everyday Victories. Not to be outdone, Pharmacia and Pfizer, the two companies that had joined together to sell the competing pain pill called Celebrex, had hired Bart Conner, a gymnast who won two gold medals in 1984. The forty-two-year-old Conner was talking to the media, politicians, and the public about how Celebrex had helped him beat the pain of his arthritis.

"It's something you can take for a long time without side effects," Conner told *People* magazine a month or so before the Sydney Olympics. That statement was false. All drugs, including Celebrex, have side effects. And regulators would have found the statement to be illegal if they had discovered it in an ad or in a corporate press release sent by Pharmacia. But the drug companies took comfort in knowing that Conner, as well as Hamill and Jenner, could claim just about anything, and there was little the FDA would do about it.

Before the introduction of Vioxx and Celebrex, sales of such anti-inflammatory pain relievers had been in decline. It was not a market that excited analysts on Wall Street. Patients with arthritis could buy a variety of cheap and effective over-the-counter medicines like aspirin or ibuprofen and ease their pain for just pennies a day.

But in 1998 news stories began to appear about the new "super-aspirins" that were coming soon. The media reports said the new drugs would offer great pain relief without the dangerous side effects of standard anti-inflammatory pain pills. The stories were the result of early corporate public relations campaigns to promote products that were still months away from gaining government approval.

The scientific theory behind the new drugs appeared to be sound. Scientists at Merck and at Searle, a company later bought by Pharmacia, developed the medicines on the basis of research into cyclooxygenase, an enzyme in the body that is often referred to as Cox. Pain relievers like aspirin and ibuprofen inhibit the Cox enzymes as they reduce pain. At the same time, these drugs often wreak havoc in the stomach and, in the worst cases, cause bleeding ulcers that kill. Merck and Searle scientists developed the new drugs on the theory that there were two kinds of Cox enzymes, Cox-1 and Cox-2. They theorized that a drug that selectively blocked only the enzyme known as Cox-2 would be far less harmful to the stomach than drugs like aspirin.

A safer anti-inflammatory drug would be an extraordinary and life-saving breakthrough. Researchers estimated in 1999 that more than sixteen thousand Americans with arthritis were dying every year from stomach ulcers caused by their anti-inflammatory pain pills, roughly the same number as those who died from AIDS.

But inside the walls of Merck and Pharmacia, scientists were worried. They were struggling to generate the scientific data that supported the "superaspirin" buzz being stirred up by their marketing colleagues. The scientists at both companies were failing to prove that the new drugs, known as Cox-2 inhibitors, relieved pain any better than the far cheaper standbys like over-the-counter ibuprofen. Also, patients taking Vioxx and Celebrex still suffered from ulcers, albeit at what appeared to be a lower rate than those using the older drugs.

At Merck, scientists were troubled by something more: they feared Vioxx might harm the hearts of some patients as it relieved their pain.

More than two years before Vioxx was approved for sale, Dr. Alise Reicin, a senior scientist at Merck, sent an e-mail to her colleagues saying that the company was in a "no-win situation" with Vioxx. She said that "the possibility of increased CV events is of great concern." The term "CV events" is scientific shorthand for cardiovascular problems like heart attacks and sudden death. In parentheses, Dr. Reicin added, "I just can't wait to be the one to present those results to senior management!"

In her e-mail, which she sent in February 1997, Dr. Reicin proposed that people with a high risk of cardiovascular problems be kept out of a proposed study in the hope that by the trial's conclusion the difference in the rate of heart complications between the Vioxx patients and those taking other pain relievers "would not be evident."

The fear that Vioxx could harm the heart continued to roil Merck's executives, scientists, and marketers in the following years, as the FDA approved the drug in May 1999, and the company began spending tens of millions of dollars a month to promote it.

In March 2000 Merck's scientists received the results of a large corporate study they had called the VIGOR trial. The study showed that patients taking Vioxx still suffered from ulcers, but at about half the rate as those patients taking a pain reliever called naproxen, which is sold under the brand name Aleve. That finding supported Merck's claim that Vioxx was at least somewhat safer on the stomach than other drugs.

Yet there was also damning evidence in the study of just the problem that Merck's scientists had feared. The company and the academic scientists it had hired to perform the study had excluded most patients with serious heart disease from the trial, the action that Dr. Reicin had suggested three years earlier. By excluding such patients, those in the study were healthier than those taking Vioxx in the real world. Even among these healthier patients in the trial, however, four times as many Vioxx patients suffered from heart attacks and other serious cardiovascular complications as those taking naproxen, the other drug tested in the study.

Dr. Edward M. Scolnick, the head of research at Merck, read the early results from the VIGOR study and sent an e-mail to his colleagues on March 9, 2000. He wrote that the cardiovascular events "are clearly there." He added that the problem was "mechanism based as we worried

it was." Scientists often refer to a drug's mechanism when they explain
how it works. They now knew there was something about how Vioxx
worked in the body that was harming some patients' hearts.

Merck's message to doctors and the American public was a different
one, however. In press releases the company explained away the heart
attacks suffered by the patients taking Vioxx in the study. Executives said
that Merck had done other studies that had not found an increased risk
of heart problems in patients taking Vioxx. They said they believed that
the new study, VIGOR, which was a comparison between patients who
took Vioxx and others who took naproxen, was not showing a problem
with Vioxx. Instead, they said, the study had uncovered a health benefit
provided by naproxen. Naproxen appeared to protect patients' hearts, the
executives said. In previous studies of naproxen, scientists had not found
it had some kind of effect like aspirin, which in some trials has appeared
to lower the risk of heart attacks. But Merck now had an explanation for
the higher number of heart attacks suffered by patients taking Vioxx in
the study. It was one the company would use for years.

THE BATTLE BETWEEN Merck and the team of Pharmacia and Pfizer
for dominance in the pain market was one of the fiercest and most expensive the industry had ever seen. The government approved Celebrex
on the last day of 1998, about five months before it approved Vioxx.

Pharmacia and Pfizer quickly made the industry's record books by
making Celebrex the first prescription drug to bring in $1 billion in sales
in its first year on the market. This only made Merck's marketers push
harder. Merck spent $160 million to advertise Vioxx to consumers in 2000,
more than any company had ever spent to advertise a prescription drug.
It was also more than was spent that year to advertise either Budweiser
or Pepsi. Many of the Vioxx ads featured Dorothy Hamill skating on a
frozen pond in the snow-covered woods to the Rascals' song "A Beautiful Morning."

"With all the great memories has come another thing I thought I'd
never experience—the pain of osteoarthritis," Ms. Hamill said in the ad.

"Vioxx is here," an announcer chimed in. "With one little pill a day . . ."

While their advertisements played during the evening news, Merck and Pharmacia were uncorking bottles of wine at thousands of dinners where they entertained the nation's doctors. In 2001 Pharmacia promoted Celebrex to medical professionals at some nine thousand dinners, meetings, and other events, while Merck hosted seventy-six hundred similar events to push Vioxx. The companies hired legions of doctors to speak at these parties, which were held in towns and cities across America at a rate of more than forty a day. The marketers of the two new drugs hired so many of the nation's rheumatologists to be speakers, consultants, or members of their advisory boards that it was hard to find one who was not on the corporate payroll. For instance, I called a national society of rheumatologists in 2000 and asked to speak to an arthritis expert for an article I was writing about Vioxx and Celebrex. I specifically requested a physician who was not being paid by either company. A staff person told me the group had many knowledgeable rheumatologists but that they all were consultants to or speakers for the sellers of the new pain pills.

For the sales reps promoting Vioxx for Merck, their every action and word, down to the way they shook hands or ordered wine when dining with physicians, were suggested by a corporate script. A training manual informed the sales reps that a handshake should start and stop "crisply," be "firm but painless," and last three seconds. In restaurants, a sales rep was expected not to "order a cheeseburger if your guest orders lobster" and to eat bread "one small bitesize piece at a time."

After Merck published the VIGOR study, some doctors began to worry about whether Vioxx might hurt their patients' hearts. To ease such concerns, Merck trained its salespeople to respond to doctors' questions with one of the corporate-approved statements listed in what it called its Obstacle Response Guide. In some cases, the reps were told to show a physician Merck's Cardiovascular Card. The card included statistics that claimed a patient taking Vioxx was eight times *less* likely to die from a cardiovascular complication than patients taking standard anti-inflammatory drugs like ibuprofen. The statistics provided in the card did not include the startling results from the VIGOR trial. Instead, the company had pooled together data from other studies it had performed, a mingling of numbers that the FDA had warned was not appropriate.

To prepare its salespeople for the increasing number of questions about the drug, Merck created a training exercise called Dodge Ball Vioxx. Each of the first dozen pages of this training document listed an "obstacle" the salespeople might encounter, like a doctor who tells them, "I am concerned about the cardiovascular effects of Vioxx." Another possible "obstacle" was described as a physician who says, "I am concerned with dose-related increases in hypertension with Vioxx." The last four pages of the training document appear to provide the response Merck expected from any salesperson encountering these "obstacles." Each page contained a single word: "DODGE!"

Yet the concern among physicians was just beginning. In the summer of 2001 three cardiologists at the Cleveland Clinic, one of the top heart centers in the nation, reported that they had found that both Vioxx and Celebrex appeared to increase the risk of heart attacks and strokes. The three doctors focused more of their concern on Vioxx, however. In an article in the *Journal of the American Medical Association*, they explained that the overall risk of heart attack when taking the drugs was low. But given that millions of Americans were taking the drugs, even a slight increase in the risk would mean that thousands of people could be harmed or even die from the pain relievers. The doctors called on Merck and Pharmacia to begin studies to prove their products were safe. Both companies rebuffed the request. By then the drugs had become megablockbuster products with combined sales of six billion dollars a year.

In the following months more articles raising questions about the safety of the new pain relievers were published. Most of them singled out Vioxx.

A group of doctors at Vanderbilt University reported in October 2002 that they had found that poor patients in Tennessee who were taking high doses of Vioxx had significantly more heart attacks and strokes than patients not using such high amounts.

Merck kept selling.

SIX

Ghostwriters and Secret Studies

> Complete honesty is of course imperative in
> scientific work.
>   —W.I.B. BEVERIDGE
>   in *The Art of Scientific Investigation*

EXECUTIVES AT NOVARTIS were in a quandary in the fall of 2002. Ritalin, the pill that had changed the way America quieted fidgety children, was no longer a big moneymaker for the company. Prescriptions had fallen so far that only a fraction of the children diagnosed with attention disorders were using the company's white and yellow tablets. The problem wasn't demand. Millions of parents, more than ever before, were giving their children pills to keep them focused and calm in school. But doctors were prescribing cheap, generic versions of the drug or new medicines made by Novartis's competitors. These newer drugs were stimulants like Ritalin. They were even made with the same chemical, a substance called methylphenidate. But scientists had transformed the new pills to work hours longer. Swallowing one of these time-released pills in the morning kept children medicated throughout the school day. Ritalin, on the other hand, worked for just a few hours, requiring the child to make an embarrassing midday march to the school nurse's office to swallow a second dose.

In an attempt to reclaim its supremacy in the market, Novartis had introduced its own new version of the drug, which it called Ritalin LA, the initials representing its longer action. The company had sent out press releases when federal regulators approved the new drug, declaring it an "important advance." But inside the company, executives knew they had a problem. Their new brand of medicine was little different from two other time-released pills already selling fast. While the old Ritalin had been an original—that is, the first methylphenidate product approved to treat inattentive children—the company's new pill was nothing more than a me-too, an imitator aiming to grab a piece of an already crowded market.

Novartis executives explained their plight in a slide show presentation to their peers. A "key challenge" in selling Ritalin LA, they said in their slides, was its "lack of significant differentiation."

"Competition is the same chemical entity!" one of the executives' slides exclaimed. Despite that problem, the company's objective, according to the presentation, was to "regain significant market share" in a product category that was "highly promotion sensitive." In other words, the executives wanted what Ritalin once had had: dominance and fast-rising sales.

But to sell a copycat pill, Novartis needed a critical element. Even as clerks were stocking drugstore shelves with Ritalin LA, the company lacked the scientific evidence that would sell its new pill. It did not have a study to show that Ritalin LA was a breakthrough—because it wasn't. Executives yearned for a published scientific report that the company's salespeople could wave in front of doctors and convince them of the new drug's greatness. For a cash-rich company like Novartis, such difficulties could be overcome. There were dozens of vendors waiting to help.

NOVARTIS HIRED INTRAMED, a division of WPP, one of the largest advertising agencies in the world, to help sell its newest medicine for children.

IntraMed had dozens of medical writers and editors at the ready to help pharmaceutical companies shape science for their corporate marketing needs. Firms like IntraMed called themselves medical education companies because their public face was one of teaching physicians about medicine and new pharmaceutical products. But these companies described their work differently when they were talking to drug executives and trying to win new accounts. "Even good science needs a little magic," said one ad placed in 2002 in *Med Ad News*, an industry magazine, by ApotheCom, one of IntraMed's competitors.

The services offered by these ad firms were part of a side of medical science that most people did not understand. It was not just independent scientists working to expand knowledge who were writing the articles published by medical journals. Often there was something else altogether going on.

Salespeople at Novartis had asked two academic scientists, John S. Markowitz and Kennerly S. Patrick, both on the faculty at the Medical University of South Carolina, to write an article for a scientific journal, describing the different medicines for attention deficit disorders and how each one worked. The scientists and executives had sent an outline of the article back and forth, but the corporate managers were not pleased with the draft the academics had recently turned in.

So on a crisp September day in Manhattan the executives and scientists met by conference call. Executives from IntraMed set up the phone call from their offices in a high-rise on Park Avenue South. The two scientists, calling in from Charleston, South Carolina, complained they were still sweltering in the summer heat. Soon joining the call was Shane Schaffer, a marketing executive at Novartis. The Swiss company ran its most profitable enterprise, that of selling prescription drugs to Americans, from offices thirty miles west of Manhattan in East Hanover, a leafy suburban town in New Jersey.

Schaffer, the Novartis executive, told the two scientists that the company really needed "a quick, down and dirty" article explaining the different medicines for ADHD and how Ritalin LA was different. Schaffer admitted that the scientific study that the company hoped would show the uniqueness of Ritalin LA had not yet begun. "Once we get the data from the study, which starts tomorrow, we'll be able to do, you know, a much more data driven result," he explained.

Schaffer asked Marcia Zabusky, a vice president at IntraMed, if she had sent the doctors a new outline of what the drug company wanted in their paper.

"No, we haven't yet, Shane," Zabusky replied. She told the doctors that employees at her agency were working on an outline that she believed would satisfy Novartis, while using some information from their first draft. But this time, she said, IntraMed wanted to write the paper.

"We would like to help draft this manuscript and then submit it to you for your—for your editing and for approval," Zabusky told the two doctors. "How does that sound?"

"That sounds fine with me," said Dr. Patrick.

"Yes, as soon as you want to send an outline or, if you've already got, you know, a draft you've worked up, we can move forward," Dr. Markowitz said.

Schaffer asked if the money Novartis had paid Dr. Markowitz for earlier work was enough to cover this paper too.

"No, not really," he replied.

"We'll take care of you then, okay?" Schaffer said.

Schaffer and Zabusky then explained more of what Novartis wanted in the paper. The paper would describe the many medicines containing methylphenidate and discuss why children needed a pill that lasted through the day. Zabusky said the paper would then describe "the ideal" pill for children who had difficulty paying attention.

"Here is a situation where it's going to be a little bit . . ."

"Theoretical," Schaffer said, completing her sentence.

"Right," she said. "Theoretical. Productive."

The paper, Zabusky said, should make a "theoretical conclusion" that a pill lasting nine hours, which Ritalin LA appeared to do, was better than one that worked for twelve hours. The leading rival in the market, a drug called Concerta, was said to last a dozen hours in children's bodies. The theory of Novartis and its marketing agency, IntraMed, was that the nine-hour stimulant would be better since it would stop working in the late afternoon, making it easier for the child to eat dinner and go to bed.

Children taking the stimulants frequently complain they aren't hungry and can't sleep.

Zabusky explained to the doctors that the paper should end by stating that more scientific data were needed but that the outlook was "very hopeful for children."

Dr. Markowitz and Dr. Patrick repeatedly agreed with the executives' suggestions. Zabusky promised to send them an outline later in the day and a new draft during the week of September 23.

"I think we're quite clear on what you want the next manuscript to look like," Dr. Patrick said, just before hanging up.

IN 1942 THE pioneering sociologist Robert K. Merton argued that scientists must be dispassionate in their quest for knowledge. He argued that such disinterestedness was one of "the norms" of science. Research should not be biased, he said, by considerations such as personal profit.

Dr. Merton, the first sociologist to receive the National Medal of Science, wrote about how there was a trend within medicine in the 1940s against patenting medical discoveries to turn them into profits. In one prominent case, Jonas Salk refused to patent his discovery of a vaccine for polio, one of the world's most feared diseases. On April 12, 1955, just hours after Dr. Salk announced his success with the vaccine, Edward R. Murrow interviewed him on the television show *See It Now*.

"Who owns the patent on this vaccine?" Murrow asked.

"Well, the people, I would say," Dr. Salk replied. "There is no patent. Could you patent the sun?"

But other scientists quickly dismissed Dr. Merton's theory that objectivity was a crucial underpinning of science. They said it was not possible to keep free of all bias. The whole notion, they said, was too idealistic. Some scientists argued that the profit motive could not be taken out of the field. For one thing, they said, many scientific discoveries could help the public only if they were turned into products that could be sold.

One of Merton's peers, John Ziman, a British physicist, argued that in the middle of the twentieth century, science was divided into two parallel cultures, one academic and the other industrial. In academia, scientists decided on their own what they would investigate and how they would go about it, Dr. Ziman wrote in a 1998 essay. Most of these university scientists desired one thing: to expand knowledge by getting their work published and supported by their peers. They were motivated by the thrill of discovery. But in industry, scientists followed the orders of their corporate employers, who were rarely scientists themselves and whose goal was to sell a product. The two cultures dealt differently with ethical issues, Dr. Ziman said.

"For most industrial scientists, an active concern about ethical issues is just asking for trouble," he wrote. "Better to treat the welfare of their firm or country as the supreme good."

For years this divide between academia and industry helped protect the public from science that was manipulated for the sake of profits. Drug companies often found they lacked certain scientific expertise and called on the university scientists for help. They frequently asked the academics for help in designing their clinical trials. The companies also counted on academic medical centers to recruit patient volunteers for their studies. The universities had strict rules for conducting research and teams of professors who monitored each trial.

But in 1980, the year Ronald Reagan was elected to the presidency, changes swept through campuses across the country. A majority in Congress was concerned that the United States was falling behind other countries in science. As an incentive to get American scientists to work harder, the lawmakers passed a measure that allowed researchers receiving federal grants to patent and profit from their discoveries. The law was known as the Bayh-Dole Act. Sponsored by the senators Birch Bayh, a Democrat from Indiana, and Robert Dole, a Republican from Kansas, it reversed decades of policy. Before this law, any discoveries made during studies paid for by the federal government had been in the public domain—that is, they had been owned and controlled by the taxpayers who had paid for them.

That same year the Supreme Court unleashed a deluge of industrial science by allowing the first patent to be placed on a living organism, a bacterium genetically engineered by a scientist at General Electric to devour oil spilled into the sea. Patents are vital to industry. They give inventors monopolies on products by preventing competitors from selling them for twenty years. The Supreme Court's ruling reversed that of the U.S. Patent Office, which had long held that living things could not be patented. The decision opened the door to the patenting of genes, cell lines, tissues, and organs. Human parts became products. Medicine became a golden business opportunity.

These two changes—the Bayh-Dole Act and the ability to patent biological things—put dollar signs in the eyes of college administrators and their faculties. Universities began to see their medical laboratories as profit centers and their professors as entrepreneurs. Between 1980 and 1995 university researchers helped start 1,633 new companies. In 1997 alone, researchers at Stanford University filed 128 new patents, created fifteen companies, and earned $52 million from licenses on products.

Hundreds of academic scientists, including many who had once looked at the pharmaceutical industry with skepticism, walked down from their ivory towers and into the boardrooms of corporate America. The role of the academic as referee to the drug companies' clinical trials became a minor one. And the moderating force that had kept scientific studies honest and impartial began to disappear.

IN THE LATE 1990s two European scientists, a husband-and-wife team from Denmark, set out to analyze the many clinical trials that had compared a new fungus-fighting drug called Diflucan with older medications. Almost all the studies had been paid for by Pfizer, which sold Diflucan, and taken together, they made the case that Diflucan was the better drug.

Pfizer advertised Diflucan to American women as the "neat" treatment for yeast infections. The company's marketing plan included a price of twenty dollars a pill and heavy use of the color pink. The tablets were pink. The ads were done up in various hues. For years Diflucan's fine sales kept Pfizer in the pink.

Doctors also used Diflucan for patients who were seriously ill. The fifteen trials that intrigued the Danish scientists involved patients who were among the most vulnerable. The volunteers suffered from cancer. Their immune systems had been so weakened by their chemotherapy that they were at severe risk for fatal infections. The cancer drugs had destroyed their disease-fighting white blood cells and caused a condition known as neutropenia. Many cancer patients beat back their disease with the cancer drugs only to die from infections. To try to help them, some doctors prescribed antifungal medicines like Diflucan with the hope they would stop microscopic bugs with names like *Candida* and *Aspergillus* from gaining a deadly hold on their weakened bodies.

The goal of Dr. Peter C. Gøtzsche and Dr. Helle Krogh Johansen was to perform a meta-analysis, a study in which statistical methods are used to combine the results of independent but similar trials of a drug. Done correctly, such an analysis can give doctors a broader view of a medicine's benefits and risks. One of Pfizer's scientists had already helped complete a meta-analysis of studies in which patients had taken either Diflucan or two older antifungal medicines, and scientists had presented the results at an international meeting. Pfizer's drug had come out significantly ahead.

As the two Danish scientists pored over many of those same studies, they grew frustrated and disturbed. Leafing through the pages of data, they began to see unusual patterns and repetitions. They found that many of the scientists leading the fifteen trials had made a similar, but strange, decision. These scientists had given one of the older drugs to these critically ill cancer patients in a way that almost assured it would not work. Patients were told to swallow the older drug, amphotericin B, even though it was well known that it must be given intravenously to fight off fungal infections. On top of that, in some trials the scientists had divided the cancer patients into three groups. The groups were assigned to take Diflucan, amphotericin B, or a drug called nystatin. The third drug, nystatin, was one of the first antifungal medicines to be discovered. It is almost insoluble, which is why it is often used as a cream for skin infections. Doctors knew that nystatin would not help cancer patients like those in the trials. But without explanation the researchers had given it to some of the patients anyway and then combined the results of that group with those for patients taking amphotericin B. The scientists then compared the results of that combined group, heavily weighed down by the sorry results of nystatin, with the group of patients taking Diflucan and concluded that Pfizer's drug was superior.

To the Danish team, the result of these odd decisions was clear. The researchers had designed the trials in such a way that the deck was stacked against amphotericin B, a cheap drug that had long ago proven it could save lives. The fifteen trials had been little more than a medical shell game.

Dr. Gøtzsche, a specialist in internal medicine, was part of an international group called the Cochrane Center, which had made meta-analysis a specialty. The goal of the nonprofit center was to summarize the results of clinical trials so that physicians had sound scientific advice at their fingertips.

Troubled by what they found in the Diflucan data, Dr. Gøtzsche and Dr. Johansen sent a letter to the Pfizer scientist who was listed as an author of one of the studies. They asked why he and the other researchers had given the older drugs to patients using such questionable methods. The corporate scientist did not respond. When they called Pfizer's large research laboratory in Sandwich, England, an employee said he was too busy to help them. He said he had passed their request to his colleagues at the company's global headquarters on Forty-second Street in Manhattan. But no one from Pfizer called back.

The Danes also wrote to the academic researchers who were named as authors of the studies but were not employees of Pfizer. Yet few of these scientists responded, and they learned nothing more to answer their questions. Two of the scientists told them that Pfizer had all the data.

In November 1999 the *Journal of the American Medical Association*, one of the world's most prestigious medical journals, published the analysis by Gøtzsche and Johansen. The Danes concluded the trials had been biased by their flawed designs. The race between the drugs was not a fair and honest one, they said. It had been fixed. And the force that had swayed the trials' outcome was apparent. There were 2,977 patients in the trials of Diflucan. In the trials accounting for 92 percent of those patients, the researchers had disclosed that Pfizer had paid for all or some of their work. In the remaining three trials, the authors failed to say who had picked up the tab, leaving the possibility that Pfizer had paid for those studies too.

The Danes' discoveries were too much for Dr. Drummond Rennie, a deputy editor at the *Journal* who had become increasingly concerned about the pharmaceutical industry's growing influence in medical research. Rennie, a bearded Englishman, had established a name for himself in scientific circles by climbing the Andes, the Alps, and the Himalayas and studying the effects of altitude on the human body. Then on an expedition to Alaska he had broken his hip as his team descended Mount McKinley. Forced to give up the expeditions, he turned to editing articles for *The New England Journal of Medicine* and later *The Journal of the American Medical Association*.

Dr. Rennie sometimes spoke about how mountaineering had taught him the essentialness of trust. When scaling thirty-foot rock walls and leaping over what appeared to be bottomless crevasses, one had to believe the rope would hold you. Climbers trust in their rope the way patients trust in the science behind the drugs their doctors prescribe. But on the basis of the discoveries by Gøtzsche and Johansen, patients should not have trusted in Pfizer's science. Rennie penned a biting editorial that appeared in the journal alongside the Danes' findings.

"When the patients agreed to take part in these trials," he asked, "were they informed that the research design was deficient?"

At that time the Diflucan trials were only the most recent case of industry experiments in which reviewers had found subtle manipulations that made products look safer and more effective than they really were. In his editorial, Rennie described how two Canadian researchers, Patricia Huston and David Moher, had tried in 1996 to do a meta-analysis of studies of Risperdal, an antipsychotic medicine sold by Johnson & Johnson. They collected twenty articles and several unpublished reports describing clinical trials of the drug. But after an analysis they described as "vexing" and "bewildering," the Canadians concluded there was far less scientific evidence about Risperdal than the articles implied. When they finally untangled the data, they found only seven small trials and two large trials of the drug, including one study that had been reported in six scientific publications with different authors for each. The repeated publications gave "an artificial impression," the researchers said, that there was wide scientific support for Risperdal's use. "It brings into question the integrity of medical research," they wrote.

Rennie also described how a British group, led by Martin R. Tramèr, a fellow at Churchill Hospital in Oxford, England, found "covert duplication" of studies of a drug called Zofran. The medicine is prescribed to prevent vomiting caused by chemotherapy or surgery. The team collected what looked like eighty-four clinical trials in which 11,980 patients had taken the drug. Many of the trials were paid for by Glaxo Wellcome, the maker of Zofran. But the researchers found that data from the trials, especially the results that most favored Zofran, had been published so many times that the drug's overall effectiveness had been overstated by 23 percent.

Rennie said the duplicate reporting of scientific data was misleading doctors into believing that new drugs were far better and safer than they actually were. "It is hard not to suspect that this practice, which serves commercial interests so well, is deliberate," he wrote, "and, because it confuses and biases information important to the care of patients, it has to stop."

Two years later, in 2001, little had changed as Rennie delivered a speech and accepted an award from the Council of Science Editors. Before a roomful of scientists, the former mountaineer talked about trust and his climbing rope. And he talked of the "corrupting influence of money on our entire scientific and editing profession."

"Clinical research is awash with money, and large amounts of money are distorting good researchers and good research," he said. His concern wasn't just with the rare cases of outright scientific misconduct, he said, but with "something infinitely more pervasive and troubling."

THE PHARMACEUTICAL INDUSTRY did not always spend so much time and money on pushing its corporate marketing agenda into the nation's libraries of medical research. The companies' strategy of using clinical trials and scientific publications to market their medicines became predominant only in the last twenty-five years. Executives realized that scientists and their data, if properly managed, could be a marketing force like no other, far more powerful than the most expensive advertising campaign.

In June 2002 two dozen executives met in Manhattan for breakfast and a roundtable discussion on this industrial trend. The group included executives from the nation's largest drug companies as well as from the advertising agencies that worked closely with the industry. The executives shared their thoughts on "the blending of science and marketing" and the best ways to get marketers and scientists to work together. One of the executives, Richard Daly, a senior vice president of marketing at Takeda Pharmaceuticals, described the trend as "the marketing approach to research."

It wasn't that the marketers were now working with test tubes and injecting drugs into human subjects. Instead, the marketers were standing beside the scientists, telling them what studies to do, what research questions to ask, what data to gather.

The trend was driven by the fact that many new drugs were not very effective and often did not work. At the same time, the industry was introducing dozens of copycat medicines that were barely distinguishable from one another. Marketers had learned it was hard to introduce yet another cholesterol-lowering statin, for example, when there were already five others like it. They found they needed data—almost any kind of data— to show that the company's medicine was somehow unique and better than the rest.

An essential part of this strategy was what many drug marketers benignly called publication planning. In industry circles, executives described this as one of their most potent marketing techniques. The goal was to flood the world's scientific medical journals with articles and clinical studies that, when taken together, would create an image of a product so effective and safe that doctors would be convinced to prescribe it. The marketers knew that the more times a drug was mentioned in a positive way in the medical literature, the more important it became in the minds of physicians. In the best-organized marketing campaigns, these corporate-sponsored research papers began appearing in medical journals years before the drug was approved for sale. The papers made certain claims over and over again until they were viewed as scientific "truth."

As the pharmaceutical companies realized the power of this marketing technique, they increased spending on what they called research and development, although it would have been more accurately described as "selling and promotion."

At the same time, they gradually took control of most of the country's medical research. In 1980 the pharmaceutical industry paid for just 32 percent of the nation's medical research. By 2000 the companies' share of total research spending had grown to 62 percent, while the percentage paid by the federal government fell.

But there was one problem the companies had to solve. They knew they could not just have their own scientists perform the clinical trials and write the research papers that promoted their products. Most doctors reading medical journals will immediately discount the results of a study conducted by industrial scientists. They will be wary that corporate bias has crept in to make the drugs appear better than they actually are.

That is why the industry aggressively recruited legions of academic scientists and private physicians to join its payrolls and help with its studies. Many of the clinical drug trials published today list four or five academics as authors, while stating in small letters at the bottom of the paper that the research was paid for by the drug company. By hiring the academics as authors and trial investigators, the companies made their studies look more credible and objective. The problem was that behind the scenes, as the clinical trial was performed and the drug was tested on patients, it was often the executives who called the shots. The industry was using the names of the professors as ornaments, hanging them on their studies like shimmering glitter on a Christmas tree.

The pharmaceutical companies outsourced much of the publication planning work to advertising firms like IntraMed, the company Novartis chose in 2002 to sell Ritalin LA. Few Americans had ever heard of Intra-Med or any of its dozens of competitors. Yet these firms were part of a fast-growing business of creating scientific publications for the marketing departments of pharmaceutical companies. By 2002 these firms had become so powerful in the practice of medicine that they could rightly claim to have helped shape what doctors and the public knew about most of the big-selling medicines introduced in the previous ten years.

The leaders of these marketing firms did not often publicly boast about their influence, however. Instead, they and the hundreds of ghostly wordsmiths the firms employed were content to stay in the shadows. A certain amount of secrecy was critical to the strategy's success.

IntraMed was one of the oldest of these firms, having opened its doors for business in 1974. It was now part of a public relations firm called Sudler & Hennessey, which promised its pharmaceutical clients that it could "produce simple, magical strategies with the power to persuade."

In a maze of a corporate structure, executives at Sudler reported to Young & Rubicam, the advertising firm that created commercials for such products as Miller beer, Dr Pepper, and Frito-Lay potato chips. All these marketing firms in turn were owned by WPP, the global advertising behemoth.

The goal of the publication planning services offered by Sudler's IntraMed and a host of other marketing firms was to create scientific "content"—articles, clinical trial reports, reviews of medicines, and just about any other type of work included in medical libraries—to boost the sales of their client's drug.

IntraMed executives explained to their corporate clients that these publications could lay the groundwork for rapid prescribing of a new drug. The firm's staff included expert medical writers and much more. Executives said the firm's staff was also skilled in the development of key messages that could be incorporated into the publications to best sell each prescription product.

The New York firm's competitors made similar promises to the drug industry. A firm called Axis Healthcare Communications offered to help pharmaceutical companies "brand the science." Part of this process was performed by an Axis subsidiary that said its expertise was in writing and editing scientific abstracts, primary data papers, and even medical textbooks that would "drive product prescriptions."

Excerpta Medica, a firm in New Jersey, said that the "highly sophisticated publication plan" it had created for a company selling a stroke medication had succeeded in getting more than 150 articles published in one year. The articles, the firm's executives explained, "ensured an extensive level of 'noise'" about the drug in the medical literature.

The marketing firms aimed to have the articles published in even the world's best medical journals, including *The New England Journal of Medicine* and *The Journal of the American Medical Association*. Readers of the published articles that resulted from this process rarely learned that the medical reports had originated inside a firm like Excerpta or IntraMed. The names of the firms and their writers rarely appeared anywhere in the text. Instead, the named "authors" of these articles were academic physicians and scientists, who were being paid by the pharmaceutical company. Often even the editors of the journals have been kept in the dark.

One of the ghostwriters working in the industry told me that some physician "authors" insisted on changing and editing much of the manuscript that the marketing firm delivered to them for their review and signature. Other doctors, the writer said, changed little or nothing at all.

An internal document prepared by a firm called Current Medical Directions listed eighty-five articles that were part of Pfizer's publication plan to promote the antidepressant Zoloft. One commercial purpose of the articles was to promote Zoloft for uses beyond depression. The proposed articles were planned to provide data on how Zoloft could be prescribed for panic, dysthymia, seasonal affective disorder, obsessive-compulsive disorder, and pedophilia. The articles also covered a range of patients. Ten of the proposed articles were planned to describe the use of Zoloft in the elderly, six would detail its use in children, and four would describe prescribing it to women.

The document by the staff at Current Medical Directions made it clear that a ghostwriter was creating some of these manuscripts. For example, the firm told Pfizer that a paper describing patients taking Zoloft for posttraumatic stress had been "completed," but that the article's "author" was "TBD." The initials appear to be short for "to be determined."

In 2002 a pair of researchers became interested in the work by Current Medical Directions and the document describing Pfizer's publication plan for Zoloft. The internal document, which had been prepared in 1999, had been uncovered in a lawsuit. The two researchers, David Healy and Dinah Cattell, both of the University of Wales in the United Kingdom, set out to find how many of the eighty-five articles proposed by Current Medical Directions were ultimately published in the world's scientific journals. They found fifty-five articles, including three that had been published in the prestigious *Journal of the American Medical Association*. The articles described twenty-five clinical trials, all of which had results that were favorable to selling Zoloft. Only two of the articles gave any hint that they had been ghostwritten by a marketing firm. Those two papers acknowledged that the "authors" had received writing assistance from a person not listed as an author.

Healy and Cattell then looked for other articles about Zoloft that had been published about the same time but were not part of Current Medical Directions's publication plan. They discovered forty-one articles. Overall, these articles had conclusions that were less favorable to Zoloft. Twenty of them reported negative findings about the drug, while eighteen reported positive results and three were ambiguous in their conclusions about the drug. Healy and Cattell said the case raised questions about the integrity of the base of scientific knowledge that was said to support the use of all prescription drugs.

THE GHOSTWRITERS WORKED hard to stay invisible and not raise suspicions that the articles were something other than the words and scientific thoughts of academic physicians.

For example, an executive at Ruder Finn, a public relations firm, warned her clients at SmithKline Beecham, the manufacturer of Paxil, that two letters composed by the firm's ghostwriters would "look fishy" if the firm used the same references in each. Sandra Stahl, the Ruder Finn executive, explained in a memo to SmithKline that the letters would be "authored" by academic psychiatrists. The key message in the letters was that patients taking antidepressants like Paxil should not worry about "discontinuation symptoms" or the nausea and sickness that many patients felt when they tried to stop taking the drugs.

"At the very least, we can't have the references appear in the same order," Stahl wrote to the SmithKline executive. "Please have a look at these and let us know how you'd like to proceed."

In another case, Dr. Troyen Brennan, of the Harvard School of Public Health, said he was perplexed when he received a phone call from an executive at Edelman Medical Communications, who offered to pay him $2,500 if he agreed to be the "author" of an editorial that had been drafted by the firm. The executive from Edelman, one of the largest public relations firms in the world, told Dr. Brennan that a pharmaceutical company was paying for the project and that he would not have to do much work for the offered fee.

Dr. Brennan said the phone call startled him. In the past, he said, he had always placed great confidence in the editorials he read in medical journals. He had believed that the editorialists were providing independent and expert reviews of the medications they described. Now a PR firm was on the phone, explaining that it was writing some of these editorials. Curious, he asked Edelman to send him more information about what the firm did. A packet soon arrived in the mail. It included examples of other published papers and editorials that Edelman had written for its pharmaceutical clients.

"We are providing these materials to you in confidence," the Edelman executive warned in an attached memo, "as we do not generally divulge the specific nature of projects conducted on behalf of our clients."

The ghostwriters had made it clear they did not want their secrets revealed. The public, they hoped, would never know who was really writing the articles that doctors staked their patients' lives on.

Turned off by the ordeal, Dr. Brennan declined the offer and later wrote about his experience in *The New England Journal of Medicine* in an article entitled "Buying Editorials."

The business of ghostwriting articles for the pharmaceutical industry was lucrative. Revenues earned from medical writing grew from $300 million in 2002 to $400 million in 2004, according to Thomson CenterWatch, a consulting firm. The ghostwriters were prolific. A firm called Complete Healthcare Communications, Inc., boasted in 2006 that it had written more than five hundred manuscripts for its pharmaceutical clients. More than 80 percent of these manuscripts had been published by the world's scientific medical journals, the firm said.

The pharmaceutical manufacturers counted on the ghostwriters to smooth and polish the articles so their products were described in the best possible light. The ghostwriters succeeded at this even if the academics who had been hired as "authors" did not find the original drafts acceptable and changed much of them to align with their thinking. With the ghostwriters and pharmaceutical executives editing the paper each step of the way, the marketers could pick certain words and phrases that helped boost the image of the product. Dangers of a medicine could be toned down. Benefits of a drug could be pumped up. A serious injury in a patient taking the drug in a trial might be referred to simply as "an event." The words "adverse reactions" might be changed to the more benign-sounding "side effects." A drug that worked only slightly better than a sugar pill might be described as having "proven efficacy." It was all a matter of degree. The ghostwriters were like photographers who airbrushed family portraits, softening blemishes and facial lines until their subjects looked far better on paper than in real life.

To help do this, Complete Healthcare Communications had developed special software to monitor the words of the final publications. With the software, the firm promised its pharmaceutical clients that they could "track and monitor the effectiveness" of their "key message strategy."

The firm's executives described an example in which a "key message" to be incorporated into published articles was a description that the drug was "well tolerated, with the majority of adverse events mild to moderate in nature." In other words, the risks of the medicine were nothing to worry about.

In a broader sense, the ghostwriting was a form of the timeworn corporate public relations strategy known to marketers as the third party technique. In 1991, Merrill Rose, executive vice president of Porter Novelli, a public relations firm, described this process as putting "your words in someone else's mouth."

Over the years pharmaceutical companies had become experts in the third party technique. They had learned how to use people as varied as patients, celebrities, government officials, and even journalists to make statements that supported their corporate interests. In 2002, Maxine Taylor, an executive with Eli Lilly, explained how drug marketers could use this technique when the corporation came under fire from critics.

"Deploy third parties to advance your cause," she advised in an article in a trade magazine. "Even though you may not have many friends, maximize the ones you have!"

The third party technique might be considered relatively harmless in other industries. For example, few people might complain if a soap manufacturer hired housewives to tell their friends about the cleaning power of a new laundry detergent they had discovered. But in the drug industry the companies were using the third party technique to create something that looked like science to sell potentially deadly medicines to patients desperate for cures.

At times the ghostwritten articles have turned out to be dangerously wrong. In the 1990s, Wyeth-Ayerst paid tens of thousands of dollars to Excerpta Medica to ghostwrite articles promoting the use of Redux, a diet pill. The drug was part of the weight loss combination known as fen-phen. According to a copy of an invoice dated in 1996, Excerpta Medica billed Wyeth more than twenty thousand dollars to write one article describing the "therapeutic effects" of Redux, also known as dexfenfluramine. Dr. Richard Atkinson, a professor at the University of Wisconsin, was to receive fifteen hundred dollars of that amount to serve as "author."

When the article was complete, Dr. Atkinson sent a letter to Excerpta, praising the ghostwriter's work. "Let me congratulate you and your writer on an excellent and thorough review of the literature, clearly written," the doctor wrote. ". . . Perhaps I can get you to write all my papers for me! My only general comment is that this piece may make dexfenfluramine sound better than it really is."

A year later, the FDA pressed Wyeth to remove Redux and a similar diet drug called Pondimin from the market after doctors reported that they were injuring the heart valves of as many as a third of the patients who took them. By then millions of Americans had taken the drugs. The pills were later linked to dozens of deaths.

SCIENTISTS RELY ON a system of self-policing to prevent science from being turned into science fiction. Most scientific journals employ this safeguard, which is known as peer review. Editors at the journals select a group of scientists to review each article before it is published. The reviewers are often some of the top academic experts in the subject, who scrutinize the study's design, statistics, and conclusions. The reviewers ask questions, demand changes, and often advise the journals' editors that the study is not worthy of being published. Physicians, scientists, and the public count on peer review to keep science honest.

Over the years, however, the pharmaceutical companies used their vast cash reserves to begin dismantling the peer review system. How? Simple. The companies hired the reviewers.

The industry has so aggressively recruited academic physicians and scientists to its payrolls that at a major medical meeting today most of the invited lecturers will be supplementing their university and physician salaries with thousands of dollars from the drug companies. At the largest annual gathering of the nation's psychiatrists in 2005, the list of speakers who disclosed they were receiving payments from the pharmaceutical industry included hundreds of physicians and spanned seventeen typed pages. Some of the speakers were working for as many as twenty-five drug companies. The list of speakers who said they did not have financial relationships with the industry was far shorter: less than four pages long.

In the legal profession, lawyers cannot take cases in which they have a conflict that could compromise their work. But in medicine, scientists and physicians regularly perform work with which they have financial conflicts.

The broad scope of the industry's academic hiring spree meant that when the editor of a scientific journal selected scientists to review the draft of a study, there was a good chance that the reviewer was also working for one or more drug companies. Even the editors at many medical journals worked as consultants to the pharmaceutical industry.

At the same time, medical journals had their own conflicts of interest with the pharmaceutical industry. When journals published favorable articles on medicines, they could earn millions of dollars from reprints purchased by the drug companies. Sales representatives distributed the glossy reprints to local physicians to highlight the new "science" supporting the use of the company's product.

By 2005 even editors of some of the world's top medical journals were admitting their controls were not strong enough to keep tainted corporate science out of their publications. "The evidence is strong that companies are getting the results they want," wrote Richard Smith, the former editor of the *British Medical Journal* in an article in 2005, "and this is especially worrisome because between two-thirds and three-quarters of the trials published in the major journals—*Annals of Internal Medicine, JAMA, Lancet,* and *New England Journal of Medicine*—are funded by the industry . . . It took me almost a quarter of a century editing for the *BMJ* to wake up to what was happening."

This means that a doctor or patient searching the scientific medical literature for the best treatment for a disease may make a decision based on reading an article that is little more than corporate marketing masquerading as science. This type of promotion is extremely effective because it appears in the guise of objective scientific fact.

"Whatever one thinks of aggressive advertising—and society appears to have become attuned to it—it does at least have the merit of being open and direct," explained Dr. Graham Dukes, a former research executive at Organon, a pharmaceutical company, in a paper in 2003. With advertising, Dr. Dukes said, a person knows he is "being subjected to a process of persuasion, and has an opportunity to resist it."

"Far more dominant and much more dangerous," Dr. Dukes wrote, "was however what I feel bound to call the corruption of truth."

WHEN ALL THESE promotional techniques came together, marketers found almost anything was possible. A clinical study that failed to show what executives had hoped and expected didn't have to be a failure. Sometimes two or three failed clinical trials of the same drug did not have to be failure. As long as the company controlled the science, failures could be repackaged as success and mediocre drugs could be turned into treasure.

Take the case of Lexapro, an antidepressant. Executives at Forest Laboratories were in a bind in 2001. They had promised investors that Lexapro, a drug still in development, would be even better than Celexa,

the fast-selling antidepressant that had turned the company into a dar-
ling of Wall Street. The drug's sales now made up more than 70 percent
of the company's revenues. But the good times were coming to an end.
Celexa's patent was set to expire in 2004, allowing other manufacturers
to sell generic versions of the drug for a fraction of the price. The Forest
executives desperately needed a new drug to replace Celexa's sales. The
value of their stock options depended on it.

The executives had earlier settled on a plan. They decided scientists
would take the active ingredient in Celexa and use a chemical process
to refine it. The company would then introduce this modified drug as a
new product. The executives had explained that the active drug ingredient in Celexa was made of two mirror images. They said that scientists
had determined that only one of the halves contributed to the drug's ability to relieve depression. By eliminating the other half, scientists would
create a drug, they said, that was more effective and had fewer adverse
effects. At least that was their theory.

By 2001 Forest Labs had spent millions of dollars on three clinical
trials to prove the executives' hypothesis. Patients in the trials took either
Celexa or the modified drug, Lexapro. All three trials came back with the
same results. Patients taking Lexapro fared no better than those taking Celexa. They suffered the same side effects, mostly nausea, sexual
dysfunction, and insomnia. The patient volunteers also found that both
drugs could take weeks to ease their depression, if they worked at all. The
executives' theory that a chemical refinement could transform Celexa
into a better drug was shown not once but three times to be wrong.

With time running out, Forest executives turned to Dr. Jack M. Gorman, a psychiatrist at Columbia University who was already on the company's payroll as a consultant. Dr. Gorman had become a popular hire
for the manufacturers of psychiatric drugs. He was the same psychiatrist
who had appeared on the morning news to tell America that Celexa
could treat "compulsive shopping disorder." He had also recently helped
boost the sales of Paxil, another antidepressant, when he provided sound
bites for television news programs while in the pay of the drug's maker,
GlaxoSmithKline. Professor Gorman's message on that corporate speak-

ing tour was that worrying too much might actually be a disease, one that was easily treatable with drugs like Paxil.

Professor Gorman was also the editor of *CNS Spectrums*, a medical journal specializing in the central nervous system. The journal was published by a small company in Manhattan called Medworks Media, which courted pharmaceutical marketers by offering to publish their corporate studies for a fee.

In April 2002, Forest paid Medworks Media to publish an article by Dr. Gorman in a supplement to *CNS Spectrums*. Dr. Gorman and his two coauthors wrote that several "provocative findings" had emerged from the first three clinical trials of Lexapro, leading them to reanalyze the data. They said they had pooled the data from the three trials and this time found that Lexapro was the better drug. Lexapro had a "superior therapeutic profile" to Celexa, they wrote, and showed "a greater magnitude of antidepressant effect." They noted that their findings were consistent with what other researchers had found when they gave the two drugs to rats.

Lexapro had lost three times in side-by-side comparative studies, but now it had suddenly been ruled the winner.

In fine print at the bottom of the first page, the article identified the affiliations of the two coauthors. One was a senior medical writer at Forest Laboratories. The other was the drug company's senior statistician.

Many physicians would tell you that such an article would not sway their prescribing decisions. They would point out that *CNS Spectrums* is not one of the respected top-tier journals that physicians count on for scientific information. In addition, they might note that Professor Gorman's article was published in a corporate-paid supplement to the journal. Doctors say they quickly throw away such articles, dismissing them as little more than paid advertisements. But that is not what happened in this case.

The study's findings went around the world as Forest Labs' agents distributed press releases quoting Professor Gorman. In the following months and years the article was used as a reference to describe Lexapro's benefits in dozens of other medical journal articles, including many that were also paid for by Forest or written by the company's academic consultants. The article was even used as a reference in at least one medical textbook.

Not content that physicians would read those articles, the company began paying for public speaking events that began even before the article was published. In May 2001, Dr. Gorman presented his findings of Lexapro's superiority to hundreds of psychiatrists at the annual meeting of the American Psychiatric Association in New Orleans, where the company's sales representatives were on hand offering free massages, Mardi Gras beads, and sugary sweet pralines. It would take more than a year for the government to approve the drug, but its promotion was already in high gear.

The company hired and trained other physicians to present the article's results to smaller groups of doctors at hundreds of dinner meetings across the country. Forest paid for so many of these parties for doctors that Dr. Richard Brown, a psychiatrist in Manhattan, was invited to two of these dinners in the course of just two months, shortly after the government approved Lexapro in August 2002. One of those dinners was organized by IntraMed, the marketing firm that was also working then to promote Ritalin LA for Novartis. The IntraMed-organized dinner was held at Daniel, one of the most expensive restaurants in Manhattan. That night waiters served the doctors *le boeuf et le foie gras* and poured glasses of 1998 Downing Family cabernet sauvignon. Worried that the fine French cuisine would not be enough to tempt physicians to attend, Forest also offered to pay each doctor five hundred dollars. Jed Beitler, the advertising executive in charge of IntraMed, later explained that the physicians had been paid as "consultants" to sit on the pharmaceutical company's "advisory board" for the evening.

But Dr. Brown said he did no consulting that night at Daniel or at any of the other dinners he was offered cash to attend. Dr. Brown said he had grown increasingly concerned that the expensive promotional dinners were corrupting the practice of medicine. Earlier he had organized a protest, complete with picket signs, outside the Four Seasons Hotel, where Forest had held yet another dinner for physicians.

"I think it's disgusting," he told me shortly after the dinner at Daniel. "This is my profession, and I hate to see this happening."

Scientists working independently from Forest Laboratories found the results from the three Lexapro trials far less convincing. In September 2002, *The Medical Letter*, a nonprofit newsletter respected for its independence from the pharmaceutical industry, reviewed the results of the same three clinical trials that Dr. Gorman had. The independent scientists concluded that Lexapro was no better than any other antidepressant, including Celexa. In 2004 two other scientists reviewed the data and concluded that the claims of Lexapro's superiority were "unwarranted." Drug regulators in Sweden and Denmark reached similar conclusions.

But these findings were drowned out by Forest's finely oiled publicity machine, which was using the academic physicians as its cogs.

Shortly after that dinner at Daniel, stock analysts at J. P. Morgan Chase declared the company's introduction of Lexapro "an instant success." Based on the number of prescriptions written for Lexapro in its first weeks on the market, the analysts said that Forest was on its way to having one of the best product launches in the pharmaceutical industry's history. Other Wall Street analysts joined in praising the company's executives during a corporate conference call on October 15, 2002.

As analyst after analyst congratulated him, Kenneth E. Goodman, Forest's president, could not hide his delight. "This market," he said, "does respond to promotion."

By 2006 Forest was earning two billion dollars a year from Lexapro, a drug that was more than twice as expensive as generic tablets of Celexa sold by other manufacturers. Patients and the nation's medical system would have saved billions of dollars in prescription drug costs if it had not been for the magical power of Forest's corporate science, which had turned three failed studies into a blockbuster of a success.

NOTHING MADE IT clearer that marketers had invaded medical science than when the global advertising agencies on Madison Avenue decided to jump into the work of performing drug experiments on humans.

By 2002 three of the world's biggest advertising firms—WPP, Omnicom, and Interpublic—all owned or had large investments in what were called contract research organizations or CROs. Pharmaceutical companies hired the CROs to do experiments they needed to gain government approval of their products or to expand their sales. The drug companies used these private research firms to avoid some of the red tape involved with paying universities to perform the clinical drug trials.

"We felt that we needed to get closer to the test tube—to actually work with clinical scientists to develop new drugs," said Thomas L. Harrison, a top executive at Omnicom, when his firm acquired an interest in a CRO called Scirex in 1999.

Omnicom and the other ad agencies had grown rich from a new stream of advertising revenue, one worth millions of dollars a year, when the FDA decided in 1997 to allow prescription drug commercials on television. At the same time, the pharmaceutical industry had been paying the ad firms to ghostwrite publications, to organize dinners and meetings for physicians, to create medical education courses, and for public relations work they called "managing the media." Now the ad firms were expanding their services to include scientific research and clinical drug trials.

"We provide services that go from the beginning of drug development all the way to the launch of your products," explained Joe Torre, an executive at Interpublic, in 2002, after his firm had bought a CRO called Target Research Associates.

The advertising firms quickly showed what potent partners their clinical research operations could be for drug companies eager to boost sales. The story of a pain reliever called Bextra provides a case in point. Pharmacia, the drug's manufacturer, had asked the FDA in 2001 to approve Bextra to treat both the chronic pain of arthritis and the more acute pain that follows surgery. The regulators agreed to approve the drug to treat arthritis but refused to allow the company to sell it for more intense pain. The regulators' decision upset Pharmacia's marketing plans. The company's executives had publicly boasted about Bextra's power, saying it relieved pain better than Celebrex, a similar pill Pharmacia was already selling with great success.

Yet most of the public did not learn that the FDA had refused the company's request to sell Bextra for acute pain. As a standard practice, the government kept such information secret, calling it confidential commercial information. Included in those secret papers were details of why FDA reviewers denied the plan. The papers described a clinical trial in which scientists had given Bextra to patients undergoing heart bypass surgery. In the experiment, patients taking Bextra and a similar pain reliever called paracoxib had "an excess of serious adverse events, including death."

At the same time, the FDA had determined that Bextra was no miracle worker when it came to relieving pain. The regulators said in the confidential papers that Pharmacia's studies had shown that Bextra relieved pain no better than cheap medicines like ibuprofen.

That was when Pharmacia turned to the advertising firm Omnicom and its research partner, Scirex. Pharmacia had paid the Scirex scientists to go to Austin, Texas, and the nearby city of San Marcos to recruit people who were to have two or more impacted molars removed during dental surgery. To ease their pain, Scirex gave the volunteers either Bextra or Percocet, a short-acting narcotic. When the study was complete, the Scirex scientists said they had found that Bextra worked just as fast as Percocet but was "superior" because it eased the patients' pain for a longer period of time. They concluded that Bextra was a "potent" reliever of moderate to severe pain resulting from oral surgery, just the conclusion Pharmacia needed for its marketing plan.

The Scirex scientists published the results of their study in the May 2002 edition of *The Journal of the American Dental Association*. Dentists reading the study had no way of knowing that the FDA had refused to let Pharmacia sell Bextra for acute pain just six months before. Omnicom, the global ad giant, and its clinical research firm had performed and published a clinical trial that would do far more to increase sales than the most creative of advertisements.

Three scientists who later reviewed the Scirex study said it was not persuasive. They pointed out that Scirex's conclusion that a dose of Bextra worked longer than a single dose of Percocet was not meaningful. Patients rarely receive just one dose of Percocet because it is well known it wears off in four to six hours. One of those scientists, Dr. Eric Topol, then the chairman of the Cleveland Clinic's department of cardiovascular medicine, called the studies "a contrived comparison." He said he found it "quite disquieting" that Scirex was partly owned by an advertising firm.

"If this is where clinical research is headed," Dr. Topol said in 2002, "that would be a terrible negative trajectory."

The Scirex study helped spur a boom in Bextra's sales. Prescriptions soared 60 percent in the three months after the trial was published. By 2004 Bextra was a billion-dollar drug.

Yet quietly, reports of injuries caused by Bextra were flowing into government offices in Maryland. In April 2005 the FDA demanded that Pfizer, which had taken over Pharmacia, remove the drug from the market. Regulators said the risks of the drug exceeded its meager benefits. By then doctors had prescribed it to millions.

ALL THIS WAS eerily reminiscent of another industry that attempted to create "science" to increase corporate sales. It is now well known that the tobacco industry hired academic scientists to sign their names as the authors of articles in medical journals that tried to refute the accumulating evidence that cigarettes were killing hundreds of thousands of Americans a year. Corporate whistle-blowers and lawsuits against the tobacco industry unearthed hundreds of internal documents that detailed the industry's covert efforts to get articles into the scientific literature that advanced its agenda.

For example, after a Japanese study in 1981 showed that secondhand smoke raised the risk of lung cancer, the tobacco companies secretly began working on their own study. They hoped to use the study to raise doubts about the original article's findings. Internal documents described how executives chose the man who would become the chief scientist for British American Tobacco to be the behind-the-scenes director of the industry's planned study, while they selected one of the tobacco companies' law firms, Covington & Burling, to be the project's manager. The plan, according to the documents, included having two Japanese professors serve as the study's authors, while the tobacco companies hid their involvement.

The public also eventually learned that the tobacco companies had a simple plan for dealing with data they were accumulating internally that showed cigarettes were addictive and deadly. They simply kept that evidence locked up in corporate file drawers.

"THERE ARE NO plans to publish data from Study 377," wrote executives at the drug company SmithKline Beecham in a memo stamped "For Internal Use Only." Almost three hundred teenagers suffering from major depression had volunteered for Study 377. The experiment was meant to test the safety and effectiveness of giving the teens the company's antidepressant Paxil. The results, however, had disappointed Smith-Kline executives. They showed that Paxil worked no better at relieving the teenagers' depression than a sugar pill.

The SmithKline executives explained in the memo, dated October 1998, why they had decided to keep the results a secret. Their "target," they wrote, was to "manage the dissemination" of data from the company's clinical trials of Paxil in teenagers "to minimise any potential negative commercial impact."

Just a year earlier executives at Bayer, the German drug company, had struggled with a similar problem. The executives had been repeatedly let down by the results of corporate studies of Baycol, its cholesterol-lowering drug. Again and again the studies paid for by Bayer failed to prove that Baycol was better at reducing cholesterol than other drugs being sold, including one promoted by Merck called Zocor.

"This paper will not be published," wrote members of a corporate committee responsible for managing the publication of scientific data about Baycol in July 1997. The study the executives were referring to was known as SN-120. They explained that Bayer executives working in the United States "did not want to publish this data" because it showed that Zocor was more effective than Baycol.

Two years later it wasn't just Baycol's lack of effectiveness that worried the Bayer executives deciding what data would get published. The company was learning about the dozens of patients who had taken Baycol and then been struck by rhabdomyolysis, the potentially fatal muscle disorder. In the minutes to the November 1, 1999, meeting of the Baycol Communications Committee, executives described how Dr. Evan Stein, a private physician who was performing some of the trials of Baycol, had told them he was worried about findings in a study called D97-008, which was testing high doses of Baycol on patients.

"Stein has been quite vocal about the lack of candor when presenting our safety data," the executives wrote in the minutes. Among the doctor's worries were patients who had tested positive for high levels of the enzyme creatine kinase, which was a sign of rhabdomyolysis. According to the written minutes, the executives dismissed Dr. Stein's concerns, saying to mention them in the published data would "draw attention to something we do not need."

Then there was the case of Propulsid, a heartburn medicine heavily promoted by Johnson & Johnson, even though repeated studies had concluded it did not work. The company had performed numerous clinical trials that attempted to show the drug helped adults with heartburn as well as children and infants who often spit up. The executives became increasingly secretive as the studies failed to show the drug helped the volunteers.

"Please note that the findings are preliminary and should not be circulated," wrote Leonard Jokubaitis, a Johnson & Johnson executive, in an e-mail to his colleagues in 1998. His message, which he labeled "STRICTLY CONFIDENTIAL," described a trial that showed Propulsid was no better at easing heartburn than the sugar pill.

The company's message to doctors was a different one. The sales reps were trained to tell doctors that Propulsid was "a unique" drug that "effectively relieves heartburn and all the motility-related symptoms such as belching, bloating and regurgitation." To make sure that message got out, the company regularly entertained doctors, especially the nation's gastroenterologists. In 1999 it held a private party for thirty-five hundred at Orlando's SeaWorld amusement park. "Physicians and their families watched in amazement as Shamu and the dolphins performed tricks and enjoyed raw fish—without a single digestive complaint," a member of the sales team later joked in an internal newsletter.

Propulsid was not even approved for use in children, but many doctors did not hesitate to prescribe it to their young patients. The company made it easier for these doctors by also offering it in the form of a cherry-flavored liquid.

Yet the executives' job of polishing Propulsid's public image became increasingly difficult. By 1999 Johnson & Johnson had received almost three hundred reports that the drug had caused serious arrhythmias and other heart problems in adults and children, including eighty-seven who had died. Federal regulators began to question whether the serious risks of taking Propulsid were worth the benefits the company claimed it provided. In a private meeting with Johnson & Johnson executives in 1998, FDA officials had shown a slide that asked, "Is it acceptable for your nighttime heartburn medicine (i.e., something for which you could take Tums) to have the potential to kill you?"

By then Johnson & Johnson was selling more than one billion dollars' worth of Propulsid each year. The executives continued to argue that the drug should not be blamed for all the reported injuries and deaths.

Not all Johnson & Johnson executives were comfortable with how the company was selectively releasing data about the drug, which was also known by its generic name, cisapride. In September 1998 an executive named Darryl Kurland e-mailed a top corporate scientist. Kurland described how he had discovered that someone at the company had rewritten reports of injuries suffered by infants who had been given Propulsid. The reports were rewritten in ways, Kurland said, that seemed intended to draw the focus away from the drug's dangers. Some important facts had been left out in the rewrite, Kurland said. The writer had also used italics to emphasize certain pieces of information in the reports. For example, if doctors had given the infant other medicines in addition to Propulsid, the writer had put the names of those drugs in italics, a change that seemed intended to raise doubt that it had been Propulsid that caused the harm.

"I don't disagree that MedWatch forms are cumbersome to review, but how we choose to portray the safety of cisapride now, especially for as delicate (and socially sensitive) a population as neonates and infants, is critical," Kurland wrote.

The reports of injuries continued to worry federal regulators, who held more private meetings with Johnson & Johnson executives. In 2000,

FDA officials decided to make their concerns public. The regulators scheduled a meeting where a panel of national experts would consider the evidence and decide whether Propulsid should continue to be sold. This was just what executives at Johnson & Johnson had been trying to avoid and had succeeded at dodging for years through what one executive later called learning to "manage the FDA."

As the company's executives prepared for the public meeting, they struggled to find data in the dozens of studies the company had paid for that showed Propulsid actually worked. "Do we want to stand in front of world & admit that we were <u>never able</u> to prove efficacy!" wrote a Johnson & Johnson executive in her notes as the company prepared for the meeting.

In the days before the meeting the executives finally relented. They decided they could no longer argue that the company's science supported the use of Propulsid. The executives announced the company would stop promoting the drug.

More than a hundred adults, children, and infants had died.

THE PUBLIC WOULD have never learned about these secret corporate studies if it had not been for whistle-blowers or lawsuits filed after people were harmed.

In the case of Paxil, Americans learned in 2004 that it had not just been Study 377 that SmithKline had kept under lock and key. The New York State attorney general, Eliot Spitzer, said in June of that year that the company had failed to publish four of five studies it had done to test the antidepressant's effectiveness in teenagers. Taken together, the five studies showed that Paxil did not ease the children's depression. Even worse, the studies showed that the drug caused a rare, but serious, complication. Twice as many teenagers taking the drug began thinking about suicide as those who had been given the placebo. The attorney general sued the company, now known as GlaxoSmithKline, for fraud. Spitzer charged that the company was earning tens of millions of dollars a year from Paxil prescriptions written for children even as it concealed studies that showed it did not help them and might even make them worse.

Spitzer pointed out that the company had schooled its legions of sales-people on the purported benefits of giving the drug to teenagers. For example, executives had sent a memo to sales representatives in 2001, telling them that "cutting-edge" research had demonstrated that Paxil had "REMARKABLE efficacy and safety in the treatment of adolescent depression." The sales reps, like the public, were kept in the dark about what SmithKline's studies were actually discovering about the blockbuster antidepressant.

No one knows how many pharmaceutical studies have been kept secret after they showed a drug did not work or caused harm. Numerous reviews have found that at least 50 percent of pharmaceutical trials have never been published. The percentage may be far higher. One group of reviewers looked at clinical trials for pain medicines known as non-steroidal anti-inflammatory drugs or NSAIDs. Their analysis found that only one of thirty-seven experiments involving the pain medicines had been published.

GlaxoSmithKline settled the lawsuit brought by Spitzer by promising to begin disclosing the results of all its clinical trials to the public. Other drug companies made similar pledges. And in the fall of 2007, Congress passed a measure requiring the government to begin keeping a registry of drug trials so that the public would not be kept in the dark. Yet Americans will never know just how many studies completed over the past decades of the medicines they take daily still sit in boxes in the dark corners of empty warehouses.

The vast corporate libraries of secret studies raised serious questions about the ethics of the pharmaceutical industry's scientific methods. Scientists have a duty to share both the negative and positive results of the studies they perform. If they disclose only positive studies, they have told only half the story. Results of the positive studies may be overturned when they are combined with trials that showed the drug did not work or had harmed its human volunteers. By publicizing the positive trials while hiding the negative ones, the companies had created a false sense of security about their products. The public and physicians believed the nation's medicine supply was far safer and more effective than it actually was.

Secrecy is contrary to the spirit of science and to the core definition of scientific research, which is the search for new knowledge. "The right to search for truth implies also a duty," Albert Einstein once said. "One must not conceal any part of what one has recognized to be true."

So what does this mean for patients? Some scientists have pointed out that only a fraction of present-day medical interventions—the drugs prescribed, tests ordered, procedures performed—are supported by sound scientific evidence. Their concern goes far beyond the studies that have been kept secret.

Dr. John P. A. Ioannidis, an epidemiologist who holds positions at Tufts University and at the University of Ioannina in Greece, said in 2005 that the conclusions of most published scientific studies are just plain wrong. In an essay, Dr. Ioannidis blamed the industrial quest for profit, the growing number of conflicts of interest among scientists, the small size of many clinical trials, as well as the manipulation of their design, for creating an era in medicine when most studies turn out to be fiction.

"There is increasing concern that in modern research, false findings may be the majority or even the vast majority of published research claims," he wrote in the journal *PLoS Medicine*. "However, this should not be surprising. It can be proven that most claimed research findings are false."

EXECUTIVES AT NOVARTIS liked to say that Ritalin was the "most studied of any drug for children."

Novartis had been selling Ritalin since 1955. At that time the Swiss company was known as Ciba, and children who could not sit still or pay attention were sometimes said to be suffering from minimal brain dysfunction. To promote the drug in those early years, the company created a plastic toy resembling the popular Mr. Potato Head dolls. The toy, which some called Ritalin Man, came in several models to teach children how the drug would help them. In one design, he was depressed and confused. In another, he was smiling, dancing, and waving his straw hat.

Since 1955, scientists had performed hundreds of studies and written thousands of papers describing how Ritalin and other stimulants could treat children unable to pay attention. Anyone taking the time to read these studies closely, however, would find that much of the work was not done independently. Instead, many of the scientists and physicians listed as authors of these papers were also being paid by the manufacturers of the children's drugs, including Novartis.

John Markowitz and Kennerly Patrick, the academics who had joined the IntraMed conference call on that September day in 2002, were just two of the dozens of scientists and physicians whom Novartis paid to help promote its new product, Ritalin LA. The company held meetings to develop these doctors into a faculty of advocates for the new drug, a group that multiplied the size and reach of its corporate public relations team. With the help of its hired hands, Novartis soon celebrated as sales of Ritalin LA overtook those of some competing medicines, including Metadate CD. The feat had not been an easy one given that Metadate CD had a head start in the market of more than a year and had been promoted with the help of an animated superhero.

In April 2003, marketers from Novartis boasted about their success in launching Ritalin LA at a meeting of the Healthcare Marketing & Communications Council, which was held at the Marriott Hotel in Hanover, New Jersey. The council's members included dozens of pharmaceutical executives.

In a presentation to the group, the Novartis marketing team detailed how they had sold the new drug. One part of their strategy, they said, had been to use advertisements to give Ritalin LA a "personality." Their goal was to portray the drug as "a young executive who is active, strong, and successful," they said. They wanted the pill to be thought of as "a man of the people—an accessible and nurturing leader who is caring and keeps the best interests of others in mind (like a shepherd)."

To expand sales, the Novartis executives had also approached the National Association of School Nurses, asking the group to distribute a corporate brochure to children, which was entitled "S.T.A.R.T. Now." The brochure warned the children not to share their medicines with others. It also made claims that clearly came from marketers and not from scientists. It said that children should not feel self-conscious about taking medication and claimed that prescription stimulants were "designed to restore the natural balance of the chemicals in the brain." The brochure went on to say that Ludwig van Beethoven, Alexander Graham Bell, and Albert Einstein all had suffered from ADHD, information the writers attributed to a website selling a nutritional supplement.

Demographically, the highest users of drugs like Ritalin are ten-year-old white boys, who had long been featured prominently in advertisements by the stimulant manufacturers. Novartis executives decided, however, they would not forget the girls. They saw girls as a market that had not yet been fully tapped.

In August 2002 a pink-colored plastic binder landed on the desks of journalists across the country. "Boys with ADHD get treated," the document began. "Girls retreat into silence." The binder claimed that 75 percent of girls suffering from attention deficit disorders had never been treated. It held a survey that had been developed with the help of Dr. Patricia Quinn, another physician who had taken a second job working for the manufacturers of stimulants, including Novartis. Dr. Quinn told the many journalists who wrote stories based on the material in the binder that far more boys than girls were being diagnosed with ADHD because the boys drew attention to themselves by running around and fidgeting in their seats, two behaviors that were said to be symptoms of the disorder. Teachers and parents were not recognizing the disorder in girls, she said, because their symptoms were different. Girls afflicted with the disorder were likely to sit quietly in their seats at school and daydream.

At the April presentation at the Marriott in New Jersey, Regina Moran, a public relations executive for Novartis, said the survey about girls was just one way the company had used "scientific data" to "make news."

What she and her colleagues did not talk about that day was that despite decades of clinical trials and thousands of scientific articles, there was relatively little known about what the company called the "most studied" of children's drugs.

In 2005 researchers at Oregon Health & Science University set out to evaluate the scientific evidence that had been published on the medicines prescribed for attention deficit disorders. The Oregon group included some of the few academic drug experts in the country who had refused to take money from the pharmaceutical industry.

The Oregon researchers combed through the medical literature dating back to the 1970s, looking for studies involving Ritalin or the other ADHD meds. They found 2,433 articles, an amazing amount of research on one type of drug. Yet the numbers were deceiving. Many of the trials were far too brief to provide reliable information. More troubling, some of the clinical studies had been designed in ways that biased their results so that the medicines appeared to be safer and more effective than they actually were.

For example, Celltech Pharmaceuticals had paid in 2002 for a study of Metadate, in which the young volunteers were tested in one trial before the main experiment began. In the first stage the Celltech researchers had removed from the study any child who became calmer and more attentive after taking nothing more than a sugar pill. Drug companies often struggle to show their drugs for mental conditions are effective because many patients improve when they are given the placebo. If scientists can remove these placebo responders from the experiment, they can increase the odds that they will ultimately show that the drug works better than the sugar pill. This is what the scientists working for Celltech had done. It raised questions about the accuracy of their conclusion that behavior had improved in 64 percent of the children taking Metadate compared with just 27 percent of those taking the placebo.

Earlier, federal regulators had found that Novartis had designed an experiment with Ritalin LA in a way that biased the final results to favor the company's drug. Novartis had provided the details of this clinical trial to the government when it applied for approval to sell Ritalin LA.

Novartis's clinical trial, known as Protocol 07, was actually two experiments in one, even though the company's main conclusions came from the second part. Novartis's scientists had first given Ritalin LA to 164 children, who ranged in age from six to twelve, for as long as four weeks. They explained this part of the trial was meant to find the dose that worked best for the child. All the children were then taken off the drug for one week, in what Novartis called a washout period. The children were then divided up. Researchers gave about half of them Ritalin LA. The other half of the group was given a daily sugar pill. This second test lasted just two weeks. The company's researchers concluded that Ritalin LA worked far better than the sugar pill in calming the children and helping them concentrate. They pointed out that few children had suffered side effects during those two weeks, even though one volunteer, an eight-year-old boy, had to be hospitalized for depression. The researchers dismissed that incident, saying the boy had a history of depression and that his hospitalization should not be blamed on the company's drug. Other studies had shown, however, that children can develop dysphoria, or feelings of sadness, when they take a drug like Ritalin.

Dr. Andrew Mosholder, a medical officer at the FDA, questioned the design of the study. He said its conclusions were limited because only the children who had tolerated Ritalin LA in the initial four-week experiment were allowed to continue to the two-week trial. Scientists had removed twenty-six children from the trial during that first phase. They had dismissed seven of those child volunteers because their behavior did not improve when they took the drug. At least four other children dropped out after they suffered ill effects. One child became extremely angry. One developed hypomania. Another suffered from anxiety and depression. A fourth developed migraines.

By removing the children whose behavior did not improve on the drug and those who got sick after taking it, Novartis had improved the odds that the kids continuing to the final phase would have good results with Ritalin LA.

The government approved Ritalin LA in June 2002 despite the flaws that Dr. Mosholder noted in the company's study. Dr. Mosholder told his colleagues that he believed that the study had provided overall evidence that Ritalin LA was an effective treatment for ADHD.

The public found out about the results of the trial when they were published in a medical journal in 2003. The scientists reported they had found that Ritalin LA was "superior" to the placebo and that its side effects were "generally mild or moderate." The lead author of the article was Dr. Joseph Biederman, a professor of psychiatry at Harvard who was considered one of the nation's leading experts in childhood attention disorders. For years Dr. Biederman had worked closely with Novartis, as well as with most of the other manufacturers of ADHD medicines. In

2006 he disclosed that he was a paid adviser to six drug companies, a paid speaker for six companies, and a paid researcher for ten companies. Dr. Biederman coauthored the article with eight other scientists, including five employees of Novartis.

In 2005, Dr. Biederman was found to be the most highly cited scientist in the field of attention deficit disorders. By then he had written 294 papers, which had been cited in other journal articles almost seven thousand times. An interviewer asked Dr. Biederman what he believed he had contributed through the hundreds of papers he had published on children and ADHD.

"Our work," he replied, "has helped to support the notion accepted today that ADHD is a treatable, serious brain disorder." He added that he believed the science in the field had advanced "dramatically" since he had begun his work.

After reviewing hundreds of the papers published by Dr. Biederman and other scientists, the Oregon researchers offered a different perspective on how much doctors actually knew about the disorder and the medicines prescribed to treat it. The Oregon group concluded that despite decades of clinical trials, there was no good scientific evidence that Ritalin or any of the other drugs were safe for treating children for longer than six months. They also said there was a dearth of information about the side effects of the pills, including whether they stunted a child's growth. Finally, they said that while scientists had proven the pills could help many children sit still, they had failed to look at whether this meant anything to them in the real world. There was little evidence of whether the medicated children had improved their grades, taken fewer risks, or gotten along better with people.

Novartis and the other manufacturers of the drugs had paid for pages and pages of science that sold millions of prescriptions to children but left much unknown.

Even Novartis was forced to admit in the official prescribing instructions for Ritalin that despite decades of research, the company didn't completely know how the drug worked.

SEVEN

"Neurontin for Everything"

DAVID FRANKLIN SAT on the Continental jetliner, smoothing the fabric of his new suit and polishing his presentation. He imagined the questions the executives would ask about his cancer research and how he would deftly answer each one.

The thirty-four-year-old scientist was almost giddy with excitement. The night before, he had rushed out to Milton's, a men's store offering rock-bottom prices, and splurged on the suit. He had no choice. When he learned that executives at Warner-Lambert wanted to fly him from his home in Boston to their corporate headquarters in New Jersey, he had panicked, remembering that not a single suit hung in his closet. In fact, it was a point of pride among some of the academic scientists he worked with at the Dana-Farber Cancer Institute not to own a suit. What scientist working twelve-hour days to find a lifesaving cure had time to think about his wardrobe?

The suit's trousers, however, had posed a problem. They were inches longer than his short legs. He had solved that dilemma with a quick self-tailoring job, done with a pair of scissors and some iron-on adhesive tape. But now, glancing at his ankles, he noticed the hem did not look quite right. The adhesive had become a rigid ring around each leg. It was fruitless to worry about it now.

Franklin was comforted by knowing he had everything he needed to make a convincing presentation. Along with the suit, he had purchased a briefcase and a portfolio bound in leather, which he thought would impress the executives if he had to take notes. He had filled the briefcase with pens, pads, résumés, as well as a slide presentation of his work, scientific articles explaining the intricacies of his field, and papers outlining the technical details of Warner-Lambert's bestselling drugs.

He had purchased everything on credit. The bill was a major investment for the scientist, who had a young daughter and was struggling to make ends meet on a salary of eighteen thousand dollars a year. Money was so tight he had even begun choosing lunch based on what menu items offered the most calories for the money, which at the time was the lo mein sold by a Chinese takeout joint near the hospital. He had decided to splurge on last night's shopping spree because he thought he might never get an opportunity like this again.

Franklin was thrilled even to have been invited for an interview at Parke-Davis, the subsidiary of Warner-Lambert that sold prescription drugs. He had sent his résumé to a dozen or more drug companies, applying for a research position in their corporate laboratories, only to be repeatedly disappointed. Then he had noticed a classified ad in *The Boston Globe* for a sales position at Parke-Davis. Franklin had no experience in sales. Becoming a pharmaceutical salesman had never been his dream. Yet he thought it would be a way into an industry where he hoped to make a long career. He could eventually work his way out of the sales department, he hoped, and into a job where he used his scientific knowledge to help bring new medicines to patients. This first job would be a means to an end.

Just days after he sent his résumé to Parke-Davis, Zona Hodge, one of the company's human resource directors, had called Franklin. She said the company wanted to learn more about Franklin, who had a Ph.D. in microbiology and had worked for three years at Dana-Farber, a hospital affiliated with Harvard. There had been a hurried meeting with a small group of the company's executives at the Ritz-Carlton Hotel in

Boston. Franklin and the executives had sat around a cocktail table in the hotel's bar. It had been more of an informal chat than an interview. He must have made a good impression because two days later Hodge had called him again. She invited him to fly to Warner-Lambert's corporate headquarters in Morris Plains, a town in north-central New Jersey, for what would be a full day of interviews. She had then offered him some advice.

"There is some question about whether your personal style is aggressive enough," he remembers her saying. "Make sure you sell yourself. Remember this is a sales position. You've got to be aggressive."

Now, looking out the windows of the plane, Franklin saw they were circling over Newark. His "performance" was about to begin.

Minutes later, as he emerged from the Jetway, Franklin saw a middle-aged man holding up a placard with his name.

"Good morning, Dr. Franklin," the man said. "I'll be your chauffeur today."

The driver took his briefcase, and Franklin followed him outside to his car. Franklin expected to find a company van or, at most, a sedan. He tried not to gasp when he saw the car was a black stretch limousine. He didn't want any word of his naïveté to get back to the executives at Parke-Davis.

The driver opened the door, and Franklin got into the back. As the driver headed the limo out of Newark, Franklin was struck by how far it was from where he sat in the back to the driver in the front. The gaping space made him feel oddly uncomfortable.

LATER ONE THING stood out in Franklin's mind about those interviews in New Jersey on March 13, 1996. He remembered how the executives had asked him curious questions.

His most important interview had been with Michael Valentino, a fast-talking executive who had climbed quickly to become the vice president of the company's sales operation in the northeastern United States. Another executive, Phil Magistro, had prepared Franklin for his interview with Valentino. Magistro had been one of the executives Franklin had met a few days before at the Ritz-Carlton. He seemed eager to help Franklin make an impression with the higher-ups.

Magistro had explained that if someone looked at the company's official organization chart, he would find that another executive, Bill Sigmund, was in charge of a group of employees known as medical liaisons. This was the position Franklin was interviewing for. Sigmund was trained as a physician. Magistro said that Sigmund had gotten a reputation among the executives for being "too conservative" when it came to promoting the company's drugs to doctors and complying with government regulations. And now, Magistro said, Sigmund's power inside Parke-Davis was fading. Valentino was really the guy in charge. He was the one Franklin needed to impress.

Franklin found Valentino just as Magistro had described. He spoke in rapid-fire precision, explaining that all the medical liaisons working in the northeastern United States reported to him. Valentino told Franklin that he needed someone for the job who was aggressive, someone who could get up early and call on doctors all day, someone who "could get a physician excited."

And then Valentino abruptly changed the subject. He asked Franklin to describe a situation in which he had been forced to "bend the rules."

Franklin remembered how he was taken aback by the question. It was not a question that one found in any of the books offering advice on how to get a job. Yet he hid his surprise from Valentino and quickly came up with a story from graduate school. As an instructor, he told Valentino, he had once had to deal with a student who had found a way of "bending the rules" in an attempt to get a better grade.

The story was not what Valentino was looking for. He had not been impressed.

It was not the only time that day Franklin was asked such a question. He remembered that at least two other executives, including Magistro, asked whether he would be willing to work in what they called "a gray area." Franklin had responded to their questions with "lots of yeses."

"I was interviewing," he said. "I wanted the job."

The eager recruit quickly put the strange questions out of his mind as the executives offered him a salary that was three times what he was making at Dana-Farber, a brand-new Chevrolet Lumina to use for both work and pleasure, and an expense account that would soon have him dining at four-star restaurants and staying at the finest hotels. Parke-Davis even had a slogan that appealed to an earnest young scientist like Franklin. On its corporate letterhead the company called itself the "People Who Care."

"I didn't really believe it," Franklin said years later, recalling the events of that day. "It was simply too easy . . . No presentation. No scientific debate. I didn't even have to ask for the job—something all of the books said I needed to do.

"I should have known."

FROM A YOUNG age David Franklin had been enthralled with science and medicine.

He traces his interest back to a summer day when he was eight years old and his father drove them from their home in Rhode Island to Fenway Park. The Red Sox that day were collecting donations for the Jimmy Fund, money that went to Dana-Farber for research aimed at finding cures for childhood cancers.

Franklin could see his father had great respect for the doctors at Dana-Farber. He kept pestering his father with questions about the hospital. His father seemed more interested, however, in talking about Carl Yastrzemski, the left fielder patrolling the grass in front of the wall known as the Green Monster.

His grandmother and three other close relatives died of cancer in the following years, and Franklin said he started to dream of finding a way to save people from the wretched disease. But he eventually realized that he could never be a physician. He found that he passed out at the sight of blood.

When he entered the University of Rhode Island in 1979, he became the first of his family to go to college. He decided to study microbiology, a scientific field that dealt more with bacteria and test tubes than with blood and needles.

One basic lesson of school never left him. He learned that science was a field where work must be done honestly and objectively. Any researcher who did otherwise would commit, in his words, "an unforgivable sin."

Thirteen years later Franklin left the university with a Ph.D., a pile of student loans, and a fellowship at Dana-Farber, where his work would be paid for by the Jimmy Fund.

He never worked harder than he did as a postdoc. The typical day at the cancer institute stretched from nine to nine, a schedule repeated six days a week. Stress came from the need to get each step of an experiment exactly right. He also found that science could be dirty and dangerous work. In the lab, his day often began by irradiating mice and rats to duplicate the effects of what might happen when children with cancer were treated with radiation. He often found himself surrounded by toxic materials like acrylamide, a carcinogen. The smell of soiled animal bedding hung in the air.

And always, he was writing applications for grants to support his research and make sure his salary did not become smaller than it already was. He often found himself exhausted. But then he would walk through the hospital's lobby and see the sick children and want to work twenty-four hours a day.

After three years at the hospital, his family's financial struggles and the crushing amount of student debt had become what he called a crisis. He began to think that a job in the pharmaceutical industry could offer a solution. He believed the industry was one of America's jewels, a powerful force for good that made money by saving people's lives. There seemed to be a way of living the good life on a corporate salary, while also feeling honorable about what you did.

"Industry," he said, "seemed like the perfect fit."

YET THERE WERE many things Franklin did not know as he began his work at Warner-Lambert and its subsidiary Parke-Davis in the spring of 1996.

Two years before he landed the job, executives had begun a series of internal meetings on what to do about the disappointing sales of a drug for epilepsy that the company's marketers had given the name Neurontin. The drug's brand name evoked an image of a chemical working to rev up the signals between the neurons in the brain. The medicine, however, was a weakling.

Based on the company's clinical studies, federal regulators had agreed that Neurontin could be sold to treat epilepsy, but only in limited cases. The company could promote it only as a second medicine for epileptics who had not been able to control their seizures with their first medication. Regulators did not want patients taking just Neurontin. That would be dangerous because the drug had not reduced the number of seizures in most volunteers in the company's clinical trials. In fact, the company had found that 5 to 10 percent of the epilepsy patients taking the drug actually got worse.

Warner-Lambert's investors were not stirred by the sales potential of the drug, which came in capsules colored white, yellow, or orange. Executives estimated Neurontin would bring in just $500 million over all the years it could be sold before its patent expired. When that happened, other companies would be able to sell a generic form of the drug at a fraction of the price charged by Warner-Lambert. The company would then watch as its sales of Neurontin plunged.

The executives decided, however, they were not satisfied in selling Neurontin for the limited use in epilepsy that the government had approved. Instead, they resolved to expand its sales greatly by promoting the drug for more than a dozen other medical conditions that had nothing to do with epilepsy, other than that they also involved the brain. The executives created an internal wish list of these other neurological conditions, each of them representing the chance for tens of thousands of additional prescriptions. Their initial targets ranged from children with attention deficit disorder to adults with sexual dysfunction. They even believed Neurontin could be sold to those who went to the doctor because their hiccups would not stop. One of the biggest potential groups of customers was those who suffered from manic depression.

The executives vowed to sell Neurontin as a treatment for these other conditions, even though the scientific evidence supporting such prescriptions consisted of little more than rumor or anecdotal reports written by physicians who had been paid by Parke-Davis. The executives agreed to follow their plan even though it violated both the law and the basic ethics at the core of science and medicine.

They laid out the details of their strategy in memorandums and written financial analyses. The operation was not driven by a bunch of rogue executives. The orders came from above. Executives at the highest levels of management, including Lodewijk J. R. de Vink, the Dutch-born businessman who was in line to become Warner-Lambert's chairman, and Anthony H. Wild, the president of its global pharmaceutical business, sat on the committee devising the plan.

This group of executives, called the New Product Committee, decided the company would not pay for the proper scientific studies needed to show that Neurontin actually worked for the other medical conditions. The executives feared the drug's patent would expire before the company could profit from the large financial investment needed for such clinical trials.

Instead, the executives resolved to promote Neurontin for these other uses anyway, which they calculated could earn the company tens of millions of dollars. A piece of the plan was laid out in a confidential memo written by John T. Boris, a senior manager from the product planning department in the company's headquarters in Morris Plains, and dated on the last day of July 1996. The memo detailed the company's plans for selling Neurontin to treat migraines, just one of fifteen experimental uses the executives talked of selling the drug for.

Boris wrote that the executives sitting on the company's New Product Committee had decided against doing the large studies needed to convince the government that Neurontin was a safe and effective treatment for migraines. Instead, the committee decided the company would pay for two smaller and cheaper trials. The company would then publish the results of these small studies, Boris explained, and use them to promote the drug to doctors treating migraine patients. But there was a catch.

The results would be published, Boris said, only if they showed that Neurontin actually worked to reduce the number of migraines the patients suffered. What was left unsaid, although strongly implied, was that any study that failed to show that Neurontin was effective for migraines would be filed away and hidden from public view.

In fact, researchers had already tested Neurontin as a treatment for migraines in two studies. One of those studies used a design considered the gold standard in medical science because it helps prevent bias that can skew results. Doctors call these experiments by the steps used in their design, which in this case was a "randomized, double-blind, placebo-controlled" trial. In simple terms, an experiment designed in this way ensures that neither the patient volunteers nor their doctors know whether a subject is receiving the drug or the sugar pill.

The trial concluded Neurontin did not work.

AT THE TIME the executives were planning their sales strategy for the epilepsy drug, Warner-Lambert was one of the nation's fastest-growing companies. Few Americans would have recognized the name Neurontin, or Warner-Lambert for that matter. They were more likely to know the company's nonmedicinal products, which included Bubblicious chewing gum, Schick razors, and Listerine.

It was not the candy or mouthwash that was making Warner-Lambert rich, however. Most of its profits came from Parke-Davis, the subsidiary selling prescription drugs. Parke-Davis had once been an independent company that had grown to be the world's largest drug manufacturer. It was founded in the 1860s, when H. C. Parke and George S. Davis took over a pharmacy in Detroit, Michigan, and expanded it into a small drug company. The two men focused their efforts on selling alkaloids, medicines made from plants.

The company's first success was the marketing of cocaine. In 1875, Parke-Davis introduced an extract made from the leaves of coca, an evergreen shrub growing on the slopes of the Andes. The plant was gaining attention among some scientists. Davis was a marketing man who had many creative ideas for expanding sales. One of his brilliant decisions was to publish booklets and magazines that targeted physicians, including a monthly newspaper titled the *Therapeutic Gazette*. The newspaper included articles detailing the benefits of the company's products, although it did not tell readers that Parke-Davis was paying for the publication.

Among the articles in the *Gazette* was a series in the 1880s on how morphine addicts could be cured with the company's elixir of cocaine. A physician writing one of the articles had quoted from the company's advertising label, which claimed that large doses of the coca elixir produced "a general excitation of the circulatory and nervous systems, imparting increased vigor to the muscles as well as to the intellect, with an indescribable feeling of satisfaction."

The articles attracted attention far and wide, including that of the Viennese physician Dr. Sigmund Freud. At the time, Dr. Freud was looking for an area of research where he could make a contribution, while also gaining the success that would permit him to marry. Dr. Freud quoted from the *Gazette*, as well as from other research, in his now famous paper "On Coca," which appeared in 1884. The paper claimed that coca could be used as a stimulant, for asthma, as an aphrodisiac, for digestive disorders, as an anesthetic, and to treat morphine addiction, just as described in George Davis's monthly. Freud concluded that "the use of coca in moderation is more likely to promote health than to impair it."

Parke-Davis then completed the circle by printing promotional materials citing Freud's writing as proof that cocaine was an effective treatment for morphine addiction. The company did not mention that Freud got the idea from the company's newspaper. Parke-Davis also paid Freud to endorse its cocaine extract, which he did when he soon wrote that the product "should have a great future."

FRANKLIN REMEMBERS HOW his first days at Parke-Davis were "surreal." His life was transformed overnight.

He went from eating cheap Chinese noodles to dining at the legendary Four Seasons Hotel. He learned that eating and drinking were part of his job description. He was told his bosses would hail him as a hero just for hanging out at the bar with a doctor the company wanted to court. Gone were the twelve-hour days in a malodorous laboratory. A Parke-Davis colleague told him he should often be able to finish his work by two o'clock in the afternoon.

Yet his elation with landing the job did not last. His thoughts kept returning to those strange questions the executives had asked him that day in New Jersey. He slowly began to understand what the executives had been trying to uncover through their queries.

As he learned more about what was expected of him, he started to worry that all was not right with what the executives were training and commanding him to do. He was told that the FDA did not allow a company to promote a drug for a medical use the government had not approved. Yet his bosses then ordered him to do exactly that in their instructions for selling Neurontin.

They told him to call on pediatricians and ask them to prescribe the epilepsy drug to children diagnosed with attention deficit disorder. They asked him to press psychiatrists to prescribe it for bipolar disorder. They told him to urge primary care doctors to prescribe it to patients debilitated by migraines.

The information that Franklin and the other medical liaisons were told to give to doctors about these experimental uses for Neurontin consisted mostly of case reports involving a few handfuls of patients at best. The stories of the patients who didn't get better on the drug—and there were thousands of them—did not get discussed.

How do you get physicians to ignore their duty to provide the best care for patients that science can offer and instead start doling out prescriptions in ways that are nothing more than an experiment? According to the executives' strategy, the company would pay them. These payments came in the form of expensive meals at the finest restaurants and stays at luxury seaside resorts. Much of the time, however, they came in the form of cold, hard cash. Franklin eventually realized that Parke-Davis had easily found a legion of physicians who were eager to help.

As the weeks passed, he also realized, to his horror, that the executives had selected him for the job because they believed he had a background that was a perfect aid to their strategy, a plan that he was coming to understand could not be legal.

Doctors had been told by the pharmaceutical industry that the medical liaisons, like Franklin, were not sales reps. They were simply employees with special training in science and medicine who could answer physicians' questions about the complex chemical products they prescribed. Franklin clearly fit the part, given his scientific training and doctorate degree. Yet his bosses seemed more excited about the initials behind his name, and the fact that he could be introduced as "Dr. Franklin," than about what he actually knew about medical science.

The executives' intentions became obvious to Franklin when rather than school him in the pharmacological intricacies of the company's products, they trained him to sell. They told him that his top responsibility as a medical liaison was to use his credentials to gain access to a neighborhood's physicians and then, once inside their offices, tell them how Neurontin could be prescribed for almost any neurological condition.

Shortly after he accepted the job, Franklin attended a corporate meeting in Parsipanny, New Jersey, where Phil Magistro described in detail how the medical liaisons should exhort doctors to experiment with Neurontin. Magistro showed the liaisons a set of slides that had been created to be part of their sales presentation to doctors. One of the slides was entitled "Anecdotal Uses of Neurontin." The list included thirteen medical conditions, including tremors, peripheral neuropathy, and Lou Gehrig's disease.

Franklin recalled how Magistro admitted to the group that some physicians might laugh when they saw the slide because it made Neurontin look like one of the quack medicines sold as cure-alls at the turn of the twentieth century. To preempt the snickers, Magistro advised the salespeople to say something like "I'm embarrassed to show you the next slide because it makes Neurontin look like snake oil, but the fact is we are seeing extraordinary results, in some cases up to 90 percent response in all of these conditions."

None of that was true.

Franklin heard similar speeches from other executives. At a meeting in Farmington, Connecticut, on April 22, 1996, John Ford, a senior marketing executive, stood in front of Franklin and the other salespeople who covered the northeastern United States for Parke-Davis and ordered them to get out there and aggressively pitch Neurontin to physicians.

"That's where we need to be, holding their hand and whispering in their ear," Ford said, "Neurontin for pain, Neurontin for monotherapy, Neurontin for bipolar, Neurontin for everything."

But Ford didn't stop there. He implored the sales team to tell doctors to prescribe the drug in doses far higher than the 1800-milligram maximum the government recommended. Getting physicians to double or nearly triple the dose would help improve the drug's image as a weak, ineffective medicine. At the same time, higher doses would make sales soar.

"I don't want to see a single patient coming off Neurontin before they've been up to at least 4800 milligrams per day," Ford ordered, as later recounted by Franklin. "I don't want to hear that safety crap either. Have you tried Neurontin? Every one of you should take one just to see there is nothing. It's a great drug."

FEDERAL LAW FORBIDS companies from promoting medicines for uses the government has not approved. The law is meant to protect patients. To gain approval, the company must show "substantial evidence" of a drug's effectiveness by performing "adequate and well-controlled investigations."

Yet the rules are different for doctors. Once a medicine is approved, it is legal for physicians to prescribe it in almost any way they believe is best for their patients. They do not need government approval, for instance, to prescribe an antiseizure medicine to a child diagnosed with attention deficit disorder. This was the loophole that Warner-Lambert set out to exploit.

A drug prescribed for an experimental use is often said to be used off label, a shorthand way of saying it was prescribed outside the FDA-approved label or prescribing instructions. There is no requirement that physicians tell their patients they are giving them a drug for an off-label use, and most patients never learn they've received such a prescription.

Some off-label uses of medications have clearly helped patients. For example, Dr. Barry Marshall's discovery that stomach ulcers could be cured with antibiotics was an unapproved use of those drugs for many years.

Sometimes doctors have found new uses for older drugs that are no longer protected by a patent. Because the medicines are so inexpensive, the manufacturers have little or no interest in paying for the clinical trials needed to get government approval for the additional uses. The class of drugs known as beta-blockers, for example, was initially approved to treat angina and high blood pressure. Years later doctors found that beta-blockers also helped patients suffering from heart failure.

Yet history has shown that drugs prescribed off label have also killed or harmed tens of thousands of patients. The deadly diet pill combination known as fen-phen was an unapproved use of the combination of two drugs. For years doctors have commonly prescribed potent drugs for schizophrenia to patients with Alzheimer's disease, even though the FDA has never approved such use. Studies have shown these antipsychotic drugs, including Zyprexa and Risperdal, do not help patients with Alzheimer's. Instead, the drugs appear to increase their risk of death.

In the late 1980s, doctors began prescribing Tambocor and Enkaid, which were approved to treat irregular heartbeats, to patients who did not have these symptoms but had suffered heart attacks. Years later a government study showed that the drugs almost tripled the death rate among such patients. In his 1995 book *Deadly Medicine*, Thomas J. Moore estimated the two drugs killed fifty thousand Americans, many who had suddenly dropped dead.

Despite such dangers, more than 90 percent of the prescriptions written for some drugs in the United States are for experimental uses. Most of the drugs that doctors prescribe to infants and children are off label. Drug companies rarely perform the studies needed to get their products approved for children. Without those studies, doctors don't understand what the medicines might do.

EXECUTIVES AT PARKE-DAVIS knew their marketing strategy was illegal. They worked hard not to leave any footprints.

The executives repeatedly told Franklin and his colleagues to avoid writing things down. Franklin later remembered how his bosses frequently urged the medical liaisons to use the corporate voice mail network, known as the Aspen system, to communicate with one another. This reduced the need for memos.

He was given similar instructions at a training seminar he was sent to in Ann Arbor, Michigan, about a month after he had joined the company. In one session an executive explained how the medical liaisons should not create written records of their work. "Most of all don't leave a paper trail," the executive told the group. "Anything you write down can be audited. So don't write anything down."

The executives then showed the group a film that portrayed the story of a company being sued. In the video an actor playing the part of a corporate executive frantically shreds a pile of documents. He and the other characters talk about how they wish they had never put their plans in writing. To Franklin, the message was clear: If you don't write things down, you won't find yourself wanting to shred the papers in your desk when the government starts asking questions.

The next day one of the instructors brought up the topic again. She told the medical liaisons that anything they wrote down could later be used against them in court. To make her point, she handed out little notepads imprinted with the headings "Ladies and gentlemen of the jury . . ." and "Your Honor, I plead . . ."

While the executives tried to avoid putting their plans in writing, they created other physical evidence meant to show they were working honestly and legally. If any authorities decided to investigate, executives would then be able to provide them with plenty of proof that they had done nothing wrong.

For example, Franklin recalled how an employee videotaped a training seminar at which executives lectured him and other medical liaisons on what they must do to stay within the lines of the government's drug marketing regulations. With the camera on, the executives leading the seminar reminded the group that the position of medical liaison was not that of a salesperson. They explained that medical liaisons could offer physicians information, but their job was not to promote the company's products. They also explained how the company could not push products for off-label uses.

At that point, the employee operating the video camera turned it off. Franklin remembered how several employees made jokes about whether the camera really was off. Then the executives told the group they should not worry about what they had just been told.

"We expect you to do your job out there and stay focused on sales," one of the executives said, according to Franklin. "Don't worry about this stuff."

"Look, without sales there is no Parke-Davis," one of the leaders explained. "We all have to sell."

FRANKLIN SOON WAS finding copies of *Selling Power* magazine in his mailbox. The subscription was a gift from the company as well as a reminder of what his bosses expected.

Before he set out to call on physicians, the company gave him what executives called precision marketing reports, which had the name and address of each doctor in the neighborhood along with details of the prescriptions they had written. Despite all the confidentiality expected in American medicine, Parke-Davis and its competitors knew down to the pill what every physician had prescribed.

These reports, which most doctors were unaware of, came from companies like IMS Health, which had created giant databases of prescription information. IMS was created in 1954 by Ludwig Wilhelm "Bill" Frohlich, the head of an advertising agency in New York. Over the years IMS built a billion-dollar business by purchasing prescription records from pharmacies and combining them with profiles of physicians purchased from the American Medical Association, the nation's largest medical society. The pharmaceutical industry gladly paid for the records, which opened up a whole new world of sales opportunities. Marketers could now spy on physicians as they treated their patients.

Franklin said Parke-Davis's sales reps used the prescription reports to determine which doctors were loyal prescribers of the company's products and therefore should be rewarded with free trips, dinners, gifts, or cash. The sales team ranked the physicians by their financial worth to the company, which was based on the number of prescriptions they wrote. The biggest prescribers received more attention from the sales reps and more of the company's marketing dollars.

The reports allowed the salespeople to tailor their pitches to each physician. If the doctor was seeing a high number of patients who suffered from pain, the salesperson could claim that Neurontin was an amazing pain reliever. If the doctor was writing dozens of prescriptions for a competitor's drug, the salesperson could prepare a speech about why Neurontin was a better choice. If a doctor suddenly switched his patients from a medicine sold by Parke-Davis to one sold by a competitor, perhaps after one of his patients had suffered an adverse reaction, the salesperson could quickly call on him, ease his fears, and offer incentives to switch his patients back.

Parke-Davis and the rest of the drug industry also used the prescription data to pay bonuses to sales representatives who succeeded in getting doctors to write more prescriptions. At some companies, the average bonus paid to each salesperson was more than his or her salary. The lure of bonuses of tens of thousands of dollars pushed the industry's sales forces to do whatever it took to win over physicians. The companies might have been training their salespeople in what they could legally do under the law, but they gave them great financial incentives to break it.

On most days, Franklin's superiors left messages for him and the other medical liaisons on the voice mail system. The messages included details of their assignments as well as exhortations to get out there and sell. The corporate bosses often sounded more like penny stock brokers than people dealing with the lives of human patients.

"What we need to do is focus on Neurontin," Phil Magistro said in a voice message he sent to the medical liaisons on an afternoon in May a couple of months after Franklin had been hired. "When we get out there, we want to kick some ass. We want to sell Neurontin on pain. All right? And monotherapy and everything that we can talk about. That's what we want to do. Cuz I'm embarrassed. I don't know if you guys are embarrassed, but I'm embarrassed with where we are with Neurontin. We've got to take it into our own hands and really kick some ass on it, all right? Let's do it up. Talk to you soon. Bye."

By that time, Franklin was worried. He knew much of what the executives were telling him to do was a criminal offense. Could he eventually find himself in jail? He bought a tape recorder and began recording the voice messages and the conference calls on which Magistro and the other executives delivered their orders to the sales force covering the northeastern United States.

In some calls, the executives seemed amazed with the power of their plan.

"Gee, just think of how we could expand the market here with Neurontin and some of these other disorders," raved John Ford to the other sales managers and medical liaisons, who had gathered by phone for a conference call. "So, I guess the sky is the limit, right?"

"Yeah, I would say," replied Magistro. "This is just unbelievable."

THE CRUX OF the illegal plan came down to finding doctors willing to be paid to tell other physicians that Neurontin was a miracle drug with uses far beyond epilepsy. The executives knew these stories would appear far more convincing if they came from physicians rather than from the company's marketers.

To aid in this part of the scheme, Parke-Davis turned to the global advertising agencies of Madison Avenue. Executives at one of these ad firms, a company called Cline Davis & Mann, sat on the committee at Parke-Davis that planned how to sell Neurontin. Executives from Cline Davis had even held what they called the Neurontin War Games, which included a day of strategizing on how to sell the drug while holed up in a conference room at the Sheraton Tara in Framingham, Massachusetts.

The drug company and its ad agencies knew that once they found doctors willing to be paid to make speeches about Neurontin, they would need to entice other doctors to listen. To do that, they planned hundreds of dinners and weekend retreats at upscale restaurants and resorts across the country, where Parke-Davis picked up the tab and also pre-

sented doctors with checks if they agreed to sit and listen to the stories
about Neurontin. The corporate goal of these events, which cost the
drug company tens of millions of dollars, was to spread the word about
the wonders of Neurontin.

An example was a meeting held at the Château Elan, a luxury resort
in the hill country north of Atlanta. The drug company and Cline Davis
planned this meeting to coincide with the final days of the 1996 Summer Olympic Games, which were held in Atlanta that year. The invited
physicians and their spouses enjoyed golf, wine tasting, horseback
riding, and the European spa at the resort, before being whisked off by
chauffeurs to watch the athletic events. Parke-Davis paid for everything,
from the couples' airfares to Atlanta to their tickets to Olympic Stadium.
The physicians and their guests could lunch on fine French cuisine on
the hotel patio, before enjoying massages and herbal wraps at the spa.
They did not need their own credit cards. All they had to do was write
"Parke-Davis" on the checks. Just in case the doctors thought five days
of expense-free luxury was not enough to sit through roughly ten hours
of lectures about Neurontin, the company also paid each of them $750.

The company spent hundreds of thousands of dollars to entertain the
physicians at the Château Elan. One Parke-Davis executive referred to
the events scheduled around the Olympic Games as the company's "$3mm
investment."

Most of the planning for the meeting at the Château Elan was done
by the advertising firm Cline Davis. In memos, the ad executives assured
Parke-Davis that some of the physicians who were being paid to lecture
at the resort had agreed to promote Neurontin for experimental uses.
Other documents explained how the advertising firm had recruited these
physician speakers and prepared the slides and lecture notes for their
presentations, just to make sure they covered the points that would help
sell more Neurontin.

The company often recorded the physicians as they spoke. It was
clear from the tape recordings that the doctors were having a good time.
Some of these physicians joked about the expanding number of uses for
Neurontin that they were promoting through their lectures.

"Good morning, everyone. I hope everybody enjoyed the cruise last night and the bright sunshine yesterday," began Dr. Steven C. Schachter, a professor of neurology at Harvard and a paid Parke-Davis consultant, as he introduced the first speaker at a three-day corporate retreat at Jupiter Beach, Florida. "Someone asked me if Neurontin was good for a sunburn . . ."

Many of the physicians speaking at these meetings made statements that would have been illegal if they had come from Parke-Davis employees, who could not promote a drug for experimental uses, or claim it had no risks, or say it worked better than studies had shown. Doctors, however, could say whatever they pleased. If the FDA questioned the statements, the company could point out that the doctor was only stating his personal opinion.

The doctors proved to be potent Neurontin promoters. For example, Parke-Davis frequently hired Dr. David Longmire, a physician from Alabama, to talk about how Neurontin could treat pain. Over two years the company paid Dr. Longmire to fly to Phoenix, Dallas, Philadelphia, and other cities to tell doctors about Neurontin.

One of those meetings was held at the Ritz-Carlton in Boston in May 1996. The company paid for a large group of physicians to travel to Boston and stay at the luxury hotel, where they also enjoyed a welcome reception, drinks, and three meals.

In his speech, Dr. Longmire told the invited physicians that he had found that the epilepsy drug relieved his patients' pain, including those with an intense, stabbinglike pain in the face called trigeminal neuralgia. The only catch, according to Dr. Longmire, was that the doctors had to prescribe Neurontin at daily doses that far exceeded the maximum recommended by the FDA, which was eighteen hundred milligrams.

"The problem with Neurontin in terms of real trigeminal neuralgia," Dr. Longmire said, according to a transcript of the speech, "is that it has to be titrated upward. And when I say 1500 milligrams, that's the target starting dose. There are colleagues in the Huntsville area who—I have people on 5400 with no side effects."

Paying Dr. Longmire and four other doctors to speak at the Ritz-Carlton proved to be a lucrative move by Parke-Davis. Records from the government's Medicaid program showed that many of the doctors who enjoyed the Ritz-Carlton wrote more prescriptions for Neurontin when they got home. For example, one doctor had never written a prescription for Neurontin before the retreat. Five days afterward, the doctor gave Neurontin to a patient with inflamed nerves in his lower back. By the end of six months, the doctor had written fifty-three Neurontin prescriptions for Medicaid patients, most of them for uses the government had not approved.

Franklin said he found that many physicians did not question even the flimsiest or most reckless claims made by the company or the physicians they hired. Everyone—both doctors and the company's employees—seemed entirely comfortable with what was going on.

"I underwent a stunning revision of my beliefs about the medical profession," Franklin later recounted. Before working at Parke-Davis, he had believed a doctor's first duty was to his patients and that no amount of money could change that. But as he went on his rounds of medical offices, he had some doctors ask him what Parke-Davis planned to do for them now that they were writing more prescriptions of Neurontin.

"You'd like to think this kind of simple scheme wouldn't work with physicians," Franklin said. "It works remarkably well."

SOMETIMES THE MARKETING executives hired a doctor to speak but later discovered the physician had no plans to provide the message about Neurontin that the company desired. Cline Davis, the global ad agency, proved to be adept at making such problems disappear.

Just such a case was laid out in a memo by Bina O'Brien, an executive who worked for Proworx, a division of Cline Davis. O'Brien wrote the memo to Allen Crook, a marketing executive at Parke-Davis. She wanted to prove to Crook and the other executives at Parke-Davis that her ad firm was worth the hundreds of thousands of dollars in fees it was charging to promote Neurontin.

In the memo, O'Brien described how Proworx had found two physicians willing to speak about Neurontin at an event to be held at the Boston Marriott in June 1997. The executives' plan was for the doctors to talk about how Neurontin eased a type of pain suffered by diabetes patients called diabetic neuropathy. The Proworx executives told the doctors what they wanted their presentations to include. They also explained to the doctors that Proworx had created slides that could be used in their presentations. The doctors told the executives they understood what the company wanted. They declined to use the slides, however, and said they would write their own speeches.

Days later, Parke-Davis executives panicked when they received the summary of the speech that one of the doctors planned to deliver. It was clear the doctor had no plans to deliver the agreed-upon message. They feared the doctor might even make negative comments about Neurontin.

That was when the Proworx executives got creative. O'Brien wrote that the executives began discussing how they could "counteract a possible 'negative' presentation."

They settled on "creating a setting," she said, where the doctor "would have no choice but to address the issues she had originally agreed to present." To do this, the executives created a list of questions that they then gave to people who would be sitting in the audience. They told them to pose the queries in the question and answer session that followed the doctor's speech. Some of the questions were designed to force the doctor to address what the company wanted her to say about Neurontin. Other questions were aimed at neutralizing any negative comments she might make about the drug.

The strategy worked. According to O'Brien, the ad firms' questions, asked by its friends in the audience, forced the doctor to address some of the "positive aspects" of Neurontin.

O'Brien promised Parke-Davis that the Proworx staff would not let such a situation happen again. The next time, she said, Proworx would do more research about the doctors who were candidates to give speeches before hiring them.

Yet that was not the only time that Parke-Davis or its advertising partners infiltrated audiences to make sure the right questions and comments were delivered to polish the image of Neurontin in the minds of physicians.

The advertising firm IntraMed planned a similar scheme at a lavish dinner for doctors that it organized for Parke-Davis at the California Culinary Academy in San Francisco. In documents, John Bayliss, an executive at IntraMed, said the night would include a reception with fine wines from Napa Valley and a meal in the academy's three-story glass-walled dining hall. Weeks before the event, Bayliss drafted a letter to one of the doctors who had frequently given speeches about Neurontin with a specific request. He offered to pay the doctor two hundred dollars if he would commit a couple of prewritten questions to memory and then bring them up in the middle of that night's dinner conversation. "The evening will be very educational and memorable," Bayliss promised the physician in the letter. Before sending the letter, Bayliss sent a draft to a Parke-Davis executive, seeking the company's approval of the plan.

"Here is a draft of the letter inviting our 'moderators,'" Bayliss wrote in a memo to the executive. "Let me know what you think."

THE AD AGENCIES and marketing firms hired by Parke-Davis had another device for promoting Neurontin: they knew how to turn the stories and rumors about the drug into medical journal articles that could be cited again and again as proof of its newfound powers.

In December 1996, a marketing firm called Medical Education Systems, Inc., wrote to executives at Parke-Davis with a proposal. For a fee of $160,500, the marketers offered to create a dozen scientific articles about Neurontin, most of them describing what they called the drug's "emerging uses." The firm proposed articles that would describe how Neurontin could allegedly treat bipolar disorder, migraines, chronic pain, and behavioral problems. The actual evidence supporting such treatment was limited to nonexistent at that time, although this did not seem to present a problem for the staff at Medical Education Systems, which worked out of offices in Philadelphia.

The marketing firm planned to recruit physicians and pay them a thousand dollars each to be the "authors" of the twelve articles. The rest of the money, which amounted to about twelve thousand dollars for each manuscript, was to go to Medical Education Systems for the article's "development."

The firm regularly sent reports of its progress to Parke-Davis. The memos made it clear that some physicians hired as "authors" were doing little of the work. The status reports also detailed how Parke-Davis executives were reviewing and editing each manuscript before it was sent to a medical journal to be published.

"DRAFT COMPLETED. WE JUST NEED AN AUTHOR," read the report for one of the articles in a memo the firm faxed to Parke-Davis. This particular article was about how drugs like Neurontin could treat children. The marketers said their "target" was to get the article published in the respected medical journal *Pediatrics.*

In its status report on another proposed article, the firm's staff wrote, "Draft 1 being reviewed internally (some rewriting being done). Will send to author and P-D by 11/17."

Parke-Davis executives were pleased with the work of Medical Education Systems and the other ghostwriting firms it employed. As article after article was published, the drug company purchased thousands of reprints and delivered boxes of them to Franklin and the other medical liaisons. The glossy pages were handed to doctors as a testament of all Neurontin could do.

THE DOCTORS CHOSEN to write articles about Neurontin or to speak about the drug at dinners and weekend retreats could increase their annual incomes by tens of thousands of dollars. The company paid one physician more than $300,000 over the course of three years to give presentations about Neurontin. Parke-Davis also paid all the bills as these speakers traveled to and stayed at some of the most luxurious resorts and hotels in the country.

"Yesterday, I was here on the beach, frolicking in the sun, and I was on a boogie board," Dr. Cynthia Harden, a physician from New York, told her audience at the meeting in Jupiter Beach, Florida. "And I was trying to ride the waves in but I noticed that I wasn't getting anywhere. In fact, I was starting to float out to Bermuda.

"Thankfully, the Parke-Davis people had been watching me, and one of their marketing people . . . saw me and came and rescued me. It was like a *Baywatch* episode."

The doctors in the audience laughed.

"And so I just want to say," Dr. Harden continued, "that Parke-Davis for me really are the people who care."

There was more laughter.

"And also, I was informed, that if this had been an Abbott conference," she added, referring to another drug company, "that they would've just let me float out to sea."

The doctors laughed some more.

Yet Warner-Lambert and its subsidiary Parke-Davis could not have succeeded in the illegal marketing campaign without the cooperation of these physicians.

Franklin soon realized that his employer had as many different ways of paying physicians as it had experimental uses for Neurontin.

Dr. Ilo Leppik, a physician at the University of Minnesota, wrote to the company, asking it to pay $303,600 to publish his book on epilepsy. The executives agreed. One doctor received $2,000 to travel to San Francisco for a seminar after a salesperson deemed him to be "a great Neurontin believer."

Dr. B. J. Wilder, professor emeritus of neurology at the University of Florida, wrote several letters to Warner-Lambert requesting money. In April 1996, Dr. Wilder asked the company to write a check for $401,350 to his private foundation to send him and 125 medical residents to the Registry Resort, a luxury hotel on the white sand beach of Naples, Florida.

Dr. Wilder's proposal aligned nicely with the company's strategy of targeting the nation's physicians in training. Executives explained in one memorandum that they spent money wooing the young doctors "to solidify Parke-Davis' role in the resident's mind as he/she evolves into a practicing physician." Such programs, they said, could "influence physicians from the bottom up."

The company paid the bill for the four-day retreat and seminar in Naples, which Dr. Wilder called the "Merritt-Putnam Epilepsy Update for Residents and Fellows in Neurology." The final tab came to more than $3,200 for each young physician.

Parke-Davis also paid doctors if they agreed to let corporate employees read their patients' medical records. Franklin learned physicians could earn fifty dollars for each patient's record, plus an additional sum to cover the doctor's cost of overhead.

In another program the company paid doctors to experiment on their patients by prescribing Neurontin in doses that were double the maximum recommended by the FDA. The executives aggressively pushed this program even though patients suffered more side effects as they took higher doses of Neurontin.

Executives called the experiment the STEPS trial. Their written plans described how the company would pay more than a thousand physicians to experiment on four thousand patients. The pay was three hundred dollars for each patient and fifty dollars more if the doctor kept the patient on Neurontin when the trial ended. The company claimed the trial was aimed at gathering research data about Neurontin, but Franklin saw it as little more than a dangerous marketing ploy.

Months after the STEPS trial began, the executives hailed it as a success. They had found that the physicians paid to put their patients in the experiment were writing higher doses of Neurontin for all their patients, which meant higher sales for Parke-Davis.

But the largest group of doctors receiving money from Parke-Davis consisted of those hired to be what the company called consultants. The company explained that it was hiring the doctors to provide advice to its marketers.

Franklin learned otherwise. He attended the dinners at which the company's consultants met. He said he did not hear the physicians offer any advice. Rather their "duties" consisted of eating, drinking, and listening to promotions of Neurontin.

Franklin found that the sales department selected the consultants on the basis of their potential to boost sales. The highest prescribers of Neurontin, he said, received the most invitations to serve as paid consultants for the night or weekend at events hosted by Parke-Davis.

The party invitations came with a caveat. The doctors had to sign a confidentiality agreement requiring them to keep quiet about much of the events' proceedings. This culture of secrecy protected both the company and physicians from scrutiny by the public. If patients learned about the financial deals, they would have worried their doctors were being corrupted.

The physicians could be quite demanding. No matter how lavish Parke-Davis made the accommodations, some doctors wanted more. "Hotel too cold inside," wrote one doctor in an evaluation he filled out after a meeting at the Sheraton Hotel in Atlantic City, the gambling mecca. "Resort places preferred." The physician was also irritated by what he viewed as another shortcoming of the weekend he had just enjoyed. Parke-Davis had paid for him to bring his entire family to Atlantic City but had failed to provide entertainment for his children.

Another doctor complained after the company paid for a three-day weekend at the Helmsley Park Lane Hotel overlooking Central Park in Manhattan. It had not been enough that Parke-Davis had paid all his expenses, including an allowance to cover his cost of driving into the city from New Jersey as well as his parking fees. The doctor said he would have rather been chauffeured. "Hired car would have been much preferable," he grumbled.

Parke-Davis carefully tracked the number of prescriptions written by its consultants. Executives asked the sales representatives to record how many Neurontin prescriptions the doctors had written in the three months leading up to the dinner or retreat they were invited to attend. Those numbers were then compared with the medicines the doctors prescribed after the party.

Yet why have your salespeople follow a doctor's prescribing habits through statistical reports when they could actually be standing inside his examining room, talking to his patients, and telling him exactly what prescriptions to write? Parke-Davis had developed another program that allowed its sales representatives to do exactly that.

The company called this its preceptorship program. Parke-Davis told physicians they could make $350 if they agreed to be preceptors for the day. The understanding was that the salesperson would follow the physician on his rounds, which the company called shadowing, to learn how the doctor worked. The executives suggested this would help the company understand how it could better meet the needs of physicians and patients.

Behind the scenes, however, Parke-Davis executives were exhorting their salespeople to sign up doctors for the program because of its potential to boost sales.

"Check this out," John Ford said as he passed on a voice mail message about the program to all the sales representatives in the Northeast. "It's on shadowing. If you're not quite sure if the doctor's telling you the whole story, if you want to drive business—shadow, preceptor him. And you'll learn what you need to learn and you'll drive business."

The message that Ford passed on was from Steve Bitman, a sales rep who had spent the day in the examination room of a neurologist in Yonkers, New York. In his message, Bitman recounted in detail the discussions he had with the doctor and her patients.

"The doctor would review the chart of each patient with me in a one-on-one fashion," he explained. "Then we would go meet the patient. The patient would be examined, and then, while the patient was dressing, the doctor and I, one-on-one, would discuss the patient and therapeutic options."

Bitman excitedly described how he had succeeded in getting the doctor to write two prescriptions of Neurontin. The first, he said, was for a thirteen-year-old girl who was having seizures. The girl was already taking Neurontin as well as a drug called Tegretol. But Bitman told the doctor that she should double the girl's dose of Neurontin and then gradually take her off Tegretol. What Bitman was suggesting was a dangerous experimental use of Neurontin. The government had agreed only that Neurontin could be prescribed to patients as an additional medicine when their primary drug was not enough to stop their seizures.

"I saw the actual prescription generated in front of me, so that was certainly nice," Bitman explained, "and I certainly felt that me being there, I had some influence on the medical decision."

The second patient Bitman boasted about was a sixty-five-year-old war veteran, who had worked as a painter. He was complaining of nerve pain in his limbs. The man had been hurt when he was exposed to lead paint, Bitman said, and had also been shot by a machine gun in the war.

The doctor had already tried to remedy the man's pain by prescribing Neurontin. When he began taking the pills, however, his vision became blurred. The doctor had stopped the prescription.

Bitman said he told the neurologist that he knew of other patients whose vision had blurred when they started to take Neurontin, but the problem went away as their bodies adjusted to the drug. On the basis of information that was accumulating about the drug, this appeared to be true for some, but not all, patients. Double vision was also a sign of the drug's toxicity.

Bitman told the doctor the man should be put back on Neurontin, but at a lower dose. She agreed.

"So again, you know, I felt like I influenced that particular situation," Bitman proudly explained. "And the patient, you know, basically agreed to give the drug a try again. So again another prescription was generated."

FRANKLIN REMEMBERS HOW his bosses justified their aggressive marketing push in internal discussions. The executives claimed that Neurontin was safe for patients, even when prescribed in very high doses. Therefore, these executives had explained, it was reasonable to tempt doctors to prescribe it for nearly any neurological condition, just to see what happened.

The executives were driven to push Neurontin by a corporate compensation system that awarded them bonuses as revenues and prescriptions rose. To get the sales force fired up, the company also sponsored internal contests that challenged employees to sell harder. Shortly after Franklin joined the company, executives announced that he and his colleagues would win a pleasure cruise in the Caribbean if sales reached a certain goal.

"I've just seen the latest weekly prescription report," Anthony Wild, the president of the company's pharmaceutical operations, reported to Franklin and the rest of the sales force in a voice mail message in the spring of 1996. "It's truly wonderful, wonderful results, with highs reached for our major products."

The potential rewards grew more lucrative as executives climbed the management ranks. Even an executive in middle management could quickly become comfortable with a salary and bonus large enough to pay for one of the biggest houses in the neighborhood, a shiny new Mercedes, and a country club membership. Everyone was making really good money. What could be wrong with that?

AS EXECUTIVES IN corporate headquarters celebrated the fast-rising prescriptions, a couple of hundred miles away in Rockville, Maryland, the FDA was receiving hundreds of reports about patients who appeared to have been harmed by Neurontin. The patients suffered from dozens of different adverse effects. Confusion. Abnormal thinking. Hallucinations. Falls. Accidents. Extreme fatigue. Increased blood pressure. Sudden death. The reports were piling up.

At the same time, more doctors were complaining the drug did not work.

"My principle exposure to Neurontin has been an attempted use for the treatment of chronic severe pain disorder," explained one neurologist. "My experience has been that it has not benefited the one or two patients I've put on it."

Warner-Lambert had paid that physician and a group of his colleagues two hundred dollars each to explain why they were not yet prescribing Neurontin, which was known generically as gabapentin. The executives hoped to learn how they could turn these doctors around.

"I tried it on two patients and I went up to 1800 mg and there were more side effects and less control," explained another neurologist in the group.

"We use it as second or third line, and it's hard to tell about efficacy," said a third. "Some epileptologists like to call it 'gaba-water' instead of gabapentin."

Yet the Neurontin marketers were unswayed by such complaints. After reading these comments, Jackie Rizzo, an executive in the company's market research department, called the doctors "slow adopters" who had simply not yet been to enough of the company's all-expense-paid events.

"If these physicians can be persuaded to attend a thought leader session, educational meeting, etc., their prescribing activities should be tracked," she wrote in a memo to other executives, "to determine their promotion responsiveness."

Franklin also began hearing about patients who had been harmed by the drug. In May 1996, Franklin called on a physician in Revere, Massachusetts, and told him, as the company had trained him to do, that Neurontin was safe for a multitude of uses.

The doctor was unconvinced. Franklin remembers that the physician responded, "You keep telling me it's a benign drug, and it's not."

The doctor then rifled through the piles of papers on his desk. He pulled one from the midst of a stack and handed it to Franklin. It was a recent medical report about Neurontin. The article described seven children who suffered from epilepsy and also had been diagnosed with attention deficit disorder or developmental problems. The doctors writing the report said that Neurontin had aggravated the children's behavior. The kids grew defiant and more hyperactive. They threw tantrums and became aggressive. The doctors said they had been forced to take the children off the drug or greatly reduce the dose.

Franklin was stunned by the report. His superiors expected him to tell doctors that Neurontin helped children with attention deficit disorder. And now a doctor had shown him a report on how Neurontin had harmed some of these kids.

He sat in his car outside the physician's office and cried. He now knew that by following his bosses' orders, he was putting patients' lives in danger. It was too much for the scientist, just starting out in the corporate world, who had believed that industrial medicine could help people.

He felt he had to do something. Somehow, he had to stop an operation that was being lauded by the company's highest executives. He cried because he knew he was not up for such a challenge. He didn't have the guts to stand up and try to stop the company he worked for.

"I froze," he said, "cried for the victim, and loathed my own limitations."

A couple of weeks later, Franklin was driving to a dinner meeting with Phil Magistro and Lisa Kellett, who also worked as a medical liaison. Franklin asked Magistro if he had read the article about children taking Neurontin.

"Yeah," Magistro replied, "but it's such a small number of kids, and they can just take them off if it happens. There's no permanent effect."

Kellett then told Franklin what to do if other doctors mentioned the article. "If they ask," she said, "just tell them there is a single report, but there are problems with it, and the kids involved had multiple problems."

"But what if it's true," Franklin asked, "and these kids start to get worse or hurt themselves in an outburst?"

"What are the chances," Magistro replied. "Besides the doctor shouldn't have been using the stuff off-label anyway."

They laughed.

"No, don't worry," Magistro said. "It will never get back to us."

FRANKLIN COULD NOT get those children out of his head.

He began to think about how he could keep himself from getting pulled deeper into the crime. That was when he started to record voice mail messages left by the executives and save the memos that crossed his desk, which described how the company was selling Neurontin.

In July 1996, only four months after being hired, Franklin decided he had to resign. He told the executives he believed the company was breaking the law and that he could no longer do what they were asking of him.

His resignation set off alarm bells in the management ranks. Phil Magistro called him, demanding that they meet to talk about what had happened. Franklin remembered how he felt threatened as Magistro yelled at him and told him he should leave quietly or face the possibility of being made a scapegoat for what had gone down.

The company's lawyers began calling him repeatedly, asking him to meet them in "a public place" to talk about why he had resigned.

"I was completely stressed out, very, very anxious about what was going on, about the phone calls I was getting," he said, "and what I was going to do next—extremely anxious and really running scared."

To protect himself, he went to talk to lawyers at Greene & Hoffman, a law firm in Boston. He told them he was frightened he could be charged with a crime for following his bosses' orders.

Eventually he and his lawyers used the evidence he had gathered to file a lawsuit against Warner-Lambert and its subsidiary Parke-Davis under the False Claims Act, a federal law passed in 1863 at the urging of

President Abraham Lincoln. The law had been directed at war profiteers who were selling the Union army guns that could not fire, horses that could not walk, and bags of "gunpowder" that contained only sawdust. The fraud by the private supply companies cost taxpayers millions of dollars and put the lives of soldiers at risk.

Congress designed the False Claims Act to encourage citizens with knowledge of a fraud against the government to file lawsuits disclosing the criminal acts. As a reward, the whistle-blowers are entitled to a percentage of the financial damages the government ultimately collects from those committing the fraud.

The law was based on qui tam actions, which were first used in thirteenth-century England. The name comes from the Latin phrase *qui tam pro domino rege quam pro sic ipso in hoc parte sequitur*, which means "he who sues for the king in this matter sues for himself as well."

In August 1996 Franklin and his lawyer, Thomas Greene, filed the lawsuit in U.S. District Court in Boston. They argued that Warner-Lambert had defrauded taxpayers of hundreds of millions of dollars, the amount paid for the experimental Neurontin prescriptions that doctors had given to thousands of poor patients covered by state Medicaid programs. They claimed the company's executives had hatched an illegal marketing scheme to promote the epilepsy drug for medical uses that were not supported by the FDA or by science. The company not only had lied about the benefits of Neurontin, they argued, but also had paid tens of millions of dollars in illegal kickbacks to doctors who agreed to experiment with Neurontin on their patients. The kickbacks included the cash the company paid to thousands of physicians, as well as the amounts spent to entertain them at hundreds of vacation retreats and gourmet dinners held around the country.

Around that same time, the federal government launched a criminal investigation into the company's promotion of the epilepsy drug. The government's inquiry eventually forced executives to turn over more than 160,000 pages of internal documents.

Yet the public did not learn about the lawsuit or the investigation for years. The law requires that a lawsuit filed under the False Claims Act be kept secret, even from those it charges with fraud, until the government has time to investigate and decide whether it wants to join in the lawsuit.

Years went by. Pfizer bought Warner-Lambert in a hostile takeover in 2000, and many executives left the company. Yet doctors across the country continued to prescribe Neurontin for everything from bipolar disorder to alcohol withdrawal. In 2000 the company's data showed that nearly 90 percent of Neurontin prescriptions had been written for uses the government had not approved.

Injury reports continued to stream into the FDA. Many of the patients who appeared to have been harmed by Neurontin had received doses much higher than the maximum approved by the FDA. These massive doses were just what Parke-Davis's aggressive marketers had urged doctors to prescribe, but they made patients drowsy and dizzy. Their vision blurred. One patient reported having five or six automobile accidents while taking a daily dose of 3,600 milligrams, twice the government's recommended maximum. A pharmacist reported that another patient taking high doses of Neurontin had suffered a concussion in an accident. A woman reported that her husband, a diabetic, had died. The forty-three-year-old man had sometimes suffered from hypoglycemia in the middle of the night, his wife had explained. Before taking Neurontin, this had not been a problem, she said. He had awakened when his blood sugar fell too low, she said, and solved the problem on his own. Hypoglycemia can be quickly remedied by drinking juice or swallowing a spoonful of honey. But Neurontin made her husband so tired, she said, that he no longer woke up. In the month that he took Neurontin, she said, an ambulance was called twice after he had fallen into a hypoglycemic coma. The last time the ambulance took her husband away, she wrote, he died.

At the same time, researchers working independently from Parke-Davis began to report that Neurontin did not work for many of the experimental uses the company had promoted it for. In some cases, the patients' conditions grew worse when they took the drug.

In one study, Dr. Jonathan Sporn, a clinical fellow in the mood and anxiety program at the National Institute of Mental Health, reported that

Neurontin worked no better than a sugar pill for patients with obsessive-compulsive disorder. Researchers at the Northwest Missouri Psychiatric Rehabilitation Center said they had found that some hospitalized patients who were given Neurontin for mania caused by bipolar disorder became more aggressive after starting the drug.

"Neurontin is being used like water for disorders where there is not much evidence it is effective," Dr. Sporn said in 2002. "Nobody even knows how it works."

The next year, Dr. Alicia Mack, a pharmacist and instructor at the University of Pittsburgh, reported that she had searched the medical literature for scientific proof that Neurontin worked for ten different conditions that Parke-Davis had promoted it for. She did not find much. Most of the articles she found described small studies that lacked the controls needed for good research. Others were little more than stories of patients who appeared to improve while taking Neurontin. Some of these were written by physicians who had been paid by Parke-Davis.

Dr. Mack cautioned doctors about prescribing Neurontin for anything more than its government-approved uses, which by then included two groups of patients. Besides its limited use in epilepsy, the government had agreed in 2002 that Neurontin could also treat patients suffering from nerve pain caused by shingles. Regulators approved the wider use of the drug after Pfizer provided studies showing it could help some patients with this kind of pain. Dr. Mack noted that there was some limited evidence that Neurontin worked for migraines and nerve pain suffered by diabetics. But she said there were no good-quality studies supporting its use for attention deficit disorder, bipolar disorder, restless leg syndrome, or four other conditions doctors were prescribing it for. As many as 95 percent of patients taking Neurontin were getting it for off-label uses, she said. The doctors writing many of those prescriptions appeared to have been swayed by marketing, she said, and not by good science.

By the time of Dr. Mack's review, Parke-Davis had finally published the results of a clinical trial in which its scientists gave Neurontin to patients with bipolar disorder. Franklin had detailed in his lawsuit how he had been trained to tell physicians that preliminary results from this trial were indicating that Neurontin helped 90 percent of patients suffering bipolar disorder. The company had completed the study by 1998 or earlier but did not publish the results until September 2000. That was the year the company had expected the drug's patent to expire, meaning it would stop promoting the drug.

The results of that long-delayed study: the sugar tablets worked better than Neurontin.

FOR MORE THAN seven years, Thomas Greene and the other lawyers on his small staff fought efforts by Warner-Lambert, and later by Pfizer, to have the case thrown out of court. The corporate lawyers argued that marketing had nothing to do with how doctors had prescribed Neurontin. Instead, physicians had independently prescribed the drug, they said, on the basis of their personal professional judgments.

The corporate lawyers also argued that the cash payments to physicians were not illegal kickbacks for prescribing Neurontin but compensation for their services to the company. They further argued that the meetings and dinners held for physicians had been educational in nature. They said these were events at which the speakers presented information based on their personal experience and scientific knowledge. They also argued that Warner-Lambert's marketing was not fraudulent but consistent with standard practices in the pharmaceutical industry.

As the case dragged on, Franklin lost hope that he could somehow stop the marketing practices that were leading doctors to prescribe medicines in ways that hurt their patients. He lost some other things as well. One day, a federal investigator working on the case told him that his friends would see him differently now that he was a corporate whistleblower. Another federal agent told him his life was over. As the years passed, he began to understand how right they were.

Warner-Lambert and Pfizer were intent on more than just winning the case. The companies wanted to keep Americans from finding out what had gone on. Their lawyers argued in court that the internal corporate papers that Franklin and his lawyers had submitted as evidence of the crime should be hidden from public view. They asked the court to place a protective seal on dozens of boxes filled with corporate memos and marketing plans. The lawyers argued the documents held confidential trade secrets that would hurt the company's business interests if they were revealed.

This had been the same argument made by other pharmaceutical companies in dozens of similar lawsuits, and in most cases the corporate lawyers had succeeded in quickly sealing the records to keep them from scrutiny. The documents detailing what may have been fraud or another crime were boxed up and sent back to the company's warehouse, never to be seen by anyone outside the company again. This has allowed some companies to continue the same practices while patients are left in the dark about the harm a drug or another product has already caused.

Greene and Franklin were not about to let that happen in the case of Warner-Lambert. Greene argued in court that the public had a right to know how the company had marketed Neurontin. In 2002 *The New York Times*, NBC, and National Public Radio joined Greene in court and also demanded that the sealed documents be released to the public. The news organizations argued that the papers would shed light on an alleged marketing scheme that may have threatened the health of thousands of people.

Federal judge Patti B. Saris later agreed that corporate lawyers had wrongly stamped "confidential" on hundreds of internal corporate documents. Gradually more evidence was revealed.

IN MAY 2004, Warner-Lambert, then a division of Pfizer, pleaded guilty to criminal charges and agreed to pay $430 million to resolve the allegations that it had illegally marketed Neurontin. The money helped repay taxpayers for part of what they had spent on experimental prescriptions for Neurontin written by doctors for patients in the government's Medicaid program.

Yet even as federal prosecutors announced the settlement, it was clear that Warner-Lambert's investment in the illegal marketing scheme had been a profitable venture. Even a fine of nearly a half billion dollars was only a fraction of the profits that Pfizer was now earning from the drug. On the day of the announcement of the settlement, experts estimated that 90 percent of Neurontin's prescriptions were for uses the government had not approved. That meant Pfizer could thank the illegal plan for most of the ten billion dollars the company had earned from sales of Neurontin since it had taken over Warner-Lambert in 2000.

No Warner-Lambert executives or the physicians they paid were indicted. And much of what Warner-Lambert did to promote Neurontin for experimental uses remains common practice in America's medical system. The drug companies continue to pay physicians to promote their corporate products for them. And many physicians continue to rely on the drug companies to support their lifestyles. In 1996, the year Franklin worked for Warner-Lambert, the drug industry paid for 151,434 dinners, retreats, meetings, or other events for America's physicians. By 2004 the number of those corporate-paid parties and events for physicians had more than tripled to 536,734. That came to 1,470 events every day, including Saturdays and Sundays. The industry paid for more dinners and events in 2004 than the nation had doctors.

It later became clear that the Neurontin case was hardly an aberration in the pharmaceutical industry. In 2005, an official in the U.S. Justice Department testified before Congress that the government had begun 180 separate investigations of the marketing practices of pharmaceutical companies. The investigations involved dozens of companies and hundreds of drugs.

"We are not seeing isolated instances of misconduct," Ronald J. Tenpas, associate deputy attorney general, told a House committee in 2007, "but repeated practices within the industry that have resulted in significant losses to federal health care programs."

Some pharmaceutical executives have brushed off these facts as much ado about nothing. "Of course there are overreaching business practices that some pharmaceutical companies sometimes utilize, such as selling too hard, charging too much, or taking advantage of consumer ignorance with overstated direct-to-consumer advertising," wrote Howard Solomon, the chairman of Forest Laboratories, in a letter to shareholders in 2002. "And, of course, it is appropriate to criticize, and in a proper case, to take action against such excesses but, at the same time, to realize that all businesses have comparable excesses. And maybe that is the way our economic system works because it is managed by a flawed species and not by saints."

Perhaps the only thing that made the Neurontin case unique was that the companies had failed in their attempts to keep the documents and the facts of the fraud a secret.

Franklin was the only employee at Warner-Lambert who publicly complained about the company's aggressive marketing practices, even though hundreds of employees appeared to be involved. How could so many other executives and salespeople go along with such a fraud, and even applaud it, when it put human lives at risk?

An answer can be found in the work of J. Scott Armstrong, a professor of marketing at the Wharton School at the University of Pennsylvania. In the 1970s Professor Armstrong set out to delve deeper into what researchers had already discovered about corporate executives: they can be expected to harm others as they go about their job. The executives make decisions that hurt people or society, the researchers found, because their foremost responsibility in America's corporate system is to maximize profits for shareholders. The interests of society are far less important.

Professor Armstrong used the case of a drug company selling a potentially lethal product to take this research a step further. He had almost two thousand college business students and executive trainees take part in a role-playing experiment in which they acted as the executives and directors of a pharmaceutical company. Armstrong told the participants that they needed to make a decision about a drug that was bringing in sales of twenty million dollars a year and was a significant contributor to the company's bottom line. Federal regulators and independent scientists had determined that the drug was needlessly causing the deaths of twenty people a year. Regulators had asked the company to take the drug off the market because there were plenty of cheap alternative medicines that did not have its deadly side effects. Armstrong gave the participants five options that ranged from immediately recalling the drug to continuing to promote it aggressively. As Armstrong explained, the numbers came down to the company's earning a million dollars for each person who died if it continued to promote the drug.

The scenario was based on an actual case in the pharmaceutical industry. In 1969 the drug company Upjohn had used its money and power in Washington to stop the FDA from removing a dangerous drug called Panalba from pharmacy shelves. Upjohn fought the FDA for years until it finally stopped selling the drug.

Armstrong presented the case study to dozens of groups of students and management trainees. As the students played the roles of the Upjohn executives and directors, not one of the groups decided to remove the drug quickly from the market to ensure that no more patients died. And 79 percent of the groups took the most socially irresponsible option of continuing to promote the drug while trying to stop the FDA from removing it from pharmacies. For these students and trainees, who were playing the roles of the executives they would soon become, profits took precedence over patients.

Armstrong's role-playing study begins to explain what motivated Warner-Lambert executives to promote Neurontin so aggressively that patients were harmed. Chief executives live in a rarefied world of limousines, corporate jets, and the finest things money can buy. They couldn't be farther away from hospital halls, morgues, and the families of people harmed by their products or actions. In some ways, the executives are like puppeteers. They are not the ones calling on doctors and proclaiming that a drug can treat just about anything. Instead, they're pulling the strings from behind the scenes and letting their aides do the dirty work.

But this still does not explain why physicians went along with Warner-Lambert's marketing scheme. The physicians had no responsibility to help the company's shareholders. Their essential duty was to their patients and to their oath: First, do no harm.

Social scientists have found that gifts as small as a cup of coffee can change the behavior of the recipient in ways that he or she does not even realize. The friendly giving of a penlight or key chain imbues a person with a sense of indebtedness. Whether he or she is conscious of it or not, the recipient feels the need to return the favor. Most doctors believe a gift can't sway their judgment, that they are somehow different from everyone else. Study after study has shown they are wrong.

If the giving of trinkets could increase sales, Warner-Lambert found that an all-expense-paid weekend at the Ritz-Carlton, with a $250 check thrown in, worked even better.

THE SETTLEMENT MADE Franklin a very wealthy man. He and his lawyers received $28 million of the total paid by Pfizer, the amount allotted to him as a whistle-blower by the False Claims Act.

When word of his case got out, he started to receive letters and calls from patients who had taken Neurontin. Some asked for advice on how to get off the drug. Some said they wanted to file suit against Warner-Lambert. A few people who were not patients also wrote him letters, including some who were furious with what he had done. Some suggested ways of killing himself.

After the settlement, Franklin and his wife purchased a small school, where he says he is trying to help gifted children who were languishing elsewhere. He said he has never been able to forgive himself for going along with his bosses' orders during the months he worked at Warner-Lambert. He said he shuddered to think that people may have been hurt by the lies he told doctors about Neurontin.

"I was encouraging doctors to experiment on patients," he said. "That's what I'm most ashamed of."

Franklin said he imagined doctors handing their patients a prescription for Neurontin and promising their troubles would disappear.

"Patients walked away," he said, "thinking they had something that could help them."

Part III

A BITTER PILL

EIGHT

Altered State

A DRY SPELL caused Iowa's rivers to run low in the fall of 2001. It was then that a crew of scientists dropped probes off the sides of bridges and waded into the murky currents to collect samples of the receding water. Tests of their specimens amazed them. They found traces of painkillers, antibiotics, antihistamines, and blood pressure medications, all of them lingering remnants of pills swallowed by the residents of cities upstream. The scientists had found striking evidence of just how extensive Iowans' use of prescription drugs had become.

Thirty percent of the water samples were laced with Tagamet, the drug that soothes heartburn and stomach complaints. Twenty percent held traces of codeine, a powerful narcotic. Another 20 percent contained tiny bits of Cardizem, a popular medicine used to control hypertension. Some samples were tinged not just with one prescription drug but with a cocktail of several.

The scientists found the vestiges of the prescription drugs downstream from wastewater treatment plants in Des Moines, Iowa City, Cedar Rapids, and seven other Iowa cities. The active chemical ingredients in the pills had gone through the bodies of the humans who took them and then flowed from toilets into the sewers. The Iowa treatment plants, just like those in cities across the country, were not designed to find and remove the pharmaceuticals before the water was released, gushing from large metal pipes, back into the rivers.

Dr. Dana Kolpin, the leader of the team and a scientist with the U.S. Geological Survey, knew most of the drugs were coming from homes in the cities because the team also tested the water upstream from the urban neighborhoods. The upstream water had trace amounts of some prescription drugs, but at far lower concentrations.

Most remarkable, the team found that about 70 percent of the downstream water samples were tainted with traces of Tegretol, a drug for epilepsy that doctors had started to prescribe for everything from pain to mood disorders.

"That just floored me," Dr. Kolpin told me, referring to the Tegretol data. "I thought there can't be that many epileptics in Iowa. It seems to be a persistent compound. It's really resilient. We don't know what that means."

This was not the first time that Dr. Kolpin, an Iowa-born hydrologist, had found prescription drugs in the state's waters. In 1999 he organized the first nationwide study that looked for pharmaceuticals in rivers and streams. The findings of that study were published in 2002. It found prescription drugs, as well as fragrances, insect repellents, disinfectants, and other household chemicals, in 80 percent of the 139 streams sampled in Iowa and twenty-nine other states.

Just what it means to be swallowing the flotsam and jetsam of thousands of medicine chests is a mystery that Dr. Kolpin says may not be solved for generations. The levels of any one drug in the rivers are so low that it would take many years of drinking the water to get even one therapeutic dose. But pharmaceuticals are different from other chemicals, including pesticides, in that they are designed to have an effect on the human body. And it's not just one drug that scientists are worried about. Americans are taking thousands of different medicines, and scientists like Kolpin are finding traces in the rivers of just about every drug they search for.

Scientists have already discovered changes in the ecosystem that they believe may be caused by the witch's brew of pharmaceuticals flowing through the nation's waters. Some species of fish may be among the first casualties.

In 2006 Dr. Vicki Blazer, a fish pathologist with the U.S. Geological Survey, reported that a team had caught dozens of bass on the Potomac River and its tributaries in Virginia and Maryland that had strange sexual deformities. The fish were males but had taken on female traits. They had immature eggs growing inside their testes. At several sites, every male smallmouth bass the team pulled from the water had eggs inside. Dr. Blazer said it appeared the fish had been harmed by a combination of pollutants. Among the suspected culprits were the traces of ethinyl estradiol, the active ingredient in birth control pills, that had been found in the Potomac's waters.

Another scientist, Dr. Marsha Black, a professor of environmental health at the University of Georgia, has studied in the laboratory what happens when fish and frogs swim in waters tainted with antidepressants. She found that mosquito fish, small and hardy creatures, became uncoordinated and lethargic when they swam in waters infused with low levels of Prozac. In another study she and her colleagues found that tadpoles took longer to turn into frogs when they lived in water tainted with small amounts of the antidepressant. Even when she reduced the level of Prozac to the minuscule amount that scientists have found in the nation's rivers, the frogs swimming in it were significantly smaller than those in clean water.

If the growth of frogs is being stunted and male fish are producing eggs, could far more subtle changes be occurring in humans? And what other environmental consequences may await us? Already scientists have traced a widespread ecological disaster of a different sort to a prescription drug.

In 2000 Dr. J. Lindsay Oaks, an assistant professor of veterinary medicine at Washington State University, began investigating a mysterious 95 percent plunge in the number of vultures in Pakistan. Three years later he had his answer.

South Asian farmers had begun to give their cattle a drug called di-clofenac, an anti-inflammatory pain reliever that is prescribed to Americans suffering from arthritis. The farmers used the drug in their cattle because it was cheap and they believed it would ward off lameness and fever. The farmers depend on vultures to eat the carcasses of cattle that die. But when the vultures ate the dead animals, they also ingested the drug, which proved to be an acute poison in their bodies that caused their kidneys to fail. Many of the birds died within days of eating the drug-tainted beef.

The case of the dying vultures showed just how quickly a single drug could devastate a species and upset the ecological balance. With the vultures no longer around to eat dead animals, the South Asians found that the population of wild dogs increased, leading to a risk that more humans could be infected with rabies. There was also a fear that the rat population would rise, bringing a heightened threat of the diseases spread by rodents, including the bubonic plague.

Despite the risks of these ecological disasters, the United States does not regulate the amount of pharmaceuticals that can be released into rivers and lakes, a fact that scientists are beginning to question as Americans take ever more pills.

"We're a chemically dependent society," Dr. Kolpin said. "We need to understand the consequences."

AMERICANS WERE WELL versed in the virtues of their daily meds. The industry had made sure of that through its almost Orwellian promotion. What the public had largely overlooked was what was happening around them as a result of the fast-rising prescriptions.

The industry's heavy marketing of prescription drugs was bringing about a great societal shift in America, not unlike that brought on by the introduction of other technologies like the Internet, electricity, or the printing press. The changes that came when a nation was fully medicated, however, were not all good as so many believed. Even those not taking medications could not escape their effects. It was becoming increasingly clear that the amazing success of the pharmaceutical industry had come at an equally amazing cost.

The medicine remnants running through the cold currents of Iowa's rivers were just the beginning.

HOOKED

A white sign posted on the street outside McCombs Middle School in Des Moines sends a warning to all who would enter. The word DRUGS is written across the sign's face. A black circle encases the word. A bold line slashes through the circle and its captured noun, a symbol marking the boundary of the drug-free school zone.

But on the morning of Wednesday, March 9, 2005, a young student did not heed the warning. The teen carried several prescription pills through the black metal doors of the brick school building and handed them to two other students. One teen swallowed some of the pills and passed out. The tablets were a medicine called clonidine that doctors prescribe to adults to lower their blood pressures and slow their hearts. Physicians also prescribe the drug to children diagnosed with attention deficit disorder, although the government has not approved it for such use.

Jean Phillips, the nursing coordinator for the Des Moines Public School District, said that incidents involving the illegal trading of medicines on school grounds had been rare. But she said the event that March day did not surprise her. She said students visit the school nurse's office frequently throughout the day, complaining of pain and asking for pills. Children had come to believe through watching advertisements on television, she said, that prescription pills swiftly cured whatever ailed them. "We're a society that looks for the quick fix and the magic pill," she said. "We're looking for the instant solution."

The incident in Des Moines was not the only one that week involving young students trading prescription drugs inside the nation's schools. Two days later, seven girls at Meadowdale Middle School in Lynnwood, Washington, were hospitalized after taking blood pressure pills that officials believed had been prescribed to one of the students' parents. School and city officials told a reporter for the *Herald* of Everett, Washington, that the girls had apparently each swallowed as many as five tablets of the drug, while hanging out in the school's restroom.

Greg Macke, the assistant fire chief, said the girls were lucky. The pills can cause a person's heart rate to plummet. A large overdose can lead to death. "We've run into this problem before," he said. "We believe there's this trend now that kids are not educated to the risk of medications that are not prescribed to them."

Teenagers for generations have been tempted to "do drugs." More of them now seemed to believe they could use prescription drugs to get a thrill without the danger that comes with taking an illegal substance like cocaine.

Three days later officials in northwestern Indiana discovered young teenagers trading powerful prescription painkillers on a school bus. Sergeant Tim Emmons of the Porter County Sheriff's Department told the *Post-Tribune* of Gary that officers had found three hydrocodone pills and five oxycodone tablets hidden in a sunglass case belonging to a fifteen-year-old boy. Both drugs are opioids, a class of painkillers that also includes the illegal drug heroin.

The boy told the authorities he had taken the narcotics from his parents' lockbox. He took them, he said, "for fun and to get high." He gave two tablets to a girl on the school bus. The fourteen-year-old girl then gave one of the pills to another eighth-grade girl inside Union Township Middle School.

The three students were arrested and taken to the county's Juvenile Detention Center. Sergeant Emmons said the boy and girl who traded the pills faced criminal charges that could result in a fifty-eight-year prison sentence if they were filed against an adult. Two other eighth graders in Porter County had been arrested just the month before. Those students had traded a generic form of Prozac during school lunch.

It was not just schoolchildren being charged with crimes involving prescription drugs that week. Two days after the incident on the Indiana school bus, Michigan authorities charged an assistant principal at West Middle School in Ypsilanti with stealing tablets of Adderall, a stimulant made of amphetamine, from a school cabinet. Students diagnosed with ADHD had legally brought the pills to school.

Officials at the Ypsilanti middle school had found more than two hundred Adderall tablets missing from the locked cupboard. Marcus Burlingame, the assistant principal, admitted to stealing fewer than twenty of the pills. He said he had become addicted to Adderall after being diagnosed with an attention disorder himself. He had taken the children's pills, he said, to add to the number provided by his own physician.

These school crimes occurred over the course of ten days. They showed how the fastest-growing danger of abuse and addiction for the nation's children in the early twenty-first century was not from cocaine flowing in from a South American drug cartel or from ecstasy, heroin, or the other illegal substances that have long been the focus of the nation's "War on Drugs." Instead, it came from prescription pills legally manufactured on U.S. soil and sitting in Americans' medicine chests.

The number of Americans who admitted in a survey that they were abusing prescription drugs nearly doubled from 1992 to 2003, according to a report in 2005 by the National Center on Addiction and Substance Abuse at Columbia University. Between those years, abuse of prescription drugs grew at a rate that was twice that involving marijuana, five times that involving cocaine, and sixty times the abuse involving heroin.

The researchers found in their surveys that more Americans admitted they had abused prescription drugs than the combined numbers of those admitting to using cocaine, hallucinogens, inhalants, or heroin. Most alarming was the 212 percent rise of prescription drug abuse found among teenagers during those years. Some parents had become unwitting drug pushers, the researchers said, by filling their bathroom cabinets with addictive prescription narcotics, depressants, and stimulants.

But there was more behind the rise in addiction than medicine chests stocked full. Today's children are the first generation to grow up with omnipresent prescription drug ads. A child turning eighteen in 2006 was nine years old in 1997, when the FDA weakened its drug advertising restrictions and allowed the companies to run ads on television. As Jean Phillips had noticed in the students in Des Moines, the children had come to believe there was a pill for any trouble. They understood that illegal street drugs could kill them, but they saw prescription drugs in a different light. The underlying message in the television ads filled with sunshine and flowers was that prescription drugs were safe and even good for you.

Some pharmaceutical companies had helped fuel the nation's epidemic of drug abuse by advertising even those products that were the most addictive, despite an international treaty that prohibited such promotion. The Convention on Psychotropic Substances was signed by dozens of countries in 1971 to limit the abuse of addictive psychoactive drugs like barbiturates, amphetamines, and LSD. Some of the most frequent violators of the treaty have been companies selling prescription stimulants to American children with attention deficit disorders.

In 2001, a company called Celltech was the first to use consumer advertisements to promote a prescription drug that had been classified as a Schedule II substance by drug enforcement officials. Drugs on Schedule II are the nation's most addictive drugs that also have a medical purpose. Only Schedule I drugs, which include cocaine, heroin, and other drugs with no legal purpose, are more tightly controlled by the Drug Enforcement Administration.

With children getting ready to return to school in August 2001, Celltech ran ads for Metadate CD, a pill made with methylphenidate, which is also the active ingredient in Ritalin. It can swiftly become a habit if it is misused. The Metadate ads ran in the back-to-school section of magazines like the *Ladies' Home Journal*, where they were tucked among the promotions for Life cereal, bologna, and Jell-O pudding. The company also targeted children by creating a Superman-like character wearing blue tights with the initials "CD" emblazoned across his chest. "A new hero for ADHD patients is here!" pronounced the company's brochure.

Celltech stopped the ads after a warning from drug enforcement officials. But it was only a brief lull in the advertising battle to sell stimulants for children. In the following years two other companies—Shire, the maker of Adderall, and Johnson & Johnson, which sells Concerta—heavily advertised their prescription stimulants to the public.

"With Concerta, I see Matt. Not his ADHD," said the tagline in an ad featuring a freckle-faced, grinning kid in *Parade* magazine in 2005. The ad promoted the pill as an academic booster, claiming it would improve math scores by "up to one full grade." In tiny print on the next page was a long list of warnings about Concerta's dangers, including that it could "lead to dependence."

That danger of dependence had already become real for tens of thousands of young Americans. In 2006, researchers estimated that seventy-five thousand American teenagers and young adults showed signs of being addicted to stimulants like Concerta, Adderall, and Ritalin. The data, culled from a survey of households in 2002, found that more than seven million Americans had misused stimulant drugs like Ritalin that year. The results confirmed reports by doctors who said that more patients were requesting stimulants for themselves or their children—not because of mental illness but to enhance their concentration and performance at work or at school.

THE MAKERS OF narcotic painkillers took a different marketing tack. Beginning in the 1990s, companies selling narcotics spent heavily to convince doctors and American consumers that their products were not as addictive or dangerous as the public believed. This campaign was led by Purdue Pharma, a private company that was selling a pill called OxyContin and had its sights set on being among the country's ten largest drugmakers.

Purdue was founded by Dr. Arthur M. Sackler, a psychiatrist from New York City, and his two brothers. Dr. Sackler is credited by many pharmaceutical and advertising executives for coming up with some of the industry's most aggressive and effective promotional techniques. In 1997, he was inducted into the industry's Medical Advertising Hall of Fame, which hailed his success in the 1960s in turning the tranquilizer Valium into the world's first $100 million drug. The Sackler family has used some of its enormous wealth to build new wings at some of the world's most prominent art museums, including the Smithsonian in Washington and Manhattan's Metropolitan Museum of Art. Dr. Sackler died in 1987, but his company continued in his tradition of using sly marketing maneuvers that were not apparent unless you knew what you were looking for.

The main message of Purdue's campaign was that many patients were needlessly suffering from chronic and serious pain because doctors were too hesitant to prescribe narcotics like OxyContin, which offered powerful relief. Purdue spent tens of millions of dollars between 1996 and 2000 flying doctors, nurses, and pharmacists to resort hotels in places like Boca Raton, Florida, and Scottsdale, Arizona, where they were wined and dined and trained as speakers to spread the word that painkillers like OxyContin were safe. By 2002 Purdue's list of trained lecturers included twenty-five hundred physicians. These speakers went back to their hometowns, where Purdue paid them to speak at local hospitals and before medical groups. The audiences at these lectures also often received checks written by Purdue.

To promote its drug to consumers, the company created a website, Partners Against Pain, where families could order a video that claimed drugs like OxyContin caused addiction in less than 1 percent of patients, a statement that federal drug regulators said was not supported by fact.

Purdue sales reps gave out coupons that allowed thousands of patients to try a thirty-day supply of OxyContin for free. The salespeople turned physicians into walking billboards for the drug by giving them OxyContin fishing hats, coffee mugs, and luggage tags. Some doctors' offices received plush stuffed toys with the OxyContin logo.

Before Purdue's campaign, doctors had prescribed opioid narcotics—that is, the dozens of different drugs containing opium or any of its derivatives—mostly to patients who were in severe pain from cancer, injuries, or other diseases. Those patients welcomed the strong pain relief that the narcotics delivered despite their many dangers. But Purdue and some of the other manufacturers were not content with selling their narcotics just to patients in severe pain. As soon as the FDA approved Oxy-Contin in 1995, executives ordered the company's battalion of sales reps to sell the drug to doctors for everything from back pain to arthritis, conditions that could be readily treated with a myriad of nonnarcotic pain relievers that did not come with the serious risk of addiction.

Purdue's own confidential documents explain that a key goal of executives was to set consumers straight on the "myths and misconceptions about addiction." These documents say that among the company's sales "targets" were obstetricians, dentists, sports doctors, nurses, or just about any health professional who might deal with someone in pain. Two other "objectives" were to increase the use of OxyContin by elderly patients and to convince doctors that they could "aggressively" treat patients with opioid narcotics, especially OxyContin.

The company instructed its sales reps to tell doctors they could "start with and stay with" OxyContin for the treatment of patients over the long term, according to the corporate documents. The reps were to say not only that OxyContin was safe but that there was "no maximum daily dose or ceiling" on the amount patients could ingest if they still suffered pain. The sales reps were also to say that few patients built up a tolerance for the drug or found themselves needing more and more pills.

For thousands of Americans this proved untrue. In fact, the aggressive marketing by Purdue and other narcotic manufacturers helped fuel a wave of drug abuse—a problem the public often associated with blighted urban neighborhoods—in dozens of rural towns and in America's middle and upper classes.

A sign of this emerged in Iowa in 2004, when the state's largest insurer noticed a surge in the number of narcotic prescriptions filled by its members, who are mostly middle-class families covered by employers' medical plans. The number of narcotic prescriptions had risen 130 percent in just five years. Some Iowans took these painkillers as directed by their doctors, to discover only too late that they were hooked.

In 1999, Chelly Griffith was a housewife and mother of two, living in the city of Davenport, when she injured her back as she picked up her infant daughter. A doctor prescribed OxyContin, telling her it was "mobility in a bottle." The pills did not relieve her pain, however, and the doctor increased the dose. It was then that she developed an intense craving for the pills. She would wake in the morning, she said, and find she couldn't wait to swallow the drug. She took another tablet, only to find that she craved the drug again within a few hours.

Her life became a blur. She found herself doing crazy things, she said, like trimming the blades of grass in her yard with scissors to make sure they all were the same length. After three years she checked into a drug treatment facility, she said, because she didn't want her kids to see what she had become.

Once patients are addicted, they change in ways that no one could have expected. Even people with families and good jobs have turned to crime to get the pills their bodies crave.

The same month that Barry Miedema, a teacher and coach at Unity Christian High School, led the boys' basketball team to the state championship in 2005, he was caught breaking into a home in search of pain pills. Miedema taught and lived in Orange City, a town in northwestern Iowa that is home to 5,600 people, a private Christian college, and a dozen churches.

A resident of a nearby town had arrived home to find Coach Miedema in his kitchen. At first Miedema explained he was looking at paint samples. Later he confessed to searching for pills. Police said Miedema also confessed to breaking into another home several times to steal medication. In August 2005 he pleaded guilty to burglary, theft, and possession of a controlled substance without a prescription. A judge required him to serve thirty days in jail. The forty-eight-year-old championship coach said he had become addicted to the painkillers after his doctor prescribed them for pain in his hip.

Other crimes have been far worse. Some of these addiction-fueled crimes were committed by teenagers only a few years older than the middle school students in Des Moines who traded pills on school grounds.

In November 2005, nineteen-year-old Ryan Ray Wichhart of North Liberty, a town in eastern Iowa, confessed to police that he had strangled a woman working the overnight shift at a drug treatment center during his attempt to steal Xanax and Klonopin pills. Police said that Wichhart, who was being treated at the center, killed Kathi Mertens, a mother of three, and left her body on the floor of the room where medications were stored. Wichhart then stole Mertens's car to get away. Officers later found the car and Wichhart, intoxicated on the pills and alcohol, at a local Hy-Vee grocery store.

Even wealth and fame offered no protection from the potent pull of the prescription narcotics. In 2003, Rush Limbaugh, the conservative talk show host, told his radio audience that he had become addicted to pain pills and was checking into a treatment center. He started taking the narcotics, he said, after surgery on his back. Florida law enforcement authorities had begun investigating Limbaugh after his maid told the *National Enquirer* that she met him in parking lots where he handed her cigar boxes filled with cash and she gave him cigar boxes filled with pills, including OxyContin. Prosecutors later charged Limbaugh with illegally obtaining prescription painkillers from more than one doctor to feed his habit. He pleaded not guilty to the charges but agreed to settle with prosecutors by submitting to random drug tests, continuing treatment for his addiction, and not owning a gun.

Tens of thousands of Americans have not outlived their addictions. Scientists at the Centers for Disease Control reported in 2006 that they had found "a national epidemic" of deaths from accidental overdoses of prescription narcotics beginning in 1990, about the same time that sales of the drugs started to take off. Between 1979 and 1990 unintentional deaths from drug poisoning had increased an average of 5.3 percent a year, the government scientists said. After that, the numbers skyrocketed, they said, matching the sharp increase in prescription opioid sales. From 1990 to 2002 the deaths increased an average of 18 percent every year.

After news reports detailed the widespread abuse of OxyContin, Purdue Pharma changed some of its marketing practices. For example, the company said it had stopped treating doctors to all-expense-paid trips to resorts in the fall of 2000. But at least some doctors and scientists continued to benefit from the largesse of Purdue's marketing department.

In April 2004 Purdue handed Dr. Gerald Gebhart, the head of the department of pharmacology at the University of Iowa, a check for fifty thousand dollars during an event at the Marriott Hotel overlooking a long strip of white sand in Grand Cayman. Doctors, scientists, and university students from all over the world had gathered at the Caribbean paradise for the Spring Pain Research Conference, which was paid for in part by Purdue and five other pharmaceutical companies.

Purdue said that Dr. Gebhart, a prominent scientist, had been selected to receive its Prize for Pain Research. Dr. Gebhart had published dozens of papers on pain and had also served as the president of the

American Pain Society, a medical group that had received hundreds of thousands of dollars from Purdue and other narcotics manufacturers over the years. The society had worked closely with its corporate backers to promote the notion that doctors should not hesitate to prescribe high doses of OxyContin or other narcotics to patients in pain.

During the conference, the doctors and academics presented their research studies on pain and then relaxed to enjoy fishing, parasailing, scuba diving, and snorkeling with the stingrays. Purdue presented Dr. Gebhart with the fifty-thousand-dollar check on the last day of the five-day conference. That night the guests and the industry executives gathered on the beach for a farewell barbecue.

THE TAB

In February 2005 David Brennan, a top executive at AstraZeneca, revealed how the pharmaceutical industry might price its medicines in the future. He had given a keynote address to a group of health care executives and academics gathered at the Park Hyatt Hotel in Philadelphia and, in answering the group's questions, provided a glimpse of what might come next.

"We'll be able to look at you and say, 'You have got a problem, and the cost of the fix should be $250,000 over your lifetime,' he said, 'but it will get you where you want to be, which is without a heart attack when you are 50.'"

"It's going to create," he added, "a different value proposition in the industry."

Brennan was talking about genomics. In essence, he was saying that a person may soon pay a quarter of a million dollars for a designer drug or treatment, one well suited for him or her on the basis of his or her personal genes, to delay serious medical conditions until an older age. But Iowans did not have to wait for the future to pay more for their medicines than they did for a median-priced home.

In 2006 a drug called Avastin could cost cancer patients as much as $100,000 a year, depending on the dose and type of cancer. When doctors added a medicine called Erbitux to the standard chemotherapy regimen for patients with advanced colon cancer, the cost of treatment rose to as much as $250,000. For patients with a rare disorder called Gaucher's disease, the needed drug, Cerezyme, could cost more than $600,000 a year.

The pharmaceutical industry had long argued that its high prices were needed to cover the cost of discovering new medicines. Yet by 2006 some companies were setting their prices so high that even this argument no longer held up. With no controls on the price of medicine in the United States, the companies were charging whatever they could get.

Every two weeks for six months, Iowan Gary Clausen received a transfusion of three drugs to treat his colon cancer at a clinic in Council Bluffs. Each time he left with another fourteen-thousand-dollar bill.

For decades, Gary and his wife, Janice, had lived in Audubon, a town in southwestern Iowa. He worked as a self-employed trucker, hauling loads of meat to California and returning with cargoes full of fresh fruits and vegetables. Yet soon after he was diagnosed with cancer in the summer of 2006, he was forced to sell his semitruck to pay for his medical care. The tab for the drugs alone came to $180,000. Then there were the doctors and hospital to pay. The bills piled up even though he and Janice had paid for their own health insurance, a plan that cost them $8,000 a year.

Six months after his chemotherapy ended, the couple did not know how they would pay the $120,000 they still owed. And Gary was scheduled for yet another surgery.

"Our savings, everything, just went," Janice said.

Wendy Sontag, who works with cancer patients at her job at the Leukemia and Lymphoma Society in Des Moines, said such stories were no longer unusual. She regularly receives calls, she said, from cancer patients who can no longer make their mortgage payments because of the cost of their drugs, doctors, and other care. One patient sent her a copy of a five-thousand-dollar bill for Thalomid, a drug for multiple myeloma. And that was for a single prescription.

She said she believes the statistics that show that getting sick in America can quickly lead to financial disaster, even for those with insurance. "We all walk a pretty thin line," she said, "between being middle class and being poor."

Going broke might be more acceptable to families if the medicines added years to their loved ones' lives. But some of these superpriced drugs barely worked at all.

Studies had shown that colon cancer patients given Avastin—at a dose priced at fifty thousand dollars a year—lived about four or five months longer on average than patients who did not receive the drug. Patients suffering from pancreatic cancer who received Tarceva, a drug that cost two thousand dollars a month in 2005, lived on average twelve days longer than other patients. Both these drugs were made by Genentech, which posted a rise in profit in 2005 and 2006 of more than 60 percent a year.

And Mr. Brennan's company, AstraZeneca, had been charging $1,800 a month for a cancer drug called Iressa when federal researchers stopped a study of the drug because it was doing nothing to lengthen lives. AstraZeneca made almost $400 million in 2004 by selling this ineffective drug, which was also blamed for killing dozens of patients with its side effects.

The pharmaceutical companies were taking advantage of the most vulnerable patients and pricing their products as if there were no limit to what society would pay for them. Even some pharmaceutical executives had begun to complain their colleagues had gone too far.

"They say, 'Here is a drug that will increase life on the average of four or five months and for that you pay $50,000,'" Dr. Ray Vagelos, the former chief executive of Merck, said in 2006. "I can't accept that."

EVEN BEFORE EXECUTIVES started charging $100,000 for a single cancer drug, it had become routine for pharmaceutical companies to raise their prices at a rate that was several times that of inflation. The industry flourished as it combined these price hikes with powerful marketing techniques that had Americans taking more and more prescriptions. But as the cost spiraled, prescription medicines became a leading reason why health insurance was no longer affordable.

Those lucky enough to have an employer paying for their insurance may not have noticed how much their medicines cost. Many of the in-

sured often paid a copayment of just ten to thirty dollars for each prescription. One had to look beyond those copays to the actual cost of the
prescriptions paid by insurance companies, government programs, and
the uninsured to understand the burden created by the industry's practice of unrestrained pricing.

Iowans paid more for the medicines they picked up at the drugstore
in 2004 than for all the items they purchased at clothing stores, shoe
stores, furniture stores, sporting goods stores, bookstores, jewelry stores,
hobby stores, and toy stores combined. The nearly $2 billion that Iowans
spent on prescriptions filled at pharmacies was approaching the $2.7 bil-
lion they spent at all the state's fast-food joints, restaurants, and bars.
And the cost of those drugs did not even include many of the highest-
priced medicines, those for cancer and other diseases that doctors administered in their clinics or the hospital, the ones the Clausens found could
cost $180,000 for treatments lasting just six months. It also didn't in-
clude the cost of drugs given to Iowans in nursing homes.

Because the bill for prescriptions was rising faster than the cost of physician services and hospitalization, drugs were accounting for an ever-
greater share of the nation's medical spending. In 1980 the nation spent
less than 5 percent of its health care bill on prescription medications. By
2002 those prescriptions were accounting for 10.5 percent of the total cost.

But all types of medical costs were soaring, creating a national crisis
that affected every American, no matter whether rich or poor, healthy or
sick. America spent nearly $2 trillion on medical care in 2005, or $6,700
for each person. With more dollars going to health care, many people had
less to spend on education, entertainment, and just about everything else.

To pay for rising health insurance premiums for employees, companies
had been forced to raise the prices of their products so that everything from
milk to machinery was more expensive. At General Motors, executives
estimated that the company's health costs in 2004 accounted for $1,500
of the cost of each vehicle it manufactured. The auto executives said rising drug costs—$1.5 billion for GM in 2004—were hurting American
automakers' ability to compete with European and Asian manufacturers.

In Iowa many workers had watched their annual pay raises shrink or
vanish altogether as employers cut their wage and salary budgets to pay

for spiraling health insurance premiums. Even as they trimmed the size of annual raises, most companies also required their workers to pay a greater share of the health care bill in the form of higher monthly premiums and copays. Real incomes for many in the middle class were starting to decline.

The consequences of the escalating medical costs did not end there. A few Iowa companies had laid off workers and delayed expansion plans as health costs swallowed more of their spending. A government study in 2004 estimated that rising medical costs had created a $500-million-a-year drag on Iowa's economy as companies raised their prices, reduced their workforces, kept wages low, invested less money in equipment and the development of new products, and still suffered from overall lower profits.

Labor unions were losing their negotiating power as companies threatened to move jobs overseas where foreign governments—not employers— paid for medical care. No one driving along Second Avenue in Des Moines in the summer of 2005 could miss the frustration of union members working in the sprawling red-brick Firestone tire factory, which sat on the city's northern edge. Workers had put up a large billboard painted with four words: EXPORT TIRES NOT JOBS.

Some unions had caved in. In Cherokee, Iowa, some six hundred workers at a plant manufacturing deli meats for Tyson Foods accepted a new contract in 2004 that slashed the starting wage for new employees from $10.69 to $9.00 an hour. As part of the deal, the union members agreed to start paying 25 percent of their medical costs, which before had been fully paid by Tyson. The workers also agreed to replace their pension plan with a 401(k) retirement plan, a step taken by a growing number of American companies to save money on one type of employee benefit while they spent ever more on health care.

The problem came down to the numbers. In 2006 an American employer paid an average health insurance premium of $11,500 for a family of four. That was an increase of 87 percent since 2000. Between those years overall inflation rose by just 18 percent.

Across the United States, many companies had stopped providing health coverage to their employees because of the soaring cost. That meant more Americans either were uninsured or had joined the ranks of those covered by Medicaid, the government program that pays the medical bills of the poor. Nearly 16 percent of the nation's population was without health insurance in 2005, according to the Census Bureau, up from 14.2 percent in 2000. Many of the uninsured were from working middle-class families who earned too much to qualify for Medicaid.

While studies have shown that people lucky enough to have medical coverage are being harmed by too many tests, medicines, and procedures, the uninsured can't get the care they need. The Institute of Medicine estimated in 2004 that as many as eighteen thousand uninsured Americans were dying every year because they did not get needed medical attention.

Even having insurance was no longer a guarantee that families would avoid medical bills that threatened to send them into bankruptcy. Almost half of all personal bankruptcy filings in 2001 resulted from an illness or medical bills, according to a study by academics at Harvard. And more than three-quarters of those people said they had been covered by insurance when illness struck.

The surging cost of medical care was limiting opportunity in the land of opportunity. Some would-be entrepreneurs stayed in jobs that offered health benefits rather than set out on their own. Other people kept working long after they were ready to retire.

George Hatzigiannakis, the owner of Mr. Filet, a restaurant in downtown Des Moines, said he desperately wanted to retire after working since age thirteen. He had operated his breakfast and lunch place for thirty-eight years. But in 2006, at age sixty-one, he had four more years until he was covered by the federal Medicare program. And so he continued to serve up lunches of steak sandwiches with potatoes on the side for the reasonable price of $6 to afford health insurance that was anything but reasonable. In 2006 the monthly premium for him and his wife, Mary, was $957, as much as he paid to rent the small restaurant on Seventh Street and up 27 percent from the year before.

"They're killing me," he said, "and everybody else who has to pay for his own. If I quit work, I wouldn't be able to pay the bill."

Even when Mr. Hatzigiannakis turns sixty-five, his problems won't be over. Analysts at Fidelity Investments estimated that a couple retiring in

2006 would need a savings account of $200,000, enough in Iowa to buy an above-average home with a big yard, to cover their prescription copays and other medical costs not covered by Medicare. This amount did not even include the cost of nursing-home care, which could mean hundreds of thousands more. The estimate was rising fast every year. A couple in their mid-forties in 2006 could expect to pay two or three times that amount.

THERE WAS, HOWEVER, one sector of Iowa's economy that was booming. More and more dollars were flowing out of Iowans' pockets and savings accounts into the amalgam of hospitals, clinics, nursing homes, laboratories, insurers, and medical companies known as the health care system. There actually didn't appear to be much that was systematic about this "system." Every one of its profit-making members seemed to be out for itself.

The good times enjoyed by this medical complex could be seen starting with the giant construction crane working above Mercy Hospital in downtown Des Moines in the summer of 2005. The crane, visible from a mile or more away to travelers on Interstate 235, was constructing a new six-story hospital wing, featuring a 123-foot glass atrium with suspended walkways. The $67 million addition was just one of Mercy's many construction projects. For years the private hospital had been opening new clinics and medical buildings all over central Iowa. Mercy was aided by the fact that it was classified as a nonprofit charity and did not need to pay taxes on any of the millions it made. It was not the only hospital constructing grand new facilities. Iowa Methodist Medical Center had broken ground on a new surgery and cardiovascular center just a mile or so away. These projects were part of the biggest boom in hospital construction in the United States since World War II.

And the physicians inside those hospitals? They were making plenty of money too. Some hospitals in Iowa paid their physicians so well that a few doctors made more than two million dollars a year, about forty-five times the average income of an Iowa family.

It was the pharmaceutical companies that provided cover for the other money-seeking members of the health care complex. When drug costs increased at a double-digit rate, the doctors and hospitals could point to the pharmaceutical companies and say, "Yes, we're making more this year than last, but just look at what *they* are raking in."

The drug companies' lust for profits could be seen at the monthly meetings held by a committee of pharmacists and physicians that oversaw how the state Medicaid program dispensed medicines to the poor. The committee reviewed data on the prescriptions paid for by Medicaid, allowing it to peer in on the prescribing habits of Iowa physicians. The committee questioned many of the practices they saw. Was it okay to give a drug for *dementia* to *children*? Should doctors be prescribing Topamax, a drug used for *epilepsy*, to patients for *weight loss*? Was it all right to give *several* different brands of epilepsy medications at a time to patients suffering from *mood swings*? Should doctors be giving the sleeping pill Ambien to patients *month after month* when the government said only the rare patient should take it for longer than *ten days*? Should physicians be prescribing *three* powerful antipsychotic medicines to a *single* patient when there was no evidence that such multiple prescriptions were safe?

Few members of the public attended these meetings, but the pharmaceutical sales representatives showed up in force. A dozen or more drug salespeople sat in on many of the meetings, watching the proceedings like the coons that had a nightly predilection for patrolling my father's chicken coop.

The sales reps and the companies that employed them had hundreds of millions of dollars in revenues to protect. Prescription drug costs were consuming more and more tax dollars in Iowa and every state in the country, a trend the pharmaceutical companies were working hard to extend.

The year 2003 marked the first time that states spent more to pay the medical bills of the poor and the disabled covered by Medicaid than they spent on elementary and secondary education. When the states added in what they paid for the medical care of government workers and inmates in the state prisons, health care consumed about a *third* of every state budget, a percentage that was rising every year.

State and local government officials across the country had been forced to raise taxes and cut services, including education and road construction, to cover the rising cost.

In Iowa, the cost of prescription drugs for patients covered by Medicaid had surged by almost 25 percent a year between 2001 and 2003. With medical costs rising much faster than inflation or state tax revenues, Iowa government officials had no choice but to reduce other services. At first, officials took hundreds of millions of dollars from a fund meant to help keep elderly Iowans living in their own homes rather than in nursing homes. When that wasn't enough, the state officials turned to college students. They sharply reduced funding to Iowa's three public universities, causing a spike in tuition and fees between 2001 and 2005 of more than 60 percent.

"Iowa used to pride itself on providing high-quality, affordable education," the editorial board of *The Des Moines Register* wrote in 2006, when a study determined that an average student at Iowa State would graduate with almost thirty thousand dollars in debt. "It's no longer affordable."

Some education officials said they feared that the high tuition costs were leading some young Iowans to skip college altogether. In a way, the state was trading away its future to throw ever more money into the bottomless pit that health care had become.

The most visible sign of the state government's struggle to pay rising medical costs was the giant Vegas-style casino that opened in Council Bluffs in 2006. The Horseshoe Casino, with chandeliers and a gambling floor bigger than a football field, was the largest of the gaming houses that the government had recently allowed to be built all over the countryside. The gambling establishments were heavily taxed, meaning that the state was paying part of its medicine bill with casino chips.

The federal government had also been forced to shift more tax dollars to pay for medical care. Washington politicians, however, had the luxury of simply adding the cost to the national debt, which would be paid by the workers of the future, the grandchildren and great grandchildren of those using the medicines today. Just the bill for the prescription drugs used by the elderly covered by Medicare, a benefit that began in 2006, was expected to rise so fast that it would account for 5 percent of the federal budget in 2020.

In all, federal, state, and local governments paid for more than 45 percent of the nation's health care in 2005. That meant that a working person without health insurance was paying taxes that covered the cost of medical care for the poor, the elderly, veterans, prison inmates, and public employees yet would be on his own if he got sick.

Analysts said there was no end in sight to the soaring costs. By 2015 America is expected to spend 20 percent of all it produces on health care.

By then Pfizer may be the biggest company on the planet, Mercy Health System may be one of the largest landowners in Des Moines and its suburbs, and Iowa will need many more casinos. A few of the luckiest gamblers may win enough to pay for that future heart medicine described by AstraZeneca's David Brennan, the $250,000 pill.

REVENGE OF THE GERMS

Just before Christmas 2003, a virulent flu swept through Iowa. Parents carried feverish children into crowded doctors' offices. Hospitals across the state filled with patients of all ages, from elderly men to the smallest of infants. Nervous Iowans stood in line at any clinic offering flu vaccine, which was hard to find across America that year.

Television stations and newspapers carried stories of the youngest Iowans who suffered. Blue-eyed Caitlin Mouw, just twenty months old, was the first Iowan to die. Her parents said the toddler was struck by both the flu and a case of pneumonia.

"They said it was a mild case of pneumonia, nothing to be concerned about," Dan Mouw, the child's father, told a reporter from KCRG-TV 9 in Cedar Rapids. "It's just an empty place in my heart where she used to be."

State officials later said they believed four Iowa children had died from the flu or its complications. Behind the scenes, however, there had been a different, even more frightening story playing out, one the public did not learn. Physicians caring for the ailing children and adults had been shaken to find that in some cases the medicines they had long counted on to fight pneumonia and other complications of the flu no longer worked.

Dr. Charles Grose wrote of the physicians' nightmare in a newsletter sent to the state's pediatricians a few months later. He said that one child had died not from the flu but from a mutant strain of staph known as MRSA that had grown resistant to many antibiotics.

Another child, Dr. Grose said, had died from a bacterial strep infection so vicious that it had killed its victim even before doctors could start treatment. Other physicians found, he said, that a powerful antibiotic called Rocephin had failed to work in three young patients. The children had developed empyema, a condition in which the lungs become surrounded by cupfuls of fluid, after their infections spread. The three appeared to get better after three to five days of Rocephin, Dr. Grose said, only to relapse a week or two later, developing fevers and suffering as their lungs were choked again by the infected pus.

The deaths and serious illnesses that holiday season were alarming evidence of another consequence of the drug companies' potent marketing campaigns. For years Iowans had responded to the industry's advertisements by asking their physicians for prescription antibiotics at the first sneeze or sign of a cold. But often the medicines worked in ways that created mutant germs that were far more powerful than those that had caused the patients' illness. In case after case, the drugs had destroyed the weak germs, while leaving the strong ones to survive and multiply. The more antibiotics Iowans used, the faster these drug-resistant superbugs spread.

Iowa's children were among the most vulnerable to these drug-resistant germs because doctors regularly gave them antibiotics. Physicians had shown no hesitation in giving these drugs even to infants. One study of Iowa children found that 75 percent had been given an antibiotic by the time of their first birthday, and 91 percent had received such a prescription by age two and a half. While parents believed they were helping their children by asking their doctors for an antibiotic for each ear infection, they may have been unknowingly setting them up for more serious problems. Numerous studies have shown that taking antibiotics increases a person's risk of later contracting powerful infections that can't be treated with the usual course of drugs. A study in Atlanta, Georgia, for example, found that white children living in the suburbs had a higher rate of drug-resistant pneumococcal infections than black children living in the city's urban core. Such infections can develop into pneumonia, meningitis, and a host of other illnesses. The researchers theorized that the white suburban children had a higher risk of harboring the drug-resistant bacteria because they had better access to health care and had taken more antibiotics.

At the same time, Iowans who heeded the advice in the drug advertisements by asking their doctors for one of the new heavily promoted antibiotics like Zithromax or Biaxin were also more at risk. These new drugs worked against a broader spectrum of germs than did older drugs like penicillin. They could knock out more of the good bacteria, or the "natural flora" in the body, as well as the bad germs, which could become even more potent if they mutated to resist the drugs. Studies had shown that patients taking these broad-spectrum antibiotics were at a higher risk of later being infected by a lethal superbug like MRSA, shorthand for methicillin-resistant *Staphylococcus aureus*.

But all Iowans, even those who did not take antibiotics, were now living with these menacing germs that could withstand even some of the most powerful modern medicines. The bugs were growing stronger, while the drugs grew weaker.

"We are facing a crisis," Dr. Richard Besser from the Centers for Disease Control told an audience of physicians in May 2000, "because doctors are pressured to prescribe antibiotics for the common cold and inner ear infection, yet we know that it is not prudent to do so."

A month later, doctors from the World Health Organization voiced a similar alarm. The group published a report that said the world risked losing its lifesaving medicines because of their overuse. The report explained how the world's major infectious diseases were slowly but surely becoming resistant to the antibiotics that had cured them.

DRUG RESISTANCE THREATENS TO REVERSE MEDICAL PROGRESS, read the headline of the press release describing the WHO's report. CURABLE DISEASES—FROM SORE THROATS AND EAR INFECTIONS TO TB

AND MALARIA—ARE IN DANGER OF BECOMING INCURABLE. The report's findings read like a futuristic thriller, although they were frighteningly true.

Iowa and the rest of the world were moving backward in time, closer to the days before the discovery of penicillin, when a scrape on the knee could mean death from runaway infection. Yet even as medical experts were growing more anxious, the corporate sellers of antibiotics were just getting warmed up.

TO SELL DRUGS to children, marketers had discovered by the year 2000 that they needed to flavor their products to taste like candy and to use whimsical, Disney-like characters as product mascots. That year, in one of the industry's biggest marketing battles, three companies were doing just that as they competed to sell antibiotics to children whose ears ached.

GlaxoSmithKline had employed a smiling amphibian named Auggie the Froggie to sell its antibiotic Augmentin. Marketers at Abbott Laboratories had created a wrinkled bulldog named Bix to represent their product, Biaxin. But marketers at Pfizer had outdone the others. They had made cherry-flavored Zithromax the top-selling antibiotic in the country with help from Max the Zebra and *Sesame Street*.

Pediatricians in Iowa and around the country opened their mailboxes that year to find medical journals wrapped in paper printed with Max's black and white stripes. Pfizer sales representatives succeeded in getting so many pediatricians to hang small plastic replicas of Max from their stethoscopes that one physician told me a family had asked if Max was the hospital's mascot. The company had even donated a real zebra to the San Francisco Zoo and invited children to a party where the beast was welcomed and named Max.

But Pfizer had not stopped there. It paid for fifteen-second advertisements that ran at the beginning and end of *Sesame Street*. The PBS show, viewers were told, had been "made possible by" a grant from Pfizer, which "brings parents the letter Z, as in Zithromax." The spot featured children frolicking with a zebra, as well as a giant wooden block with the letter Z painted on its side.

Pfizer even put Elmo, the show's furry Muppet star, on its corporate payroll. It paid the Children's Television Workshop, which produced *Sesame Street*, to make a video featuring Elmo going to the doctor with an ear infection. As part of the deal, Pfizer featured Elmo on its website (kidsears.com), where it gave away five thousand of those videos and promoted Zithromax. The company also held the How to Get to Sesame Street Sweepstakes. The family winning the grand prize was whisked off to Manhattan on a free trip to see a live taping of the Muppet show.

A poster created by Pfizer told Elmo's story this way: "The doctor looked in Elmo's ears and in Elmo's throat—'say aaahh'—and listened to Elmo's little, red monster heart go thump—thump, thump—thump. Ha ha ha—that tickles! The doctor gave Elmo medicine to take until it was all gone. The doctor helped Elmo feel better. The doctor can help you feel better too!"

No doubt many parents appreciated the story. Its basic message to children was that medicine would take their troubles away. "We used something kids love," Patrick Kelly, Pfizer's vice president of worldwide marketing, said in 2000, "to get them past something they don't like."

One problem with selling Zithromax or any antibiotic as if it were a box of sugar-coated Frosted Flakes is that most ear infections go away without drugs. When a doctor gives children prescriptions they do not need, they risk all its potentially serious side effects, but gain no benefit.

Pfizer had continued its aggressive marketing of Zithromax even after pediatric experts and the federal government warned physicians in 1999 that most children with earaches did not need an antibiotic and that the minority that required one should be given a cheaper drug called amoxicillin, which doctors had used for years.

But many doctors in Iowa and across the country did not heed the experts' advice on limiting their antibiotic prescriptions to only patients who needed them. Wellmark, the large health insurer, found that prescriptions for Zithromax and other similar drugs known as macrolide antibiotics soared by 35 percent in Iowa between 2000 and 2002. The use of the drugs varied from town to town, with the residents of some Iowa communities filling macrolide prescriptions at more than double the national rate. It wasn't that the towns with high numbers of Zithromax prescriptions were plagued by more illness. It was more likely that these towns were in the territory of a particularly aggressive pharmaceutical sales rep, or perhaps they simply had physicians who gave in too easily to patients' requests for a Z-pak, the popular nickname for a box of Pfizer's drug.

"We see Zithromax being prescribed like water," Dr. Randel Cardott, the medical director at a group of clinics in Davenport, said in 2003, when Wellmark issued its report on the fast-rising use of antibiotics. Iowa's doctors were frequently prescribing Pfizer's drug, Dr. Cardott said, even for acute bronchitis, an illness that is most often caused by a virus that can't be treated with antibiotics.

Doctors appeared to be overusing Zithromax all over the country. In 2002 a group of researchers announced that they had found that 48 percent of the children with strep throat at a private school in Pittsburgh could not be treated with a drug called erythromycin, an antibiotic similar to Zithromax. The researchers blamed the children's drug-resistant infections on physicians' rising use of Zithromax for patients with all types of illness.

But it was not just strep throat that was getting harder to treat. Nor was Zithromax the only antibiotic that doctors overprescribed. America's list of drug-resistant infections was getting longer all the time.

No one knows how many Americans are dying from these mutant germs. There are no national reporting requirements. In 2005 Iowa government officials weren't trying to track the numbers of people who died. If they had tried to trace these deaths, they could expect the state's hospitals to protest. Hospitals around the country have lobbied to keep the public from finding out how many patients contract potentially deadly infections while in their care. The hospitals don't want people to know that they may be lax in preventing infections from spreading or that their doctors often forget to wash their hands.

There are only rough calculations of the actual toll. The federal government estimates that each year roughly two million Americans get infections while staying in the hospital. More than 70 percent of the bacteria causing those infections, the government says, are resistant to at least one of the antibiotics that once easily treated them. Experts estimate that ninety thousand Americans who acquired infections in the hospital die every year. That is about 250 deaths every day, and an escalation from 1992, when the infections were believed to kill thirteen thousand Americans each year.

Those numbers do not include the deaths from drug-resistant bacteria that now live outside hospitals, an invisible threat with the potential to cause pandemics that scientists are only beginning to comprehend.

IN 1999 DOCTORS reported that four children from Minnesota and North Dakota had died from the virulent mutant bug MRSA. That wasn't the part of the news that had disturbed physicians. Thousands of Americans had been dying from that drug-resistant staph bacterium every year. But until the report on the deaths of the four children, scientists had believed that people could get the lethal strain only during a stay in the hospital. These four children had been healthy and had not been in the hospital until they suddenly fell violently ill.

One was a sixteen-month-old American Indian girl from rural North Dakota who arrived at the hospital in shock and with a fever of 105 degrees. Doctors gave her a drug called ceftriaxone, but within two hours she was dead. Just the month before, a doctor had given the child an antibiotic for an ear infection.

Another victim was a seven-year-old black girl from an urban area of Minnesota. She had been admitted to the hospital with an infection in the joint of her right hip. Doctors gave her an antibiotic, but the infection spread through her bloodstream to her lungs. She soon developed pneumonia and empyema. She died after five weeks in the hospital.

The other two children were a twelve-month-old white boy from rural North Dakota and a thirteen-year-old white girl from Minnesota. Both had suddenly developed ferocious lung infections. Doctors gave them vancomycin, an extremely powerful antibiotic that is considered a medicine of last resort. But the infection had continued to eat away their lungs.

Soon cases of community-acquired MRSA—that is, one in which a person had been infected with the germ somewhere outside the hospital—

were surfacing all over the country. The superbug had moved into homes, locker rooms, gyms, day care centers, or just about anywhere bacteria grow.

As the drug-resistant pathogen spread, it attacked both the weak and the strong. Football players and wrestlers were among its first victims.

In 2001 Iowa health officials reported that high school wrestlers in the state had been infected by an outbreak of MRSA. The drug-resistant staph lives on the skin, which puts wrestlers at higher risk because of their close contact with competitors and the frequent scrapes they suffer.

Similar MRSA infections hit five players for the St. Louis Rams in 2003. The football players were linemen or linebackers who suffered turf burns on their elbows, forearms, or knees. The players' abrasions rapidly became large abscesses up to seven centimeters across that required surgical incisions to drain them. The researchers who wrote about the Rams' infections found that each player had received an average of 2.6 prescriptions for antibiotics during the past year, about ten times the number taken by the average American.

In some rare cases, MRSA has developed into necrotizing fasciitis, known to the public as flesh-eating bacteria. The bacteria release a toxin that rapidly destroys the skin and flesh. Left untreated, the person soon goes into shock and dies. In 2005 doctors in Los Angeles reported that they had treated fourteen patients with MRSA who had developed necrotizing fasciitis. None of the patients died, but they had serious complications, including long stays in the intensive care unit. Some required reconstructive surgery because the bacteria had eaten away so much of their skin.

MRSA doesn't just prey on those who have taken antibiotics. It can infect anyone. A study in 2005 estimated that two million Americans have MRSA living in their nostrils. Most of these people have no symptoms but can pass the infectious bacteria on to others. Illness can begin when the skin is cut or scraped or when a person's immune system is weakened.

One of the strains of MRSA that has rapidly spread across America is especially virulent and deadly in children, as doctors found that Christmas season in 2003. This particular strain is capable of producing a toxin called Panton-Valentine leukocidin. At its worst the toxin can cause a serious form of pneumonia that can destroy the lungs of a child in twenty-four hours. Officials from the Centers for Disease Control warned that December that it was the first time they had seen so many cases in which the drug-resistant staph killed children who had been healthy until stricken by a bout of the flu.

MRSA was just one of the mutant germs now everywhere, waiting for their next opportunity to grow more lethal with the help of an unnecessary prescription.

UNDER THE INFLUENCE

Specialist Dustin Colby and Staff Sergeant Bruce Pollema were traveling in the third National Guard convoy to leave Camp Dodge that August morning. A crowd had gathered to bid farewell to the soldiers of the 2168th Transportation Company, who would soon be running supplies in Iraq.

Colby drove the semitruck assigned to the pair. He waved at a television news crew at the side of the road that was filming the troops' departure. A Black Hawk military helicopter flying nearby carried a Humvee in a sling.

The soldiers had just passed through the main gate when the right wheel of the truck went gently off the edge of the narrow road. If Colby tried to get the tire back on the road, he moved far too slowly. The truck rolled as it went into the steep ditch, killing both men. It took a crane and two hours of work by a rescue crew to remove their bodies from the crushed cab.

At first it was a mystery why the twenty-year-old soldier, who had been trained as a heavy equipment operator, would drive off the road. The pavement was dry. The truck left no skid marks.

Later military and police investigators had their answer: Colby had been taking three different prescription pain pills, a regimen he had begun after a dentist pulled his tooth. After a five-month probe, investigators said they believed the powerful cocktail of Darvon, Vicodin, and Tylenol with codeine may have slowed Colby's reaction time.

The soldier perhaps never realized the danger in the prescription pills, which eased the intense pain threatening to get in the way of his tour of duty in Iraq. Colby had been a determined soul, who often spoke the words that had become his personal motto: "Get 'er done."

His mother explained that her son had gone to the dentist at his commander's request to have the tooth pulled before leaving for the Middle East. But Colby had suffered what is called a dry socket, in which the hole left when a tooth comes out does not heal. The excruciating pain can last for weeks.

Colby had started taking one of the painkillers before his tooth was pulled. Five days after a dentist pulled the tooth, the soldier went to the emergency room, where a doctor prescribed a second drug. Two days later another dentist gave him the third prescription. The label for each of these drugs comes with a warning against driving because each one can make people dizzy and drowsy. Some patients become sedated. These effects were clear in one simulated driving test that found that young people taking codeine went off the road more and had nearly ten times the number of collisions as people not taking the drug. Taking three different narcotics at the same time would have only heightened that risk.

After the crash in the summer of 2004, Iowa National Guard officials said they would begin asking military truck drivers before a trip whether they were taking medications. But that was too late for Colby and his passenger, Bruce Pollema, who had grown up and lived in Hull, a small town in northwestern Iowa. The thirty-year-old Pollema had loved to camp, fish, and golf. He also had enjoyed his civilian job as an enforcement officer for the state Department of Transportation, a job that had helped keep Iowa's roads safe.

THE GOVERNMENT DOES not know how many Americans die every year in accidents caused by drivers impaired by prescription drugs. Crash investigators rarely consider the possibility that the adverse effects of a medication could be to blame. A doctor in the state medical examiner's office in Iowa told me in 2005 that investigators often test the blood of drivers killed in automobile crashes for illegal drugs like heroin or cocaine but rarely look for prescription drugs. Nationally only the blood of pilots killed in air crashes is regularly tested for prescription medications.

It is clear, however, that medications have long been causing thousands of motor vehicle accidents every year and killing innocent people in their wake.

Concerned that medications were sedating older drivers, Dr. Wayne A. Ray, a professor at Vanderbilt University, compared the prescription records of Medicaid patients in Tennessee with police reports of motor vehicle accidents. On the basis of those data, he estimated that psychoactive drugs taken by older drivers were to blame for sixteen thousand motor vehicle accidents causing injuries every year in America. That is about forty-four injury accidents every day, just for drivers ages sixty-five and older.

The medications that Dr. Ray and his colleagues found the most dangerous were benzodiazepines such as Valium and tricyclic antidepressants such as Elavil. They also determined that the possibility of a crash increased quickly as drivers took higher doses of these drugs. An older person taking 125 milligrams or more of Elavil had a much higher risk of an injury accident than if he or she was taking only 25 milligrams. The risk also rose significantly for those who took two or more of these drugs at a time.

Dr. Ray's study, published in 1992, used records from the late 1980s. Other studies have found that barbiturates, opioid pain relievers, and sedating antihistamines hurt drivers' performance. More recent studies have tied motor vehicle accidents to sleeping pills such as Ambien and muscle relaxants like Soma and Miltown. Some medications are worse than alcohol in that they can incapacitate a driver without warning.

A group of physicians in New York reported in 1999 that nine patients taking a certain type of medicine used to treat Parkinson's disease had crashed after falling asleep at the wheel. Four of those patients had also suddenly fallen asleep during business meetings or halfway through phone calls. Other researchers looked at these same drugs in 2005. They found that 22 percent of the Parkinson's patients taking these drugs— Mirapex, Requip, and Permax—reported suffering from sudden, uncontrollable attacks of sleep.

Police investigators and medical researchers have also documented dozens of cases where people taking medicines have driven in a kind of semiconscious state.

For example, in 2005 forensic toxicologists in Wisconsin described cases in which people taking Ambien had driven into mailboxes, parked cars, and other stationary objects. The drivers could not stay in their lanes, the Wisconsin scientists said, and there had been many near head-on collisions. Officers who stopped these drivers often found them disoriented and unable to stand up. Some of these people later said they had no recollection of what they had done.

One Ambien-impaired driver in Wisconsin drove against traffic six times and just missed causing three head-on collisions. The driver, not described as a man or a woman, drove in and out of the ditch until finally hitting a wooden sign. The officer reported that the driver had stumbled onto the highway to see the flattened sign and had a glassy, blank stare. Another driver plowed down a light pole and then drove onto the sidewalk. When stopped, the driver appeared to "look right through" the officer trying to talk to him.

But Ambien was not the only drug that could lead to what some had begun to call sleep driving.

NICHOLAS LITTLE ARRIVED home from his overnight shift at Kalona Plastics in southeastern Iowa at seven o'clock in the morning on February 17, 2004. He drank one twenty-four-ounce can of beer, used mouthwash containing alcohol, and took his prescription pills. He took Zoloft, an antidepressant; Zyprexa, an antipsychotic; and two one-milligram tablets of Xanax, an antianxiety medicine, and then went to bed. A short time later he got into his car and began driving.

Just before 10:00 a.m., Mr. Little ran his car into a vehicle stopped at a stop sign. When he got out of his car to talk to the other driver, his vehicle began rolling forward and nearly hit the other car again. According to the driver of the other car, Mr. Little had trouble climbing out of his car. He hung on to the car door for support.

Minutes after the first accident, Mr. Little was back in his car and soon collided with another vehicle at an intersection. When the driver of that car asked Mr. Little to move his car so that she could look for damage to her bumper, he backed up but then pulled forward and hit her car two more times. Mr. Little asked her not to call the police and offered her money to pay for any damage. According to that driver, Mr. Little was slurring his words. He seemed nervous, she said, and his eyes looked unusually small. When she tried to move her car out of traffic, Mr. Little followed her, nearly hit her again, and then drove away.

Sergeant Mike Clark of the Washington township police force stopped Mr. Little a short time later. Mr. Little told Sergeant Clark that his name was Nick Price. He also said he had drunk five or six beers and was on his way home from picking up a prescription. He was not wearing a coat despite the winter weather. When Mr. Little failed a field sobriety test, Sergeant Clark took him to the police station, where he continued to say things that did not make sense, including that he had last worked at Kalona Plastics in 1993. At one point Mr. Little fell off his chair.

A breath test showed Mr. Little's blood alcohol to be 0.071 percent, below the legal limit in Iowa of 0.08 percent. That blood alcohol level also did not seem to support Mr. Little's claim of drinking "five or six beers." To Sergeant Clark, Mr. Little appeared to be far more impaired than the alcohol breath test had revealed, so he requested a urine sample. That sample also came up below the legal limit for blood alcohol. But it helped solve the puzzle of Mr. Little's impairment when it also tested positive for Xanax and Zoloft.

Mr. Little later testified that he did not remember anything he had done between going to bed and waking up in the police station. Mr. Little's physician, Dr. Alfred Savage, told the court he had not told his patient not to drink while taking the Xanax, only that he should not drink as much. Dr. Savage also did not tell Mr. Little not to drive while taking Xanax, even though the written instructions for the medicine warn against driving.

THE FEW STATES that have tried to track motor vehicle accidents caused by prescription drugs have found the numbers to be rising. For example, the number of impaired drivers found to have taken Klonopin, an anxiety pill, in Wisconsin increased by about 90 percent between 2004 and 2005, according to Laura J. Liddicoat, supervisor of forensic toxicology at the state's laboratory of hygiene. Similarly, the number of impaired drivers found to be on Valium increased by about 30 percent between those years. The increase, she said, is partly due to officers' testing more drivers for prescription drugs, but it also corresponds with the public's rising use of medication.

"The number of drugs we find in tests of drivers and the concentration of these drugs," she said, "keeps getting higher every year."

The true scope of the problem is unknown, she said, because states lack money for testing and because there is little awareness about the dangers of heavily medicated drivers. Of the drivers stopped by officers in Wisconsin, she said, only about 10 percent are tested for medications because of the cost.

West Virginia is one of the few states that regularly test for drugs, both legal and illegal, in traffic accidents in which drivers are killed. In an analysis of these fatalities, officials discovered that in 2004 and 2005 roughly the same percentage of drivers who died had drugs in their bodies as those who had blood alcohol levels that exceeded the legal limit. They also found that among the deceased drivers testing positive for drugs, more had been taking prescription drugs than illegal drugs like marijuana or cocaine.

A national study of crashes involving semitrailers and other large trucks also found evidence that prescriptions may be causing far more accidents than the public knows. In a report to Congress, researchers said they had found that prescription drugs were a possible factor in an estimated 26 percent of the truck crashes that caused death or injury between 2001 and 2003. The researchers had catalogued about a thousand different "associative factors"—that is, things investigators believed may have contributed to the crash—as they dug more deeply into a large sample of these accidents. Prescription medications ranked at the top of their list. On a national level, the study's estimate meant that prescriptions may have played a role in tens of thousands of serious truck crashes during those years.

Said Scott Falb, a safety specialist in Iowa's Office of Driver Services: "We're just waking up to the breadth of the effect medications are having."

EVEN HIGHLY PUBLICIZED, gruesome fatal accidents have failed to make the public understand that prescription medicines can impair drivers just as alcohol can.

In 1998 a Greyhound bus, traveling from New York to Pittsburgh, drove off the Pennsylvania Turnpike and struck the rear of a parked semi-trailer. The crash killed the bus driver and six passengers. Investigators said a probable cause of the accident was the driver's use of Benadryl, a sedating antihistamine available over the counter in pharmacies.

On a winter evening in 2004, Anna Bik killed a thirteen-year-old boy on a motorscooter while driving after she took her migraine medicine. Bik said she had taken large amounts of the drug Fioricet, a barbiturate, because she had grown tolerant to its effects. She told the judge in Bucks County, Pennsylvania, that she left the scene of the accident because she thought she had only hit a pothole.

A Mack semitruck became airborne and landed on top of a Chevrolet Silverado pickup, parked in the driveway of a house in Pine Bluff, Arkansas, in 1997. All four people in the pickup and the driver of the semitruck were killed. Investigators said the probable cause of the accident was a painkiller called tramadol, which was found in the truck driver's blood. The drug is known to cause sleepiness, dizziness, and seizures.

That same painkiller was blamed in 2003, when a ferry in New York Harbor cruised full speed into a pier on Staten Island. Eleven passengers were killed, and many more were maimed. The pilot of the ferry, Richard Smith, had passed out at the helm.

Smith later said he had been taking tramadol for back pain, as well as Flomax, for prostate problems, and dyphenhydramine, the active ingredient in both Benadryl and Tylenol PM. Prosecutors also found that Smith had lied on his medical exam form in 2000 when he said he was not taking any medication. He had actually been using pills for insomnia, cholesterol, high blood pressure, back pain, and his prostate. Smith's doctor was indicted on charges of knowingly signing that medical report, which he knew was false. Smith pleaded guilty to eleven counts of seaman's manslaughter.

"You are no better than a drunk driver," Deborah Palamara, the sister of a man who died on the ferry, told Smith in court as a judge sentenced him to an eighteen-month prison term. Ms. Palamara said her brother's body had been so torn apart that it could be identified only by the tattoo on his arm.

STATES CAN FIND it difficult to prosecute people for driving under the influence of prescription drugs. Unlike the case with alcohol, states do not have standard limits on the amount of medication a driver can use before being impaired. Some states, like Iowa, have laws that can let drivers on prescribed medications off the hook. Iowa law states that a driver who has a prescription for a drug cannot be prosecuted for driving while impaired if the doctor failed to warn him about the dangers of driving while taking it.

Often drivers causing fatal accidents have pleaded for leniency, saying they should not be found guilty because the drugs were prescribed by a physician.

In December 2004 Brian Hust drove to a Safeway pharmacy in Napa, California, to pick up his prescription for Vicodin. He downed thirty of the pills and began driving back home. He drove his Toyota 4Runner erratically, going onto the dirt shoulder to pass other cars. He lost control and plowed into a sedan driven by Luz Lopez Martinez, a grandmother who was on her way to Wal-Mart. The sixty-year-old Martinez was killed.

Hust explained he had become addicted to the pills after an accident at the Anheuser-Busch plant where he worked. Two pallets had fallen on his head, requiring three surgeries and a host of medications. In early 2006 a jury decided against convicting him of second-degree murder. Instead, it found him guilty of involuntary manslaughter. A judge sentenced him to four years in state prison rather than the fifteen years to life he could have received for the murder charge. The jury's verdict upset the members of the Martinez family, who consoled one another outside the courtroom.

"It's not fair," Martinez's son, Jose, told *The Napa Valley Register*, just after the jury's decision. "Justice has not been served."

Yet the punishment was even less for another overmedicated driver in Napa County, who killed a motorcyclist just three months after Hust was sentenced. Linda Grassi crossed the centerline in her van and ran head-on into Timothy Fitzpatrick, a sixty-year-old grandfather. Investigators found traces of nine prescription drugs and marijuana in Grassi's blood. She asked the judge for mercy, pointing out that a physician had prescribed the pills. She had taken high amounts of the painkillers and antidepressants, she said, because she had grown tolerant of their effects. She pleaded guilty to manslaughter, and a judge sent her to jail for six months.

ON A SUNNY fall day in Iowa in 2005 the parents of Staff Sergeant Bruce Pollema greeted the 2168th Transportation Company as the soldiers returned from Iraq. Betty and Wilmar Pollema sat in the football bleachers at Sheldon High School, among a crowd of hundreds, who cheered and waved flags as they caught sight of loved ones they had not seen for more than a year.

"Bruce was very dear to us," Betty Pollema later said, remembering that bright October day when the troops came home. "It was very, very hard for us to know that our son was not coming off that bus."

NINE

Deadly Doses

THE LETTER ARRIVED in Jerry Houk's mailbox in 1996. It looked official. It was typed on plain white paper and addressed to him by name. It had been sent by a company named Parke-Davis. The letter said the company was soon introducing a new medicine called Rezulin to help people with diabetes, a problem Jerry just happened to be struggling with.

He remembers thinking, "Well, maybe this will help."

Jerry ran a forklift at the big meatpacking plant in his hometown of Ottumwa, Iowa. His wages were enough to support his wife, Sadie, and their four sons and still pay for things like an annual trout fishing trip to Colorado. A burly guy, he had also worked construction and built roads, bridges, or, in his words, "just about anything." But that year he had not felt well. Three years earlier doctors had diagnosed him with Type 2 diabetes. The disease allows excess sugar to build in the blood. If not controlled, diabetes exacts a terrific toll on the body, causing disabling complications like blindness and even early death.

Type 2 diabetes can often be managed, even cured, by exercising more and eating less. But many doctors don't explain this to their patients. They assume Americans don't have the willpower. It is much easier for doctors, in the fifteen to twenty minutes they take to see a patient, quickly to prescribe a pill and send the afflicted on his or her way. The drug companies could not be happier with this situation. When the government approved Rezulin in January 1997, the company's chief executive told investors he believed it would be a "billion-dollar blockbuster."

Jerry took the letter to his doctor, who told him he had not even heard of the drug it was so new. Eventually, however, Jerry got his prescription.

AFTER NINE MONTHS of taking Rezulin, Jerry felt nothing like the smiling people he saw in the drug ads. He felt nauseated, as if he had the flu. When the malaise lingered and grew worse, he began to fear he had cancer. People told him his skin had a strange bright yellow tint.

On an early spring day in 1998 he was settling in to watch television when a disabling pain swept through him. "It was like someone hit me in the chest with a baseball bat," he said.

He thought he was having a heart attack. He called his mother, asking her to come from her nearby home and drive him to the emergency room. He was only thirty-six.

The physicians in the emergency room told him that they too believed it was his heart. But as they performed more tests, the doctors discovered that it wasn't his heart at all. He remembers one doctor told him it was "the medicine." Fighting for his life, he had little time to contemplate then what the doctor had meant.

Jerry spent almost all of the next three months in the hospital. When he finally went home, he had another person's liver.

Few illnesses are as dramatic or as devastating as when the liver fails. The patient can go from good health to near death in two to ten days. A general feeling of fatigue and nausea is followed by jaundice. In the most severe cases, patients suffer from altered mental states and coma. About 80 percent of those suffering from acute liver failure die.

Weighing about three pounds, the dark reddish brown liver is the body's largest internal organ. Among its numerous functions is to act as a filter and remove harmful substances like drugs, insecticides, food additives, and other chemicals from the blood.

The public hears much about the dangers of viral hepatitis infections, which can lead to liver failure. But viruses such as hepatitis A are not the leading cause of this organ's failure in the United States. Not by far. Instead, most Americans who suffer from liver failure have been poisoned by their medications.

Researchers reported that 51 percent of the cases of liver failure at some two dozen American medical centers in 2003 were caused by a single drug, acetaminophen, which is sold under the brand name of Tylenol and also included in a wide array of other medicines. But dozens of other drugs can cause the liver to fail, as Jerry Houk found out.

Jerry said months after he left the hospital he heard a report that Rezulin had been pulled from the market because of its propensity to ravage the liver. That's when he finally understood what had happened to him.

"I was sitting on the couch, watching the *World News*," he said. "I said, 'Hell, that's the pill I took.'"

Jerry still doesn't understand how the marketers at Parke-Davis obtained his name and address, which allowed them to send him that promotional letter back in 1996. He doesn't know how the drug executives knew he had diabetes. For years, however, pharmaceutical companies have been paying pharmacies, doctors, and other health care providers to send personal letters to patients promoting their new medicines.

For example, in 2002 one of my colleagues at the *Times* received a letter from Duane Reade, a pharmacy chain in Manhattan, after he had picked up the allergy medicine Claritin, then available only by prescription. The letter promoted a new drug called Clarinex, sold by Schering-Plough. Schering also sold Claritin, but the patent on that product would soon be running out, allowing other companies to sell it in a low-priced generic form. Schering marketers were working desperately to switch patients taking Claritin to the company's new product, Clarinex, although the two drugs were almost indistinguishable. The letter said that Duane Reade "felt it was our responsibility to make you aware" of the new Clarinex. Typed in small letters at the bottom of the letter were the words "Funding for this mailing was provided by Schering Corporation, the makers of Clarinex."

Sales representatives from Eli Lilly took these marketing tactics a step further in 2002. They arranged, with help from a group of physicians, the mailing of free samples of a new long-acting version of the antidepressant Prozac to dozens of patients in Florida. The patients had not requested the pills. The family of one sixteen-year-old boy who received a one-month supply of Prozac in the mail said he had never been diagnosed with depression. The pills had arrived in a Walgreens drugstore package with a form letter signed by local physicians.

Given these marketing partnerships among pharmaceutical companies, pharmacies, and physicians, it is plausible that a health care provider shared Jerry's medical history and address with Parke-Davis, the company that was purchased by Pfizer in 2000 and no longer exists independently.

Another troubling fact is that Jerry said he received the letter from Parke-Davis in 1996, before Rezulin was approved by the government in January 1997. Jerry remembers how the letter had explained that Rezulin would soon be in pharmacies, similar to how moviegoers see previews of films that are "coming soon." Federal law prohibits drug companies from promoting products before government approval.

Jerry said he doesn't blame his doctor for prescribing Rezulin. After all, he took the letter to the physician and asked him to prescribe the drug, the very action pharmaceutical companies try to provoke through their advertisements. "It was my bright idea to try it," he said.

Years after getting a new liver, Jerry and scores of other patients who were harmed by Rezulin, as well as the families of those who died after taking it, received financial settlements from Pfizer. But the money won't bring back Jerry's old life. He says he tires easily and can no longer hunt pheasants and deer as he used to. It seems he is always at the doctor's office. He has arthritis, he said, and "holes in my spine" because of the prednisone, a steroid drug, he had to take for five years as part of his liver transplant. In fact, now he has no choice but to be a lifelong customer of the companies making pharmaceuticals. In all, he takes five or six different meds. The pills he takes to keep his body from rejecting his new liver come with warnings that they can cause cancer.

"I was ticked off what it done to me," he said of Rezulin. He remembers how he once listened to the drug ads on television, thinking that the list of side effects mentioned in each one was not worth worrying about. "Now I tell people it would be smart to stay away."

MEDICINES WORK AND provide their benefits by interfering in some way with the chemical makeup of the body's cells. Scientists design drug molecules to have a certain desired biological effect, but every one has unplanned and unpredictable effects as well. A basic lesson of pharmacology is that there is a thin line between where a drug works as a medicine and where it becomes a poison.

All over Iowa, as the state's physicians busily diagnosed disease and wrote prescriptions, they were unintentionally creating a different kind of illness, one that few of them wanted to talk to about. In the medical literature, these maladies are broadly called "drug-induced disorders" or "adverse drug reactions." Industry scientists writing in medical journals often refer to them simply as "events." Many physicians and pharmacists prefer to call them "medical misadventures," as if someone had suffered an unlucky mishap like wandering off a path in the woods. The euphemism has helped create a false perception that these are unfortunate occurrences in the practice of medicine that no one can do anything about. Stripped of all such embellishments, these "events" are the serious injuries and deaths caused by prescription drugs.

Emergency rooms, like the one where Jerry Houk ended up, are first to see many of those harmed. Dr. Mark A. Graber, a professor at the University of Iowa and an emergency room physician at the university's hospital in Iowa City, said he sees patients whose stomachs are bleeding because of pain relievers and others whose hearts are failing because their diabetes meds or pain pills have caused dangerous buildups of fluids. Other patients, he said, have suffered severe and sudden allergic reactions to antibiotics.

The university does not keep track of the numbers of patients rushed to the emergency room because of injuries caused by their medications, Dr. Graber said. "My sense is that we're seeing more drug interactions and more adverse effects," he said.

Doctors treat drug-induced injuries every day in emergency rooms all over the country. One study found that as many as 28 percent of all emergency visits were related to medications. And the most vulnerable group of patients are, not surprisingly, older people.

Roughly half of Americans ages sixty-five and older take five or more different drugs or supplements every week. Twelve percent use ten or more different brands of pills every week. In part, the elderly use more drugs because they have more chronic illnesses.

Dr. Jerry H. Gurwitz, an expert in geriatric medicine, explains this to his students in this way: "As older patients move through time, often from physician to physician, they are at increasing risk of accumulating layer upon layer of drug therapy, as a reef accumulates layer upon layer of coral."

There's another factor at work too. Older people and the families who care for them are particularly susceptible to the marketers' manipulation. The underlying message in many drug advertisements is basic and frightening: you will soon die if you don't ask your doctor for a prescription.

Every one of the medications added to an elderly person's regimen, however, increases the chance of a dangerous drug interaction. At the same time, the very process of aging makes seniors more susceptible to the drugs' adverse effects. Older bodies struggle to excrete medicines because livers and kidneys don't work as they once did. Aging physiques retain less water and have more fat and less muscle mass, meaning that the recommended adult dosages for many drugs are too strong.

Gloria Fisher, eighty-one, said that she hears frequent stories about medications from the elderly residents of Davenport, an Iowa city of about a hundred thousand that sits on the banks of the Mississippi. Gloria meets with more than a hundred older residents a week as part of her work for a group called Senior Voice. She listens to the people and reports back to the city with their concerns. She often drops in on groups gathered to play cards, among whom a leading topic of conversation has become prescription drugs.

Gloria said some of the older people she talks to are on so many drugs that they have lost track of what they are taking them for. Doctors have prescribed drugs to some people, she said, not because the person has a new illness but to remedy the side effects of the first medicine they prescribed. A good geriatrician would explain that such a practice, which can quickly lead to a cascade of pills, should almost never be done.

"Pretty soon they are taking all kinds of prescriptions," Gloria said. "They wonder why they feel ill right now."

Knowing that older people can easily be harmed, drug companies have excluded them from many of the clinical trials they perform to show their products are safe. That means there are few studies looking at what happens when a seventy-five-year-old man takes a single drug and no studies looking at the consequences when he takes that drug along with five other medications. With no science backing their decisions, doctors don't know what harm they might be causing with their prescription pads.

In 1991 a group of academics created a list of dozens of drugs that should not be prescribed for older people. The list of dangerous medicines was updated in 1997 and again in 2003. "If you have no idea what this drug is likely to do in this particular patient, you have no right prescribing it," explained Dr. Mark H. Beers, the lead author of the list, in 2004. "This is not a trivial part of what we do—it may be the most important."

But many physicians, dependent on the pharmaceutical industry for their education, have not been taught what medicines to avoid prescribing to the elderly or simply choose to ignore the advice. In a study in Iowa, researchers found that 13 percent of the 729 medicines prescribed to sixty Iowans living in a nursing home were dangerously inappropriate and included in the list of dangerous medicines, which is known as the Beers Criteria. The government has found an even higher rate. In 1995 the General Accounting Office said that almost 18 percent of all Medicare patients were taking medicines that are not safe for older people.

The medicines can cause adverse effects that are subtle but potentially deadly, for instance, when they cause dizziness, weaken muscles, and lead to falls. A study back in 1987 estimated that psychotropic medications, such as sleeping pills and antidepressants, were causing more than thirty-two thousand elderly Americans to fall and break a hip each year. About 20 percent of people fracturing a hip die within five years. This problem appears to be escalating as people take more pills. The death

rate from falls among Americans age sixty-five or older spiked by 55 percent between 1993 and 2003.

In recent years, various drug companies have publicized this danger
of falling, but they have not made it clear that medicines are often to
blame. Instead, the companies have used the statistics on falls to create
a new blockbuster pharmaceutical market for drugs they claim will reduce the chance of breaking a bone. In 2003 this global market for osteoporosis drugs such as Fosamax and Actonel was worth five billion dollars,
and analysts said then that they expected it to reach ten billion dollars by
2011. The sellers of the osteoporosis drugs had discovered that the side
effects from some medicines can open up billion-dollar sales opportunities for other types of pills.

The harm caused by medications may not be apparent for years, and
even then it may be so subtle that scientists find it only when they look
for trends among large groups of patients. In 2003, for example, researchers published a study that showed that older Iowa women who were taking high doses of the sleeping pills known as benzodiazepines suffered
faster physical declines and were less able to get around their own
homes than those who did not take the drugs.

The researchers first visited these women living in southeastern Iowa
in 1988. They measured how fast they walked, how easily they got up from
their chairs, and how stable they were while standing. The scientists returned four years later to perform the same tests. They found that the
longer the women took the sleeping pills, and the higher the doses, the
more their bodies failed them. In other words, the women using high
amounts of the drugs aged faster than those not using the tablets or taking them for only a short time.

IN THEIR HASTE to see patients and write prescriptions, doctors
can easily confuse the harm caused by a medicine with the onset of a
new disease. Drug-induced dementia masquerades as Alzheimer's disease. Drug-induced tremors look like the beginning of Parkinson's
disease. Physicians learn about the latest treatments for Alzheimer's and
Parkinson's from the pharmaceutical sales representatives, but they have

not been trained to recognize when an affliction is actually caused by medicines.

No one knows how many patients suffering from such drug-induced disorders die every year without knowing it was their medicines that caused their mental or physical decline. Any one of these cases is a tragedy because the symptoms will often subside—memories will return and tremors will ease—if the patient stops taking the offending drug.

The chance of such a misdiagnosis is high and increasing fast as the elderly take more and more medications. One study found that more than 10 percent of the people experiencing a sharp decline in memory had dementia caused by drugs. Similarly, as many as 30 percent of people developing the tremors and uncontrollable shaking that mimic the symptoms of Parkinson's disease are instead suffering from their medications.

Studies show that physicians are missing the true cause of a patient's suffering in many of these cases. A group of researchers found that some doctors in New Jersey appeared to be misdiagnosing Parkinson's disease in patients who began to suffer from irrepressible tremors after taking a drug called Reglan. The drug, which is prescribed for gastrointestinal reflux disorders and to prevent nausea after surgery, is just one of many medicines known for causing such tremors. But rather than stop the patients' doses of Reglan, the physicians added a prescription for levodopa, a medicine for Parkinson's disease.

In Iowa, a group of scientists found that the state's doctors may have failed to recognize dozens of cases of drug-induced dementia in just a few years. Dr. Ryan Carnahan, a fellow of psychopharmacology at the University of Iowa, and his colleagues searched prescription data from the state's Medicaid program to find older Iowans who filled their first prescription for Aricept, a medicine for Alzheimer's, in 1997, 1998, or 1999. They then looked at what medicines these patients had been taking in the three months before that initial Aricept prescription. They found that 30 percent of these Iowans had been taking drugs that were well known for causing dementia. These drugs included Ditropan, a medicine prescribed for incontinence; Elavil, an antidepressant; and antihistamines such as diphenhydramine, the active ingredient in many over-the-counter products, including Benadryl and Tylenol PM.

Dr. Carnahan, who left Iowa in 2004 to teach at the University of Oklahoma, said that on the basis of the group's findings, he feared that medicines had caused the dementia in many of the patients. He said doctors had been told since 1991 that they should not prescribe medicines known to have anticholinergic properties to patients who begin to lose their memory. These anticholinergic drugs can cause dementia or can make an older person's mild memory problems far worse.

But in dozens of cases the Iowa doctors had failed to heed this basic and critical advice. Instead, they appeared to be following the advice of the drug salespeople who had visited their offices to tell them about Aricept, the new medicine available for all those patients whose memories were failing.

And then there are those who have died.

EVERY DAY A stream of death certificates crosses the desk of Jerry McDowell.

As the state's nosologist, McDowell translates deaths into data, corpses into codes. From his office near the gold-domed state capitol in Des Moines, he processes each death certificate filed in Iowa, some twenty-seven thousand a year. Since he took the job in 1972, McDowell has sorted and classified hundreds of thousands of deaths so that statistics on the cause of each one can be sent to the federal government.

Malignant neoplasm. Diabetes mellitus. Acute myocardial infarction. Influenza. Asthma. Automobile accident. The rare assault. The death certificates keep coming and coming, about five hundred every week. McDowell, a short man with a wide mind for details, says the endless reports on the dead have never bothered him. He rarely looks at the names.

A computer helps catalog the deceased. The machine spits out cases that don't fit the federal government's classification rules. McDowell processes these cases—about a hundred each week—by hand, often calling the physician who signed the certificate if something doesn't make sense. Among the cases spewed from the machine are deaths caused by prescription drugs.

In a world dominated by the pharmaceutical companies and their cash, few researchers have tried to compile these deaths or estimate how many Americans are dying from their medications every year. A study that is often cited by the government was published in 1998 by a group at the University of Toronto. The academics estimated that 106,000 Americans had died in 1994 from the adverse effects of their medications. That amounted to nearly 5 percent of all the deaths in the United States that year. It made prescription drugs the country's fourth leading cause of death, after heart disease, cancer, and stroke. According to the study, another two million Americans were seriously injured by their medicines, but did not die.

The researchers had been selective as they set out to estimate the number of drug-induced deaths. They excluded injuries caused by medication errors made by doctors and pharmacists. They also left out overdoses and cases where patients died after abusing the medications. In other words, they looked at people who were harmed by medicines that had been properly prescribed and taken exactly as directed.

They also limited their study to hospitalized patients—that is, those who died from medications administered in the hospital and those who died after being hospitalized because a medicine prescribed in an outside clinic had made them sick. This meant that anyone who died outside the hospital would not have been included. It also excluded people who died from medicines in nursing homes.

Given this conservative estimate and the fact that Iowa's population represents about 1 percent of the nation, one could conclude that more than a thousand Iowans are dying each year from medications they took according to their doctors' instructions. This is the equivalent of ten airliners crashing on their approach to Des Moines International. It is also two hundred more people than live in my hometown.

I mentioned this estimate to McDowell. He said he was not finding that many prescription drug deaths among the certificates. In fact, by the time Iowa's death certificates were logged in the final statistics kept by the federal Centers for Disease Control, the adverse effects of medications were said to have killed only five Iowans in 2002.

What's more, in all of the United States in 2002, officials attributed just 247 deaths to the side effects of medications. Where were the other

100,000 Americans that the Toronto researchers had conservatively estimated to be dying from medications taken as prescribed? Could drugs
be killing people but escaping all blame, leaving them to harm even more
Americans until someone, finally, catches on?

It was one of those hot summer days when the perspiring cornfields
surrounding Iowa's towns and cities make the air so sultry that lungs ache
for drier air. I had found some relief inside Iowa's morgue, where John
Kraemer, the director of forensic operations, was showing me around.
The corpse of a middle-aged man with a dark beard lay on a metal table
in one of the room-size coolers. A white sheet covered most of the body.
Only his ashen-colored feet and face were exposed.

The state's new morgue had opened only a few months before. It
smelled not of death but of new carpet. Kraemer took me down a hall to
the receiving area and the main autopsy room with its chrome examination tables. The temperature in the room was turned so low that goose
bumps formed on my arms.

"You can see a gunshot wound, but you can't see the mechanism of
which a person dies from drugs," Kraemer explained when I asked whether
the morgue's doctors were discovering more medication-related deaths
as Iowans swallowed more pills. "If a person was taking the drugs appro-
priately, there would be no reason for us to concentrate on whether the
drugs were the problem."

Kraemer is an earnest-looking young man with reddish brown hair
and wire-rim glasses. Trained as a physician assistant, he helps three pathologists operate the state morgue.

I asked him what would be written on a death certificate if a person
with cancer died from the drugs prescribed as treatment rather than from
the disease. Such a death, he said, would most likely be classified as a
"natural" death and attributed to the cancer. "Because if it would not have
been for the cancer," he explained, "they would not have gone through
the treatment." Many medical examiners, he said, use a rule of thumb
that could be described as "the 'if not for' clause." If it had not been for
the disease, the theory goes, the person would not be taking the meds.

Therefore, the underlying cause of death is the disease. In rare cases, he said, doctors may list a medicine as "contributing" to the death.

This is the same theory that I later found in articles that instructed physicians how to fill out death certificates and determine the cause of death. The articles and advice emphasized attributing most deaths to an underlying illness or disorder, even when a medicine or a medical procedure was the immediate cause of death.

For example, an article written in 1997 to instruct the ninety thousand members of the American Academy of Family Physicians on filling out death certificates explained that a "therapeutic misadventure"—where a medical procedure had killed a patient—can be called a "natural" death. "In many cases, the procedure is not the cause of death even though the death immediately follows the procedure," the authors explained.

Another example of how this works was detailed in a 2005 study by pathologists in Vermont. The doctors had pored through the medical charts of fifty patients who had died in an academic medical center. They used their expertise in forensics to determine what they believed caused the patients to die and then compared their finding with what doctors at the medical center had written on the death certificate. They found that 96 percent of death certificates contained some kind of error. About 34 percent of the death certificates had such serious errors, the pathologists said, that doctors had written the wrong causes or manners of death.

But even these Vermont pathologists, who were concerned that doctors lacked the training to determine the true causes of deaths, disregarded the harm caused by prescription drugs. In one of the cases they wrote about, a patient died after the diuretic pills prescribed for congestive heart failure caused hyponatremia, a dangerous condition in which there is not enough sodium in the blood. Such an electrolyte imbalance is a known risk of diuretic treatment. The patient's doctors had listed hyponatremia as the cause of death on the death certificate. The pathologists said this was wrong. They said the underlying cause of death should have been listed as the atherosclerotic cardiovascular disease that had caused the congestive heart failure. They said nothing about noting the harm caused by the diuretic pills on the death certificate even though they had concluded that the medicine brought on the death. This line of reasoning takes all blame off the medicine and the doctor, who may have prescribed a dose of diuretics that was too high. The doctor also may have failed to monitor the levels of sodium in the patient's body, even though such tests might have found the problem before it became life-threatening.

At Iowa's morgue, Dr. Dennis Klein, a tall pathologist who serves as the state's deputy medical examiner, reiterated Kraemer's points on how hard it is for even an expert schooled in forensics to link a death to a prescription drug. Dr. Klein said that if a middle-aged person were taking several drugs and had a sudden heart attack, the pathologist would most likely determine the death to be a natural one. "If the drugs are at the therapeutic level," he said, "it would be hard for us to question whether they were a cause of death."

When a doctor determines a death to be a natural one, there is a presumption that the death would be almost impossible to prevent. But if a prescription drug or another medical procedure hastens a death and cuts off years from a life, it is hard to understand what is still natural about it.

Even when medical examiners determine that a drug caused a death, they can face pressure from physicians to change their conclusion. In March 2000, Dr. Ljubisa Dragovic, the medical examiner in Oakland County, Michigan, was asked to examine the body of a fourteen-year-old boy who had collapsed while riding his skateboard. Officials believed the boy, Matthew Smith, had died by falling and hitting his head. But Dr. Dragovic found that Matthew had not hit his head hard enough to die. Instead, the autopsy revealed that Matthew's heart had given out after being damaged by seven years of Ritalin use. The drug increases the heart rate and raises blood pressure, which had very slowly taken a toll. The young teenager's heart, Dr. Dragovic said, looked like that of a longtime cocaine addict. He wrote on the death certificate that Matthew died from "long term use of methylphenidate (Ritalin)." His decision did not sit well with several psychiatrists.

"They kept calling me and saying, 'Couldn't you find some other cause?'" Dr. Dragovic said. The physicians told him that studies had not found that Ritalin could damage a child's heart.

The pleas failed to sway Dr. Dragovic to change the outcome of his autopsy and investigation. "I'm in the business of fact-finding," he said. "A death investigation is not a democratic process."

Seven years later, after a review of similar deaths among those taking drugs like Ritalin, the FDA required the manufacturers to warn doctors and patients that the products could harm the heart and, in rare cases, lead to sudden death.

STATE MEDICAL EXAMINERS are the best authorities on why people die. They are independent investigators of death and not connected to hospitals or clinics. But most families do not benefit from their forensic skills when a loved one dies. The medical examiners step in to perform an autopsy and investigate a death only when someone dies suddenly, violently, suspiciously, or unexpectedly. They may be called on to do an autopsy of a forty-year-old woman found dead in her living room but not of an eighty-year-old man who dies in his sleep.

In most cases, a person's own physician determines the cause of death. If one dies in the hospital, the physician or another member of the hospital staff prepares the death certificate. This practice leaves doctors and hospitals sitting in judgment of the treatment they personally delivered, which is like letting a motorist involved in a crash review his own driving. Was it his excessive speed or the rain-slicked road that caused him to hit the other car? The driver, like the doctor, would hesitate to take the blame. That is human nature.

Also hampering efforts to understand how many people die from their medicines is the fact that hospitals no longer perform autopsies on most patients. That means the evidence of the true causes of patients' deaths is buried right along with them.

The autopsy rate in the nation's hospitals has plummeted, from 50 percent after World War II to less than 8 percent today. Some hospitals perform no autopsies despite the many patients who die within their walls. No one knows how many patients who die in nursing homes are autopsied, although the estimates range from one in one hundred to one in one thousand.

That decline in the rate of autopsies, which are considered one of the most powerful tools in the history of medicine, has had tragic consequences. Without an autopsy to verify what a doctor writes on the death certificate, diagnoses like "cardiac disease" or "Alzheimer's disease" have become death causes of convenience.

For more than two centuries, autopsies were responsible for most of our knowledge of disease. Autopsies, for example, played a major role in linking smoking to lung cancer. Autopsies can find mistakes and keep doctors from making them again. But with no autopsy, it is often unclear why someone has died. Studies have consistently found a 40 percent difference between what the physician said was the cause of death and the actual cause learned from an autopsy.

With such a high rate of error, it is clear that we don't really understand why Americans are dying today. We lack knowledge that could help prevent more of these deaths. We also do not understand where modern medicine is helping Americans live longer lives and where it is actually killing them.

"Medical interventions have to be based on better science and in medicine that means investigating when something goes wrong," Dr. George D. Lundberg, the former editor of *The Journal of the American Medical Association*, wrote in his 2000 book *Severed Trust*. "The place to begin is the autopsy."

A backlash against the autopsy began in the 1970s, he said, as more physicians became annoyed with what pathologists were discovering in autopsies. "They didn't want the pathologist to see the outcome of their work," Lundberg wrote, "and they didn't want anyone else to see it either."

A hint of just how many hospital patients killed by medicines were being buried before the truth could be revealed came in a report published in 2002. Researchers in Norway said they had studied every death occurring in a hospital over two years. In many cases, they performed an autopsy to try to verify the initial death determination. They found that 9 percent of the deaths were directly caused by drugs, while another 9 percent were indirectly caused by medications. In all, the researchers tied almost one of every five deaths at the hospital to prescription drugs. Few of these cases, they said, had initially been blamed on a medication. This report and a handful of similar studies show that the closer scientists look at what is happening inside hospitals, the more drug-induced deaths they find.

American doctors and hospitals have added to the unknowns by successfully lobbying for state and national laws that veil their actions in secrecy. In Iowa, doctors and hospitals do not have to report deaths caused by medical errors, unless the doctor who was at fault is considered by his peers to be seriously incompetent. In other words, if other physicians and the hospital's chief believe the death was caused by an honest mistake, it can remain a secret. Even if the medical error is reported to Iowa regulators, the information is kept from the public. Only if the state eventually takes action against the doctor does the public learn the briefest of details about the death. By then, many years have likely passed since the patient died.

If the family of the patient who dies files a lawsuit, doctors and their lawyers often demand that the court papers be kept confidential. There is a federal law that requires insurance companies to report settlements in malpractice cases to a federally funded data bank, but the public has little access to this information. Many hospitals have avoided even this reporting requirement by removing the doctor's name from the malpractice lawsuit. This secrecy is systemic, and it works to protect bad doctors and bad drugs, just as today's medical industry has shown it prefers.

But there is one system, woefully underfunded and weak, that collects deaths and injuries from prescription drugs. The system, called Med-Watch, runs on a voluntary basis. The government encourages doctors to file a MedWatch report whenever a patient is harmed by a drug, but there is no law requiring them to do so. The FDA, which operates the system, has no way of knowing how many of the injuries caused by drugs actually get recorded. Regulators say that they may get reports of as few as 1 percent of the actual injuries and deaths caused by medications.

But for all its inadequacies, MedWatch has helped uncover some deadly medicines, and one Iowan, a nurse who was not one to easily give up, remembered its significance as she came to understand why her sister had died.

The floor of Rosemary Rahm's den was almost covered with the papers she'd collected since that day back in October 2000 when she received word of a death. Knowing that I was coming, she had arranged the letters and news clippings in piles on the rug. The death had been one that paralyzed her with grief and that she came to believe was hastened by years. For much of the past five years it had consumed her thoughts.

"There's just so much," she said, shaking her head, her eyes scanning the stacks of papers. "It's so sad. It killed her. She would have had a longer life."

They had called that autumn day to say her older sister, Virginia, had been found dead in the bedroom of her home. The firefighters had broken in and found her sister's body after her colleagues reported that the always dependable Virginia had not shown up for work on Monday and Tuesday. In fact, Friday was the last time anyone had heard from the pretty, petite fifty-nine-year-old woman with bright brown eyes, who lived alone after being twice divorced.

Almost from the moment she learned of Virginia's death, Rosemary believed she knew why her sister had died. She remembered that Virginia had started taking a new, heavily advertised pain reliever called Vioxx for the arthritis in her hands. Just a month before she died, Virginia had sent Rosemary a letter and package. Inside the bundle, tucked among some cooking tips from Martha Stewart, was a report written by the rheumatologist who had prescribed the Vioxx tablets for her pain. Rosemary remembered how she had thought it was odd for Virginia, out of the blue, to mail her personal medical records. Her sister had never done such a thing before. It was almost as if she had felt something was coming.

Unable to go out because of her grief, Rosemary sent her husband to Bauder Pharmacy, an independent drugstore near their home in Des Moines, to get the lengthy FDA-approved prescribing instructions for Vioxx. The government counts on this document to warn doctors and the public about the risks of a medicine, but allows the manufacturer to write it using medical terminology that most Americans can't comprehend.

Aided by knowledge gained over more than thirty years of working as a registered nurse, Rosemary understood much of the information. But she found almost no information on Vioxx's effect on the heart. She began to fear, she said, that Vioxx came with a serious risk that doctors and patients did not yet understand.

VIRGINIA, ROSEMARY, AND the rest of the Marshall clan grew up in Des Moines not far from where Rosemary and her husband now live in a tidy house with lace curtains in a neighborhood distinguished by its towering old oak trees. The Marshalls have a long history in the city. Their grandfather and great-grandfather bottled and sold horseradish through a business started in the nineteenth century. "Grown & put up by Marshall's," reads the label of one of the old horseradish jars that Rosemary keeps in her kitchen. "Since 1872."

Virginia was the first member of the Marshall family to leave Iowa. She moved with her husband, who taught history, to the orange groves of Southern California in the 1960s. Virginia had the mind of a meticulous scientist and had won a chemistry prize in her college coursework. She did not earn enough credits for a degree because she had taken time off from her studies to have two daughters. She proved, however, that she did not need a degree. She worked her way up to become an analyst for Boeing, the aircraft manufacturer, and, by many accounts, did the work of a far more educated engineer.

Her family says she was a complicated, rather private woman, who found great joy in her daughters and three grandchildren. She had an infectious laugh, they say, and drove them crazy with the snapshots she took at family gatherings. She loved to listen to the piano and was fond of cross-stitch needlework and reading historical novels, including Tolstoy's *War and Peace*.

Virginia was five years older than Rosemary. The younger sister remembers that she had been fifteen when she made Virginia's wedding gown. A few weeks before I visited her, Rosemary had passed her sister in age, bringing the ache back again.

"She could have been saved," Rosemary said, the pain after five years still evident on her face. "All of this was known before."

A COUPLE OF months after Virginia died, Rosemary drove to Iowa's State Medical Library in downtown Des Moines to find what had been published on Vioxx in the scientific journals. It was on her second trip to the library that she discovered a study published in *The New England Journal of Medicine* in November 2000 and completed months before Virginia started taking Vioxx in August of that year. The study had been paid for by Merck and was published under the names of thirteen physicians, who called themselves the VIGOR Study Group. Eleven of those doctors were academics, but they all had financial relationships with Merck, including consulting contracts or positions on the company's "advisory board." The other two scientists, including a doctor named Alise Reicin, were employed directly by Merck. By the end of the study four out of every one thousand patients taking Vioxx had suffered heart attacks. This was four times the number of heart attacks suffered by patients in the study who had taken a different drug called naproxen. The researchers, however, had dismissed the heart attacks and deaths, saying the safety of both drugs was comparable. To Rosemary, however, the study was evidence that Vioxx was harming patients' hearts.

She called the rheumatologist in California who had prescribed Vioxx to her sister. She told him she was concerned that physicians did not fully understand the risks of Vioxx and asked him to file a report with the FDA's MedWatch program to inform the government that a patient taking Vioxx had died.

The rheumatologist assured Rosemary he would report Virginia's death to the regulators. About a month later she called him back to make sure he had.

"He said, 'I'm very interested in your sister, but I've talked to some people and I've decided not to file a report,'" Rosemary said, remembering the call. "I just sat there stunned. I said, 'Who did you talk to—people at Merck?' And he said, 'Yes.'"

ROSEMARY DECIDED TO file the MedWatch report herself. The government allows and encourages anyone to report injuries or deaths he or she suspects were caused by a medicine. After she sent the report, Rosemary asked the FDA to send her information on the other cases the agency had received about patients taking Vioxx. In August 2001 she received a package from the government. Inside was a computer disk. It took her several tries and help from her son to determine how to open the contents on the disk, but once she did, she was stunned by what she found. She began writing out in longhand the basic facts from each case on the disk but did not get far before giving up. Cardiac arrest and death in a thirty-five-year-old woman. A similar death report had been filed for a thirty-three-year-old man. Sudden death, unexplained, in a sixty-seven-year-old man. Even though Vioxx had been sold for only two years, the reports of injuries and deaths numbered in the thousands.

"I felt overwhelmed," she said.

About that same time, Rosemary went to a continuing education class for nurses at a hotel in Des Moines. As in many such classes she had been to, the pharmaceutical companies had paid to place their sales booths in the room where the nurses could get refreshments. Rosemary stopped at Merck's booth. She remembers how the table was covered with brochures advertising Vioxx, as well as piles of pens and other trinkets engraved with the drug's brand name.

She told the Merck sales representative that her sister had died suddenly and that she believed Vioxx was harming patients' hearts.

"Right away he said, 'We need to step aside,'" she said. The two walked away from the booth and talked. He asked if someone from Merck could contact her to find out more about Virginia. And then he asked how she knew that Vioxx might have an effect on the heart. "We don't talk about that," he said.

ALMOST FOUR YEARS after Virginia died, Merck pulled Vioxx from pharmacy shelves, saying that a study had shown that Vioxx doubled the risk of heart attacks and strokes in patients who took it for eighteen months or longer.

"When they pulled the drug," Rosemary said, "I grieved again."

Rosemary knows her sister might not have had a long life. Virginia had smoked, and even though a doctor never diagnosed her with heart disease, the coroner found her arteries filled with plaque. But Rosemary believes Virginia would have lived years longer if she had never taken Vioxx. "Vioxx killed her," she said.

In November 2004 a scientist at the FDA testified before the Senate Finance Committee that Vioxx may have caused heart attacks in as many as 139,000 Americans. He estimated that 30 to 40 percent of these people had died.

Rosemary heard those estimates of death and did the figures in her head. "It's a Vietnam."

Epilogue

AMERICANS SPEND MORE on medical care today than they do on housing, food, transportation, or anything else. This was not the case in 1980, when medical costs barely made the list of a household's top five expenses.

Few Americans understand they are spending so much on medical care. They write big checks each month for their mortgage, rent, and car payments. The true financial burden of health care is hidden. Most people have health insurance paid for by an employer, which covers the majority of their medical bills. They don't realize how many thousands of dollars of their taxes are funneled to the medical system. Taxpayers covered nearly half the country's health care tab in 2005. At the same time, medical spending is concentrated with the minority of Americans suffering from chronic or serious illnesses, even though everyone pitches in to pay the fast-rising cost.

By the time all the medical bills had been tallied in 2005, the nation had spent an average of $6,700 for each person, or $26,800 for a household of four. Economists say the cost of medical treatment will continue on this tear, eating up more and more of what people have to spend. By 2015 Americans are expected to surrender one dollar of every five dollars they produce to the pharmaceutical industry and the rest of the nation's medical system.

Pharmaceutical executives have said over and over that Americans should be delighted by this. Their logic, as explained in a press release from the industry's trade group, is that the escalating cost is "good news" because it means that "more people are getting more and better medicines." Americans should stop complaining about the high cost, the drug executives say, and consider how much they have gained by spending more of their incomes on medical treatment.

"The current dilemma we face as a nation is not about the failures of our healthcare system, but rather about its success," David Brennan, a top executive at AstraZeneca, told the Detroit Economic Club in 2004. "Yes, its success—success in helping Americans live longer and healthier lives. In the past 25 years, especially in the past decade, there has been a revolution in medical breakthroughs.

"We need to ask ourselves a key question," he continued. "Would we accept 1980's-era medicines in exchange for 1980's pricing? I know I would not, and I doubt sincerely that there are many in this room who would."

Indeed, American medicine of 1980 has little resemblance to that of today. In 1980 the pharmaceutical industry did not promote its products on television. It was also a time when medicines were often introduced in other nations before they were in the United States, in part because the FDA spent more time making sure they were safe before agreeing they could be sold. It was also a time when most medical research was done by academic or government scientists with few ties to the pharmaceutical industry.

Today Americans regularly try out new medicines before anyone else in the world. The pharmaceutical industry controls most medical research in the United States. And Americans frequently take medications even when they suffer no real illness. Many have come to believe the industry's claim that utopia can be encapsulated.

The rising revenues of the pharmaceutical companies show how much has changed. Between 1980 and 2003 the amount spent yearly by Americans on prescription drugs rose from $12 billion to $197 billion, creating growth rarely seen in such a long-established business. While

Americans doubled their spending on new autos between those years and tripled what they paid for clothing, they increased their spending on prescription drugs by seventeen times.

The drug companies have created reams of data to detail the value of the medicines they sell. These studies paint a picture of prescription drugs being the most cost-effective part of America's medical system. The papers say that medicines are not only saving lives but saving money by keeping people out of the hospital and eliminating the need for surgeries.

But the cost-saving potential of most medicines is not so apparent. Most of these studies, known as pharmacoeconomic reports, suffer from the same bias as other research the industry has paid for. Many were written by academics who work as consultants to the industry. Almost always left out of these analyses is the cost of caring for patients who are injured by their medications, an expense that may exceed what was paid for the drugs in the first place. The studies touted by the industry also don't look at how many lives could be extended and money saved if the nation invested in keeping people healthy and actually preventing disease rather than spending ever more on expensive pills.

Another way of looking at the value of all these new medicines the industry has sold in the last twenty-five years is to take a global view.

In 1980 a sixty-five-year-old American woman could be comforted by the fact that her expected life span was longer than that of her contemporaries living almost anywhere else in the world. Now, with access to an almost unlimited supply of the pharmaceutical industry's newest and most expensive medicines, an American woman of sixty-five has lost her place among the women in the world with the longest lives. By 2002, in a list of the longevity in thirty nations, sixty-five-year-old American women came in seventeenth.

American men have also fallen in the international rankings of life expectancy. The average sixty-five-year-old American man can now expect a shorter life than a man his age living in Mexico.

No one knows exactly why the United States is falling behind in the international rankings of longevity despite spending far more on medical care per person than any other country on the planet.

American life expectancies haven't been helped by the fact that many people now believe they can eat whatever they want and not suffer the consequences since they can just take a prescription pill. One only has to look at the pharmaceutical industry's ads for heartburn drugs and cholesterol-reducing medicines to see how marketers have pushed this idea in their attempt to sell more medicines.

An ad for the heartburn drug Pepcid assured revelers during the winter holidays that they could "eat, drink and be merry." Indeed, the industry has ads promoting overindulgence for just about every change in the seasons. In the summer of 2006, marketers of the heartburn drug Prilosec sponsored a concert by the hard-partying country-rock duo Big & Rich at the Iowa State Fair. Fairgoers were even offered a guide to eating the fat-laden snacks offered by vendors on the midway.

"Pace yourself," the Prilosec guide warned. "If you just polished off a funnel cake, don't immediately chase it with a chili-cheese dog."

As Americans have gained weight, the drug industry has made more money by selling pills that treat diabetes and heart disease. But the pills are not the quick fix the industry says they are. Obesity can take more than a decade off a person's life span. Researchers reported in 2005 that the nation's growing epidemic of obesity may soon cause life expectancies to decline.

Or are the nation's disappointing expectancy rankings due in part to the deaths and serious injuries caused by the increasing number of prescription pills we take?

With the drug companies now controlling medical science, it can take decades before the truth is revealed about how their products may cause an early death. This is especially true when a drug causes harmful effects that masquerade as disease. In 2006 this became clear when another chapter was added to the story of Prempro and the other estrogen pills, which the industry has promoted to women as age-defying elixirs since the 1940s.

More than 40 percent of American women between the ages of fifty and seventy-four were taking Prempro or a similar drug in 2002, when a large government study found that the pills raised a woman's risk of breast cancer, heart attack, and stroke. Upon learning of the study's results, millions of women threw away their pill bottles. The number of prescriptions written for Prempro fell by more than 65 percent. But that was not the end of the tale.

In December 2006 researchers tracking the incidence of cancer in the United States announced that they were astonished by statistics they had pulled together for 2003. After rising steadily for decades, the number of women diagnosed with breast cancer had suddenly plummeted in 2003 by 7 percent. Some fourteen thousand fewer women, they said, had been diagnosed with breast cancer in 2003 than in the previous year. This was the first full year after women had stopped taking Prempro in droves.

Researchers said they finally understood why women in some of the most affluent areas of the country, places like Marin County, California, had for years suffered from higher rates of breast cancer than places not as wealthy. The affluent women, they said, had been more likely to take the prescription hormones. For decades, doctors had been unwittingly fueling the rate of breast cancer in the United States by writing prescriptions for the estrogen pills.

It can take a hundred years before all the risks of a medicine are known, explained Dr. Janet Woodcock, a top FDA official, in a presentation to a panel of experts who were reviewing the safety of the nation's drug supply in 2005.

And in a stunning admission, Dr. Woodcock said that the FDA could no longer count on the nation's physicians to understand even the *known* risks of medicines. "The keystone of the current drug safety system is the prescriber," she explained, "and that learned intermediary is charged with determining for the individual patient whether the benefits outweigh the risks.

"Now this system," she said, "has obviously broken down."

This failure has created a crisis for all patients, whether they are rich or poor, young or old. Even Americans who don't take prescription drugs are suffering the consequences of the industry's ruthless promotional push.

More Americans now abuse prescription drugs than they do cocaine. The roads have become less safe as more drivers are impaired by the effects of the prescription drugs they take. Doctors are finding that lifesaving antibiotics no longer work for some patients dying from infections because the products have been overprescribed to those who did not need them. America's rivers and streams are flowing with the invisible traces of medications swallowed by people upstream. And children trade prescription pills in the schoolyard the way students of an earlier generation traded cigarettes.

The pharmaceutical companies have become so wealthy and powerful that the whole medical system has become unbalanced. Inside hospitals and medical offices, corporate marketers are now calling the shots. They decide how patients will be treated, and the doctors follow along.

How else can you describe a system where doctors now prescribe a pill called Detrol for a disease called overactive bladder, a malady the manufacturer of the drug takes credit for creating? Why else did hundreds of doctors prescribe Neurontin, a drug for epilepsy, to children with attention deficit disorder and adults with bipolar disorder, even though there was no scientific evidence the drug would help them? These cases only begin to describe the scope and danger of the industry's increasingly hard sell.

As the pharmaceutical industry has devoted itself to aggressive promotion, it has been transformed from one with the ability to do great good to one that is causing far too much needless harm. And it is not just a few companies involved. The profiteering has become routine.

Executives want the public to believe their companies are all about science and education. "We call it a sales force," Hank McKinnell, the chief executive of Pfizer, once told me, "but our sales force doesn't sell. It transmits knowledge."

Yet startling disclosures about the risks of heavily hyped medicines have continued to come one after another.

In 2007 popular and expensive drugs for anemia, sold to cancer patients as energy-boosting pick-me-ups, were found to increase the risk of death. A drug for Parkinson's disease called Permax, which had been sold for almost two decades, was pulled from pharmacy shelves after scientists found it could kill patients by damaging the valves in their hearts. And the overmedication of the American public was confirmed again by a study that estimated one of every four people diagnosed with depression was not clinically depressed or mentally ill but temporarily saddened by recent life experiences like a divorce.

These new reports on excessive prescribing and the dangers of medicines were published even as the industry spent more on marketing than ever before and used advertisements like one in 2006 for a sleeping pill, Rozerem, that featured a beaver chatting with Abraham Lincoln. Yet another campaign, this one for the antiviral drug Tamiflu, targeted children by showing the tap-dancing penguins from the movie *Happy Feet*.

There is a kind of madness in it. The drug companies pay hundreds of millions of dollars in government fines for promoting their products illegally and hundreds of millions of dollars more to the families of the victims who suffered or died, then raise their prices and promote their products even harder.

Much of the blame must be put on the nation's physicians, who have enjoyed the industry's gifts as their profession has been corrupted and patients have suffered.

Marketing has no place in medicine. But in America marketing has replaced the science, honesty, and caring that the best medicine requires. Money rules. Patients come second. There's a moral imperative that the medical industry's marketers be stopped before many more lives are lost.

This is what must be done:

Listen to the dead. They have stories to tell.

No one knows how many Americans are buried without their families knowing they were killed by prescription drugs. By the best estimates, however, there appear to be scores of these cases *every day* in the United States. Consider the case of Karen Garcia, a thirty-four-year-old woman with long dark hair and coffee-colored eyes, who worked as a disc jockey at KUZZ, the popular country music radio station in Bakersfield, California.

On a chilly night in November 2005, Karen did not show up for her all-request show, which went on the air each night at seven. The police later found her body in her bedroom, sprawled on the floor, next to her desk.

Detectives found signs she had put up a struggle. Her computer monitor and lamp had been pulled from her desk onto the seat of her chair. A pathologist working for the coroner discovered bruises on her neck and cuts on her lip and the bridge of her nose. After a four-week investigation, the coroner ruled Karen had been strangled.

Determined to find her killer, detectives questioned dozens of Karen's friends, neighbors, and family. They repeatedly watched the videotapes taken by surveillance cameras outside her apartment building, looking for vehicles that had arrived around the time Karen had died. The radio station offered a ten-thousand-dollar reward for information leading to her killers. No one had any idea who would have wanted the pretty young woman dead.

The coroner decided to have two other forensic experts review the facts of the case. That was when the truth began to emerge.

A year after Karen's body was found, the coroner changed his decision. Karen had not been strangled after all, he said. She appeared to have been working at her computer when she suffered a severe seizure. The seizure had been brought on, he said, by the antidepressant she was taking, a drug called Wellbutrin.

When her body began to convulse, Karen appeared to have fallen from her chair, pulling the computer and fan from her desk. She struck her head on the desk and the frame of her bed. When she landed unconscious on the floor, the coroner said, her neck was at such an awkward angle that she could not breathe.

The investigators determined Karen had been taking 150 milligrams of Wellbutrin for three weeks but had increased her dose to 300 milligrams a few days before she died. These doses were not out of the ordinary. Karen was taking the drug just as directed by GlaxoSmithKline, the drug's manufacturer. The company's thirty-six-page prescribing instructions advised that the usual adult dose is 300 milligrams, which can be increased to as much as 450 milligrams. On page nine of those instructions, GlaxoSmithKline also warned the drug can cause seizures, even at the doses Karen was taking. The company added that the risk of seizures rose as the dose was increased.

GlaxoSmithKline included these instructions on a website where it promoted Wellbutrin with a brand logo resembling a shining yellow sun. The website also featured the photo of a smiling woman, who appeared about Karen's age, standing next to a tranquil lake. The tagline: "I'm ready to experience life."

Wellbutrin had killed Karen Garcia and almost got away scot-free.

It took three independent forensic experts and a yearlong investigation to determine what had really killed Karen. Most families don't get the benefit of such careful determination of what caused their loved one's death. Instead, they are handed a death certificate hastily filled out by a physician who may have written the deadly prescription. It's far too easy for the doctor to scribble "cardiac, other" or some other common medical condition onto the line on the certificate that asks for the cause of death.

If we don't know how many people are dying from their medicines, there is no way to keep people safe.

Hospitals were once required to do autopsies on at least 20 percent of patients who died within their walls. They should be required to do so again. Families should request an autopsy if they wonder about the true cause of a loved one's death. Medicare pays for an autopsy when someone over the age of sixty-five dies. The cost is built into the overall rates that the government pays the hospital to care for patients. Even though hospitals no longer do autopsies, they still get this money but spend it on something else.

Doctors must be trained to determine the actual cause of a person's death. They should be required to look specifically at whether a drug may have caused the death or had a part in it.

The standard death certificate should be redesigned to ask specifically whether a drug or medical procedure was involved, with an additional line where the physician identifies which one. This would help doctors understand which treatments are more dangerous than they have believed. New York City has attempted to do this by adding "therapeutic complication" to the options on the death certificate that a physician can choose as the manner of death. Most states now have only five possibilities for the manner of death: natural, accident, suicide, homicide, or undetermined. This makes it too easy to attribute a death caused by a medicine to "natural" causes.

At the same time, laws should be changed so that doctors and hospitals can no longer keep secret the details of deaths where they may be at fault.

Finally, doctors should be required to report to the FDA's program known as MedWatch any serious injury or death that is suspected to have been caused by a drug. Doctors now rarely file these reports because the system is voluntary. The reports should be filed directly with the FDA, not with the drug's manufacturer. The companies are required to give the FDA details of the injury reports they receive, but they have been sometimes found to tone down the language of the facts to make the case sound less severe or raise questions about whether it was the company's product that caused the harm. The FDA has found cases in which companies have failed to submit the reports to the government, including some where patients had died.

No drug company would deny that people are dying from prescription medications. But there is a widespread impression among the companies and the public that these deaths are rare and that medicines save far more people than they harm. Unfortunately, for some drugs, especially the newest ones, it is impossible to know whether this theory is true.

Stop physicians from taking the drug money.

While it is illegal for radio disc jockeys to accept money from music companies trying to get songs on the air, doctors can take money and gifts from any number of pharmaceutical companies attempting to sell prescriptions. With no restrictions, nearly 95 percent of American physicians now line their pockets with corporate lucre.

The nation needs a law that bans doctors from taking cash and gifts from any medical company, while also prohibiting companies from giving these handouts. The law must specifically stop physicians from working as the industry's so-called consultants.

Lawmakers should also ban the industry from paying for physicians' education. With the pharmaceutical industry paying for most continuing medical education today, physicians learn to prescribe new medicines but fail to provide some of the most basic care their patients require. At the same time, doctors prescribe the industry's heavily promoted products when nondrug treatment may help their patients more. They diagnose patients with the industry's disease of the moment, while missing the true causes of their patients' problems.

America's physicians need to be trained by the best independent medical minds rather than by speakers trained by Madison Avenue advertising firms to promote the latest pharmaceutical products. Doctors are some of the highest-paid professionals in the country. There is no reason they can't afford to pay for their own education.

At the least, doctors should be required to give patients a list of everything they have received from medical companies in the last two years. The receptionist could hand patients this list when they checked in. The list would describe the gift and its financial value. It might begin like this: Dr. Jones regularly meets with sales representatives from companies selling products he prescribes. These are the gifts and payments he has received from these companies in the last two years: January 17, dinner and drinks at Daniel, compliments of Forest Labs, value three hundred dollars; January 23, fee for speaking about a new asthma drug, compliments of GlaxoSmithKline, two thousand dollars; February 12 to 15, educational conference in Aspen, Colorado, sponsored by Pfizer, Merck, and Bristol-Myers Squibb, value of the corporate subsidies to Dr. Jones, twenty-five hundred dollars; and so on.

If patients grew uncomfortable as they read through the gift list, they could find another physician. Patients would also know to ask more questions of a doctor who hands them prescriptions for some of the drugs heavily promoted by companies on the list.

States must also make sure they have strong medical boards, which are the agencies that license and regulate physicians. The boards should not be run by physicians for physicians. They need to be organized so that they protect patients and are not afraid to take action against doctors who violate laws or recklessly harm people.

Finally, the drug companies should be stopped from paying their sales representatives bonuses and commissions that are calculated on the basis of the number of prescriptions written by doctors they call on. These financial incentives encourage sales reps to do whatever it takes to get a doctor to prescribe, even if it breaks the law.

Make science honest again.

As David Franklin, the scientist who worked at Warner-Lambert, once explained, "You can design an experiment to prove anything you want."

Over the past twenty-five years the pharmaceutical companies have created a vast scientific library of clinical trials and articles to help them sell more drugs. In the process, they have transformed medical science into what some doctors now call propaganda. For Americans, this means that their doctors are prescribing drugs on the basis of studies that may be dangerously wrong.

We desperately need more scientists who are working for the public's interest rather than for that of the pharmaceutical companies. The National Institutes of Health, which distribute billions of dollars in grants each year, could help increase the number of independent researchers by prohibiting any scientist who wins a government contract from also accepting industry money. At the same time, state legislatures should stop professors and scientists at public universities from taking cash and gifts from corporations. And the universities should fire professors who say they are the authors of papers that were actually written by ghost-writers working for the industry. Students are expelled for plagiarizing another's work. Professors should suffer the same consequences.

Some medical researchers have called for the government to create a national scientific agency that would pore through the industry's clinical trial reports, throw out the biased research, and determine what drugs actually work. Such an agency, designed in the right way, could transform America's medical system. To be effective, the agency must limit its staff to those medical experts who are free of ties to corporate America. The agency should be funded by the government but not run by the government. The pharmaceutical companies are so politically powerful that it would be easy for them to manipulate the process if it were managed by the government.

The agency would review classes of medicine to determine what drugs were the most effective and had the fewest side effects and, on the other hand, what products should be avoided. It could organize new clinical trials in areas where there was a gap in understanding, for instance, what happens when a medication is taken for longer than six months. The pharmaceutical companies rarely perform these expensive, long-term trials.

The new agency would almost surely pay for itself as doctors received unbiased scientific information and stopped prescribing expensive pills that did not work or those that caused more harm than good. The agency might even save money, which could then be invested in research aimed at finding drugs the public desperately needs, like those for rare illnesses such as Lou Gehrig's disease or aggressive cancers that kill children and young adults.

Tell patients the truth about drugs before they are prescribed.

If you knew a drug worked for only 40 percent of those who took it, which was about the same result patients got by taking a sugar pill, would you take it? Now consider that this same drug came with a small but real risk of causing serious harm, even death. What would you do?

Those facts describe a drug that has been sold to millions of Americans. Many people would hesitate to take such a pill, especially if there were other medications that were safer and more effective, if lifestyle changes could eliminate the need for medication altogether, or if the drug was not for a life-threatening condition. Yet patients today don't get this information. Instead, they learn just about everything they know about drugs from television ads, which imply the pills always work and have risks of little significance.

Doctors have a legal and professional duty to warn patients about the risks of a drug before it is prescribed. They can be sued for malpractice if they fail to do so. But surveys of patients show that doctors often don't tell people about the dangers.

The FDA should make it easier for doctors to go over the risks and benefits of a drug with their patients. The agency could require easy-to-read brochures for every drug on the market. Doctors could download the brochures from a government website and go over the facts with the patient *before* the prescription was written. The brochures could be written by the same national agency that independently evaluated drugs.

The brochures must say what chance there is that the drug will actually work as well as provide a list of its risks, beginning with those that are the most life-threatening. The brochures should show too how this drug's safety and effectiveness compare with other medications and with treatment that doesn't involve drugs. They should also warn patients about drug products that have not yet been sold for five years, which means that doctors still know little about them.

The government now requires written medication guides for some drugs, but the information is incomplete and difficult to understand. Doctors rarely have these guides available in their offices. Instead, some patients get them from pharmacists after the prescription is written.

Lawmakers should also require doctors to tell patients when they are prescribing a drug for an off-label use that has not been approved by the FDA. Doctors rarely give their patients this information, even though these prescriptions may have no basis in science.

As for drug advertisements, the FDA should return to the rules in place before they were changed in 1997. The previous advertising rules required the companies to detail the many risks of the product, impossible to do in a thirty-second television commercial.

The agency should go further still by setting stricter limits for ads in newspapers and magazines. These print ads, just like those on television today, imply that prescription drugs are safer and more effective than they actually are by showing scenes of people enjoying hikes in the woods and cartoon characters cracking jokes. The only appropriate way to advertise these products is to have black-and-white ads, with few illustrations, that read like the FDA-approved patient brochures. The ads should include the probability that the drug will actually work and emphasize the more serious risks. They should also describe brief facts on how lifestyle changes, like losing weight and exercise, might eliminate the need for drug treatment altogether.

The advertisements should include the average price of the drug in pharmacies so that both patients and the public paying the bill know the financial cost. Disclosing the drug's price would put pressure on the company to charge prices more in line with the drug's benefits rather than whatever executives believe they can get away with. It would be hard for a company to charge two hundred dollars a month for a drug that worked little better than a placebo, let alone fifty thousand dollars for a cancer drug that might hurt many patients more than help them.

Overall, there must be more honesty from scientists and physicians about the limits of modern medicine and the uncertainty of present medical knowledge. By exaggerating the benefits and minimizing the risks of treatment, the health care establishment has spread an undoubting belief in medicines, a confidence that is unwarranted and hurting people far more than they know.

Strengthen the FDA.

If a drug doesn't work, it can only harm. That is why Dr. Michael Elashoff, a biostatistician at the FDA, recommended that his agency not approve a drug for the flu called Relenza.

The team of government scientists working with Elashoff agreed with him that the drug offered little or no relief to patients suffering from the flu. So did the panel of experts that the FDA convened to review the drug. By a vote of 13 to 4, the panel said Relenza should not be approved.

Dr. Elashoff said he had combed through the studies done by the drug's manufacturer, Glaxo Wellcome, searching for evidence that Relenza might help even a subgroup of people.

"In analysis after analysis, the drug wasn't giving any benefit," he said. "It's really the same as giving patients nothing."

Actually, it may have been worse than giving them nothing. Relenza is a powder that must be inhaled, and it came with risks, especially for people with asthma and other lung disorders.

Elashoff's review of Relenza infuriated executives at Glaxo. Days after the panel voted against the drug, an executive sent a fiery letter to the director of the FDA's antiviral drugs division. The executive said the decision not to support the drug was "completely at odds with the will of Congress that drug development and approval proceed swiftly and surely."

The executive was referring to a 1992 law, passed at the urging of the industry's lobbyists, which allowed drug companies to pay "user fees" to the FDA to have their products approved more quickly. The law turned the relationship between the FDA and the drug companies on its head. The FDA began providing a service to the industry that now paid it. Drug companies became the agency's customers. Prior to the law, the sole duty of the FDA had been to police companies and protect consumers.

Glaxo's threatening letter worked. Shortly after receiving it, Elashoff's superiors approved Relenza. The company then began promoting the drug with television ads featuring a flu-stricken woman inhaling a dose of the drug and then booting a personification of the flu out her door. Americans seeing the ads believed they could wipe out the flu with a whiff from a Relenza inhaler. Glaxo was soon selling tens of thousands of prescriptions of a drug that its own studies had shown barely worked.

"I felt the entire process had been compromised," Elashoff said, recounting the experience six years after the drug was approved in 1999. Frustrated by the influence the industry had inside the government offices, he left the FDA soon after Relenza was approved. "The whole thing," he said, "still seems rather bizarre."

The case was not an isolated one. The FDA has approved many drugs it should have rejected. By 2007 more than a dozen drugs approved since 1992 had been pulled from the market or had steep restrictions put on their use. The agency said it could no longer argue that the products helped patients more than harmed them. These drugs were taken by millions of people, and killed hundreds, before they were withdrawn.

The law should be changed so that the industry no longer pays fees to the FDA. America needs regulators who can do their work without feeling a need to please the companies that are paying their salaries.

Stop the covert marketing of drugs, which is far more effective than the industry's advertisements.

The FDA must change the drug marketing rules to stop companies from hiring celebrities to endorse their products or talk about health matters with the public. Americans' fascination with celebrities makes it impossible for a Hollywood star or a sports hero to talk about a drug without leaving an impression that it is some kind of panacea.

Nonprofit groups should also be prevented from promoting medicines to the public without disclosing they have received money from the drugs' manufacturers. Charities should be forced to disclose on their websites and in their annual reports how much each company has given them. Some of this information is available in forms filed with the Internal Revenue Service, but the documents are not easily accessible to the public and do not include a detailed list of the group's donors. The charities should also disclose the names of companies funding their activities in each of their press releases and publications. The organizations should face the loss of their nonprofit status if they fail to disclose the corporate donations. Some of these groups, which pay no taxes, have become little more than marketing arms of the drug industry.

Public schools and universities should scrutinize any group offering to educate students about health or screen them for medical problems. The public should also be wary of health fairs or conferences sponsored by the pharmaceutical industry. The money for these events comes from companies' marketing departments. At the same time, legislatures should question the appropriateness of the financial grants the industry gives to state health departments and the agencies that operate the Medicaid program.

Newspapers and television stations must stop turning the press releases and videos they receive from drug marketers into news stories. The resulting news reports often quote physicians who are being paid by the manufacturer of the featured drug but fail to disclose the doctors' conflicts of interest. The news stories almost always exaggerate the possible benefits of a drug while ignoring its risks, just the outcome the company's public relations team was aiming for.

Prevent automobile accidents caused by drivers impaired by the effects of their medications.

The FDA should require a clear, bold warning against driving on the bottles of prescription or over-the-counter medications that cause drowsiness, dizziness, or any other side effect that can make it dangerous to drive. The warning should include a prominent symbol, like a bright red triangle, that patients can't miss.

States also need tough penalties for physicians who fail to warn patients not to drive after taking these medications as well as for patients who don't heed their doctors' warnings.

Traffic officers should be trained to recognize drivers who have been impaired by their medications. Any driver involved in an accident that causes fatalities or serious injury should be tested for prescription drugs. The federal government should collect statistics on the number of accidents caused by each type of prescription medication and warn the public about those causing the most danger on the roads.

Stop the fraud.

By 2007 just about every major pharmaceutical company was under investigation for fraudulent marketing or other illegal business practices. Prosecutors have tried to discourage the fraud by imposing fines of nearly a billion dollars on some drug companies. The pharmaceutical executives appear to consider these fines as little more than a cost of doing business. With no limits on drug prices in America, the companies have simply raised their prices to cover the penalties.

Congress must change the law so that pharmaceutical crimes result in harsh penalties for the executives who plan and direct them. Executives should face prison time if they are found to have ordered their employees to engage in illegal practices that put patients' lives at risk.

Spend less money on pills and more on keeping people from getting sick in the first place.

Despite estimates that 15 percent of American deaths are caused by inactivity or a poor diet, doctors do little to encourage healthier habits. Only about half of Americans age fifty or above say their doctors have asked whether they were active. Physicians are even more lax in telling children about the benefits of exercise. In one study, less than a quarter of all children or their parents were told by their doctors that exercise could keep them healthy.

At the same time, the skies over many cities remain polluted even though scientists have shown that people living in the worst smog die at higher rates than those breathing cleaner air. Americans also continue to use toys, cosmetics, and pesticides containing industrial chemicals that have been banned in other countries because of their potential to harm human health.

Much could be done to prevent disease, but keeping people healthy is not a priority in America's profit-driven medical system, which thrives when people are ill.

Protect yourself.

Find a physician who refuses to take the pharmaceutical industry's hand-outs and instead works only to give patients the best care. A small but growing number of doctors have refused to let sales reps into their offices. They throw away the invitations to the industry's dinner parties. Always aware of the potential bias, they do their best to unravel the industry's studies they read in medical journals. They hesitate to prescribe the newest drugs that their patients ask about after seeing ads on TV. They prescribe drugs only when necessary and make sure patients understand all the potential risks.

Look inside a physician's waiting room to see how friendly he or she is with the industry. Are there sales brochures for drugs displayed on the tables? Are there sharply dressed sales representatives bringing lunch for the doctor's entire staff? Are the clocks and tissue boxes displaying ads for medications? If you like your physician but can see that the drug companies have his ear, tell him it worries you.

Before taking any drug, ask yourself and your doctor whether you really need it. Are there ways you could solve your problem without taking medication? If your blood pressure is too high, for instance, perhaps limiting the salt in your diet would bring it back down.

Don't take any drug before you know all the risks. Get a copy of the drug's label. The pharmaceutical companies write this document in language that even most doctors can't understand, but it contains all the information the FDA believes is needed to use the drug safely. The label lists all the known risks of the drug, and the drug companies use it to escape legal liability. If a patient dies or is injured, executives point out that they listed the risk in the label and that it was not their fault the patient took the drug anyway.

Be skeptical if a doctor suggests that you take a drug for symptoms that are not actually disease. The drug marketers have learned to expand their markets by getting doctors to prescribe pills for things like "prediabetes," "subclinical thyroid disease," and "prehypertension." While such diagnoses don't meet the threshold of disease, the marketers urge doctors to prescribe pills to these patients anyway, claiming it will ward off real illness or somehow help the patient by providing "early treatment." Many doctors have followed the marketers' pleas, perhaps because each new diagnosis provides them with a stream of revenue from continuing office visits.

All drugs have risks, even when prescribed exactly as approved by the FDA. That is why it is hard to justify giving prescriptions to someone who is not sick. A healthy person gains no benefit from the drug but still suffers all the harm.

If you start taking a drug but find yourself suffering from another health problem, always consider that it might be a side effect. Never stop taking a medicine without talking to your doctor, however. Some drugs need to be stopped slowly. Some may be necessary even if they bother you with side effects.

Beware of any drug you see advertised on television or that your doctor hands you in the form of a free sample. These are the newest products, the ones that scientists know the least about. You want the medicine that has the best chance of helping you with the least amount of risk. You don't want a drug just because the sales representative has dropped off samples with the doctor's receptionist.

Start a revolution.

This is your medical system. You're paying dearly for it, whether you use it or not. At some point, you or someone you care about will have to use it, and your lives will depend on it.

Write or talk to your state and federal lawmakers. Vote for those political candidates who promise to take on the pharmaceutical industry and change the system so that patients once again come first.

There's too much at stake.

NOTES
BIBLIOGRAPHY
ACKNOWLEDGMENTS
INDEX

NOTES

Abbreviations

BMJ   *British Medical Journal*
JAMA *The Journal of the American Medical Association*
NEJM *The New England Journal of Medicine*

Introduction

4   **Vaniqa:** Bristol-Myers Squibb began selling Vaniqa as a facial hair removal cream in 2000 through an aggressive marketing campaign that included ads on television and in magazines like *Cosmopolitan*. Controversy erupted when the public realized a drug being used to minimize the mustaches of American women was not available to people dying of sleeping sickness in Africa. Eventually the French drug company Aventis, which held the rights to the drug, signed a deal to provide it for free for five years to the World Health Organization to treat poor patients suffering from sleeping sickness. Bristol-Myers contributed to this program. See "Aventis to Donate Sleeping-Sickness Drugs," *The New York Times*, May 4, 2001. Also see description of the industry's lack of interest in selling drugs for sleeping sickness by Donald G. McNeil, Jr., "Medicine Merchants: Drug Makers and 3rd World: Study in Neglect," *The New York Times*, May 21, 2000.

4   **transformation in the . . . industry over the last twenty-five years:** This is described in detail in chapters 4 and 5. Also see comments by pharmaceutical execu-

tives about how the industry has entered an era of marketing and me-too drugs in "Viewpoint: In Your Own Words," *Pharmaceutical Executive*, Aug. 2006.

4 **"pearlescent pigments":** Andrew Bridges, "FDA OKs Pearly Pigments to Color Pills," The Associated Press, July 20, 2006.

5 **"can look beautiful":** "Ortho Evra Joins Rosa Cha by Amir Slama for Mercedes-Benz Fashion Week Spring 2004," Press release from Johnson & Johnson, Sept. 2003.

5 **free tips on your golf game:** "New PGA Tour Partner Cialis Debuts Consumer Golf Plans at the Honda Classic," Press release from Lilly ICOS, March 11, 2004.

5 **Americans spent more on prescription drugs in 2004:** According to IMS Health, a consulting firm, Americans spent $251.8 billion on prescription drugs in 2005 and $238.9 billion in 2004. See IMS National Sales Perspectives, Jan. 2006. Gross domestic product in 2005 in U.S. dollars for Argentina ($172.1 billion) and Peru ($72.9 billion) is from *World Economic Outlook Database*, Apr. 2005. Accessed from International Monetary Fund website (imf.org) in Apr. 2006. Year 2004 consumer spending figures are from U.S. Department of Commerce's Bureau of Economic Analysis "Table 2.4.5U. Personal Consumption Expenditures by Type of Product." In 2004, Americans spent $227.2 billion on gasoline and other motor fuel, $200 billion on "meals at limited service eating places," $117.7 billion on higher education, and $97.5 billion on new automobiles. Americans spent $213.7 billion on prescription drugs in 2004, according to Table 2.4.5U, but this amount does not include drugs used in hospitals and other such facilities.

5 **Americans spend more on medicines than do all the people of Japan:** According to statistics from IMS Health's "Retail Drug Monitor: 12 months to Feb. 2005." Available at imshealth.com.

5 **65 percent of the nation now takes:** "Outpatient Prescription Drug Expenses in the U.S. Community Population, 2003," Medical Expenditure Panel Survey Chartbook No. 16. Available at meps.ahrq.gov.

5 **build their laboratories on . . . public universities:** For example, Eli Lilly operated a clinical research lab in 2004 on the campus of Indiana University School of Medicine.

6 **average American collected more than twelve prescriptions . . . in 2006:** "Prescription Drug Trends," Kaiser Family Foundation, May 2007.

6 **Older Americans take . . . an average of thirty prescriptions:** See "Cost Overdose: Growth in Drug Spending for the Elderly," a report by Families USA, July 2000.

6 **"do you use sleeping tablets":** Transcript of interview of Secretary Powell by Abdul Rahman al-Rashed, Nov. 5, 2003. Accessed from state.gov in July 2006.

6   **hundred thousand Americans die each year:** Lazarou et al., "Incidence of Adverse Drug Reactions in Hospitalized Patients," *JAMA*, Apr. 15, 1998.

7   **twice as many as . . . automobile accidents:** In 2005, 43,442 Americans died in highway accidents, according to press release of Sept. 18, 2006, from National Transportation Safety Board.

7   **more Americans than . . . diabetes:** In 2004, 73,138 Americans died of diabetes, while 65,965 died from Alzheimer's disease. See Table 31, "Health, United States, 2006," U.S. Department of Health and Human Services. Available at cdc.gov.

7   **"grossly overprescribed nation":** Interview with Dr. Arthur Relman, July 29, 2002.

7   **may now pay as much to care for patients . . . harmed by their prescriptions:** A study by Ernst and Grizzle estimated that drug-related problems (adverse reactions, overdoses, failure to receive a needed drug, etc.) cost the nation more than $177 billion in 2000. That cost was for emergency room visits, hospital stays, nursing home care, and other expenses needed by those hurt or killed by prescription drugs. That year Americans spent $120 billion on prescription drugs, according to the Centers for Medicare & Medicaid Services. See Ernst and Grizzle, "Drug-Related Morbidity and Mortality: Updating the Cost-of-Illness Model," *Journal of the American Pharmaceutical Association*, March 2001. This study did not include the cost of caring for patients harmed by drugs they received in the hospital, which would have added tens of billions of dollars.

7   **prescription spending rose faster for children:** See "2004 Drug Trend Report," published by Medco. Also see Bergstrom et al., "The Growing Pediatrics Market," *Pharmaceutical Executive*, Aug. 2004.

8   **More than 750 . . . children died:** Moore et al., "Reported Adverse Drug Events in Infants and Children Under 2 Years of Age," *Pediatrics*, Nov. 2002.

8   **vast majority of the industry's marketing . . . at physicians:** 85 percent is directed at doctors, according to "Lifetime Customer Value in the Pharmaceutical Industry: Compliance, Disease Management and CRM," a report by Cutting Edge Information in 2002, p. 29.

8   **an army of . . . sales representatives:** The pharmaceutical industry employed 101,531 sales reps in 2004, according to Verispan, a consulting firm. These statistics were quoted in an article by Ed Silverman, "Pfizer Bucks Sales-Force Trend," *The Star-Ledger*, Apr. 17, 2005. Physicians and surgeons held about 567,000 jobs in 2004, according to the *Occupational Outlook Handbook, 2006–7 Edition*, published by U.S. Department of Labor, Bureau of Labor Statistics, accessed at bls.gov, Apr. 2006. In 1995 the industry employed about 38,000 sales reps, according to Verispan's Pharmaceutical Sales Force Structures & Strategies. That report's statistics were presented by Kelly Sborlini on Jan. 21, 2004, to the Healthcare Marketing & Communications Council.

8   **virtually every . . . physician now takes these handouts:** Campbell et al., "A National Survey of Physician-Industry Relationships," *NEJM*, Apr. 26, 2007.

8   **Tap Pharmaceutical:** Description of the company's gifts to physicians is from facts uncovered by federal investigators and used as evidence of criminal fraud in the case, *United States of America v. Tap Pharmaceutical Products*, filed in U.S. District Court in Boston. The company pleaded guilty to conspiracy and agreed to pay $875 million to settle the case in 2001. Also see evidence filed in a related criminal case in the same court, *United States of America v. Joseph Spinella*. Dr. Spinella pleaded guilty to health care fraud in 2001.

8   **"It's nice after an exhausting day":** Identical letters sent by Dr. Nancy Sika and Dr. Colleen Heniff in 2002 to the Office of Inspector General, U.S. Department of Health and Human Services, in response to a request for public comment on whether new restrictions should be put on the marketing efforts of pharmaceutical companies.

9   **"We were helpless":** Letter written by Mrs. Albert F. Rust on Oct. 1, 2002, and sent to the Office of Inspector General in response to the same request for public comment.

9   **10 percent of the price . . . raw chemicals and manufacturing:** Melody Petersen, "Lifting the Curtain on the Real Costs of Making AIDS Drugs," *The New York Times*, Apr. 24, 2001.

9   **sixteen cents of each dollar of revenue into profit:** Exhibit 1.21: Profitability Among Pharmaceutical Manufacturers Compared to Other Industries, *Trends and Indicators in the Changing Health Care Marketplace*, Kaiser Family Foundation. Accessed at kff.org.

10   **spent more on lobbying . . . than any other industry:** M. Asif Ismail, "Drug Lobby Second to None," The Center for Public Integrity, July 7, 2005. The report said the drug industry had 1,291 registered lobbyists in 2004, more than twice the 535 members of Congress.

10   **pay far lower taxes . . . than other major industries:** "Memorandum: Federal Taxation of the Drug Industry from 1990 to 1996," Congressional Research Service, Dec. 13, 1999.

11   **"Sell them their dreams":** Quoted in William Leach, *Land of Desire* (New York: Pantheon, 1993), p. 298.

ONE: Creating Disease

15   **affecting . . . one in every four American adults:** Press release from Pharmacia, "One in Four Adults Report Symptoms of Overactive Bladder," May 28, 1998.

15   **Wolf was preparing to reveal:** Speech entitled "Positioning Detrol (Creating a Disease)," at the Pharmaceutical Marketing Global Summit, Philadelphia, Pa.,

Jan. 13, 2003. Information is from my notes taken while listening to the presentation as well as from the slides Mr. Wolf prepared to accompany his talk. Permission to use this material was obtained in 2003 from Mr. Wolf and from the Strategic Research Institute, which organized the Global Summit.

16 **giant pill capsules on the midways:** Brochure entitled *The Competitive Edge, on and off the Track,* from HomeMed Pharmacy and Kelley Racing.

16 **promote prescription pills at . . . malls:** Brochure entitled *Healthcare Solutions: The Mall Is the Medium,* from Simon Brand Ventures.

17 **profits at . . . twice the rate of the broader market:** According to an analysis by Bernstein Research in 2002, big drug companies increased their earnings per share at a rate of 11.4 percent a year over the previous two decades compared with 5.6 percent for all companies in the S&P 500. Bernstein Research, "Pharmaceutical Quarterly," Apr. 2002.

17 **send more than eighty-eight thousand American students:** In 2004 the average total annual cost, including room and board, for an in-state student at a four-year public college was $11,354, according to "Trends in College Pricing 2004," a survey by the College Board.

18 **pill's color had become a marketing tool:** See "Pharma Brands Capture Minds and Hearts," by IMS Health consultants, Sept. 25, 2001. Accessed at imshealth.com, Dec. 2004.

19 **benchmark of one billion dollars in sales:** See "Blockbusters Blast a Highway Through Pharma Sales," by IMS Health consultants, Feb. 1, 2000. Accessed at imshealth.com, Oct. 2004.

19 **"You create a desire":** Interview with Daniel Vasella, Sept. 5, 2000.

21 **Her hallucinations began:** This patient is described in Jack W. Tsao and Kenneth M. Heilman, "Transient Memory Impairment and Hallucinations Associated with Tolterodine Use," *NEJM,* Dec. 4, 2003.

21 **"branding a condition":** Vince Parry, "The Art of Branding a Condition," *Medical Marketing & Media,* May 2003.

22 **market for Listerine . . . halitosis:** James Harvey Young, *The Medical Messiahs: A Social History of Health Quackery in Twentieth-Century America* (Princeton, N.J.: Princeton University Press, 1992).

22 **few people knew . . . generalized anxiety disorder:** See Brendan I. Koerner, "Disorders Made to Order," *Mother Jones,* July/Aug. 2002.

22 **Sarafem . . . television ads:** See letter addressed to Gregory T. Brophy, an executive at Eli Lilly, and written by Lisa L. Stockbridge at the FDA. Released Nov. 16, 2000.

23   **European regulators . . . "not a well-established disease":** See Dec. 2003 let-
      ter written by Eli Lilly executives in Basingstoke, England, which was distrib-
      uted to British doctors.

23   **no real definition of disease:** For a discussion of this, as well as a list of the
      expanding number of things considered disease, see Richard Smith, "In Search
      of Non-disease," *BMJ*, Apr. 13, 2002.

23   **"in general use without formal definition":** J. G. Scadding, "Diagnosis: The
      Clinician and the Computer," *The Lancet*, Oct. 21, 1967.

24   **"gnaw away at our self-confidence":** Lynn Payer, *Disease-Mongers: How Doctors,
      Drug Companies, and Insurers Are Making You Feel Sick* (New York: John Wiley
      & Sons, 1992), p. 6.

24   **Even the tests . . . can harm:** For an example, see Christopher Windham,
      "Study Warns of CT Scans' Risks," *The Wall Street Journal*, Aug. 31, 2004.

24   **40 percent of tests . . . not needed:** Gortmaker et al., "A Successful Experi-
      ment to Reduce Unnecessary Laboratory Use in a Community Hospital," *Medical
      Care*, 1988.

24   **three-act play titled *Knock*:** Jules Romains, *Knock, ou Le triomphe de la
      médecine* (Paris: Gallimard, 1924). Also see I. Bamforth, "Knock: A Study of
      Medical Cynicism," *Medical Humanities*, June 2002.

25   **Watching their salaries stall:** See Hoangmai Pham, et al., "Financial Pressures
      Spur Physician Entrepreneurialism," *Health Affairs*, March–Apr. 2004. Also see
      Deborah Borfitz, "Make Your Practices More Profitable," *Medical Economics*,
      Jan. 8, 2001.

25   **Dr. Martin Keller . . . at Brown:** Alison Bass, "Drug Companies Enrich Brown
      Professor," *The Boston Globe*, Oct. 4, 1999.

25   **Dr. Arnold Klein, a Beverly Hills dermatologist:** See Gina Piccalo, "A Glam-
      orous Drug, an Illness, a Very Public Battle," *Los Angeles Times*, Sept. 22, 2004.

26   **Dr. P. Trey Sunderland, an expert on Alzheimer's:** See stories by David Will-
      man in the *Los Angeles Times* in 2004 and 2005, including "NIH Seeks Outside
      Inquiry of Scientist," Jan. 28, 2005. The NIH later banned its employees from
      taking gifts and fees from the pharmaceutical industry.

26   **Merck, doctors could . . . make travel reservations:** From information at
      merckservices.com. Accessed Feb. 28, 2005.

26   **"a lot of hay about nothing":** Interview with Charles Nemeroff in July 2003.
      Also see Melody Petersen, "Undisclosed Financial Ties Prompt Reproval of
      Doctor," *The New York Times*, Aug. 3, 2003. Dr. Nemeroff's financial ties to the
      industry were disclosed in Nemeroff and Gutman, "Preclinical and Clinical Stud-
      ies of Novel Antidepressants," which was available on medscape.com in 2003.

26   **word-of-mouth marketing:** George Silverman and Eve Zukergood, "How to Harness Word of Mouth in the Pharmaceutical Industry," 2000. Accessed Feb. 2005 on website of Market Navigation (mnav.com). Article is a revision of one first published in *Medical Marketing & Media*. Also see profile of Silverman at mnav.com.

27   **signed up more than twenty thousand physicians:** *Unleashing the Power of Medical Education*, a brochure distributed by Thomson Physicians World in 2002.

28   **"We work with the second-tier":** My notes from a panel discussion called "Pre-Launch Marketing Strategies: Improving Product Uptake" at the Pharmaceutical Marketing Congress in Philadelphia on Oct. 1, 2002.

28   **Pharmacia paid to gather its physicians:** Pharmacia provided a grant to pay for two symposia held in London. It also paid to have the proceedings of these symposia published in two supplements in *Urology*, a medical journal. See "The Overactive Bladder: From Basic Science to Clinical Management: Consensus Conference," ed. Paul Abrams and Alan J. Wein, *Urology*, Dec. 1997. Also see "Overactive Bladder and Its Treatments: Consensus Conference," ed. Paul Abrams and Alan J. Wein, *Urology*, May 2000. Both Dr. Abrams, of the Bristol Urological Institute, and Dr. Wein, of the University of Pennsylvania's School of Medicine, worked as consultants to Pharmacia for many years.

28   **Pharmacia's urologists . . . eventually agreed with the drug company:** Wolf told the audience in Philadelphia on Jan. 13, 2003, that Pharmacia had won "a major coup" at the symposium in July 1999 when the urologists agreed that a patient did not have to actually be incontinent to have the disease.

28   **The doctors talked about . . . "profound" effect:** Wolf explained during his 2003 presentation that one of Pharmacia's "critical success factors" in its process of creating a disease was to "establish OAB as a serious medical condition with profound negative impact on people's quality of life." The company began this process by recruiting doctors to talk and write about how an overactive bladder could hinder one's life. Some of this work was done by doctors affiliated with the Bristol Urological Institute in the United Kingdom. For example, an early article was written by Simon Jackson, a doctor connected with the institute, and published in the 1997 supplement to *Urology*. See Simon Jackson, "The Patient with an Overactive Bladder—Symptoms and Quality-of-Life Issues," *Urology*, Dec. 1997. A similar article was by Dr. Abrams. See Paul Abrams et al., "Overactive Bladder Significantly Affects Quality of Life," *The American Journal of Managed Care*, July 2000. Dr. Abrams is also from the Bristol institute. The website for the Bristol Urological Institute explains that Pharmacia gave "generous donations" to help pay for a new building that began construction in 2003. See bui.ac.uk. Accessed Aug. 2006.

29   **Elsevier . . . had a "pharmaceutical division":** See int.elsevierhealth.com.
      Accessed Dec. 2004.

29   **The names of these doctors are in . . . articles:** At a meeting in New York City
      in December 1999, Dr. Paul Abrams said he and other doctors at the meeting
      had reached a consensus on the definition of overactive bladder. This meeting
      was also organized and paid for by Pharmacia. Many of the doctors attend-
      ing also worked for Pharmacia as consultants. The company then paid to have
      the meeting's proceedings published in "Overactive Bladder: Examining the Bur-
      den of Disease," a supplement to the *American Journal of Managed Care*, July
      2000. The supplement included a lengthy article by Dr. Alan J. Wein on how
      overactive bladder should be defined. Two years later, Dr. Abrams and Dr. Wein
      were among the authors of the 2002 article that was often cited as providing the
      official definition of overactive bladder. See Abrams et al., "The standardization
      of terminology of lower urinary tract function: report from the standardization
      subcommittee of the International Continence Society," *Neurourology and Uro-
      dynamics*, 2002. Later, Wein explained in a presentation that there was no real
      definition of the disorder before 2002 and that the term had originated with the
      package of information that Pharmacia had submitted to the FDA in its attempt
      to get Detrol approved. See Alan J. Wein, "Overactive Bladder Terminology, Di-
      agnosis and Treatment Options," a slide presentation available at urotoday.com.
      Accessed in Nov. 2004.

30   **"helped coin the term":** Rebecca Gardyn, "Detrol: Neil Wolf," *Advertising Age*,
      June 28, 1999.

31   **Lauren Bacall:** Melody Petersen, "Heartfelt Advice, Hefty Fees," *The New York
      Times*, Aug. 11, 2002.

31   **On an episode of *ER*:** Hill & Knowlton, a public relations firm hired by Pfizer,
      suggested to producers at NBC that Aricept, a drug for Alzheimer's, be put into
      the show's script. Described in "Alzheimer's Campaign Peaks [*sic*] Public and
      Media Interest," *PR News*, May 21, 2001.

31   **"I can go into a room":** "Secrets of a Supermodel: Lauren Hutton Talks About
      Menopause," transcript of a webcast video recorded on Dec. 18, 2000, by
      Healthology. See healthology.com. At the time Hutton was the celebrity spokes-
      person for a campaign paid for by Wyeth-Ayerst, the maker of Prempro.

32   **"appear to be spontaneous":** Robert Chandler and Gianfranco Chicco, "Cre-
      ating a Pharma Buzz," *PharmaVOICE*, Jan.–Feb. 2002.

32   **The "ultimate goal":** From *Prime Cut*, a newsletter written by Chandler and
      Chicco, Spring 2004.

32   **Debbie Reynolds:** Patrick Perry, "On Tour with Debbie Reynolds," *The Satur-
      day Evening Post*, Jan.–Feb. 2003. Also see Pharmacia's press release "Hollywood
      Icon Debbie Reynolds Brings Overactive Bladder into the Spotlight," Apr. 25,
      2002.

33 **"For the last decade":** Jane E. Brody, "Treatments Offer Promise for Embarrassing Ailment," *The New York Times*, Dec. 8, 1998.

33 **bladder problems and sex lives:** See press release dated June 8, 2001, "Harris Interactive Survey Examines a Not-So-Talked-About Health Issue Affecting Intimacy for Many."

33 **FDA sent a warning letter:** See letter from FDA to Kathleen Day at Pharmacia & Upjohn, Dec. 7, 2000.

33 **16 percent of the American population:** See Stewart et al., "Prevalence and Burden of Overactive Bladder in the United States," *World Journal of Urology*, May 2003. Pharmacia paid for this survey according to a press release dated May 2000 and entitled, "National Screening of More than 80,000 Americans Sheds New Light on Nation's Bladder Health."

34 **market . . . growing by 30 percent:** See press release "Novartis to buy Enablex," March 18, 2003.

34 **Competitors tried to imitate:** See "Pharmacia Corp. Promotes Overactive Bladder Awareness Through the American Society of Travel Agents," *Med Ad News*, June 1, 2001, as well as a March 28, 2001, press release, "Pharmacia Corp. and the American Society of Travel Agents Announce Partnership." Also see press release "Professional Golfers Drive Awareness on and off the Links for Bladder Health," June 5, 2001. And see press release "National Association of Female Executives Launches Healthcare Initiative to Educate About Overactive Bladder," Jan. 25, 2005. (In 2005, Alza was known as Ortho-McNeil, a subsidiary of Johnson & Johnson.)

34 **five-question screening guide:** Wolf presentation in Jan. 2003.

35 **Mary Lou Retton:** See press release "Gold-Medal Winner Reveals Struggle with Serious Health Condition That Affects Millions of Americans," Sept. 29, 2004.

35 **One of Retton's first stops . . . Cincinnati:** From promotional description of the event by radio station 96.5 The Star (WYGY-FM).

35 **"I wish I hadn't waited":** Retton's quote is from a Pfizer press release of Sept. 29, 2004.

35 **FDA pointed out:** Letter from Mark W. Askine of the FDA to Kathleen J. Day at Pharmacia, sent Apr. 13, 1999.

35 **FDA said Alza had broken the law:** Letter from Mark Askine to Stephen W. Sherman at Alza, sent Apr. 2, 1999.

36 **She was only forty-six:** Described in Kyle Womack and Kenneth Heilman, "Tolterodine and Memory: Dry but Forgetful," *Archives of Neurology*, May 2003.

36 **Another woman, age seventy-three:** Described in Tsao and Heilman, "Transient Memory Impairment and Hallucinations Associated with Tolterodine Use," *NEJM*, Dec. 4, 2003.

37   **"pushes them over the edge"**: Interview with Dr. Jack Tsao in 2005.

37   **researchers at Emory University**: Jewart et al., "Cognitive, Behavioral and Physiological Changes in Alzheimer Disease Patients as a Function of Incontinence Medications," *American Journal of Geriatric Psychiatry*, Apr. 2005.

37   **British researchers studied the brains**: See Elaine Perry et al., "Increased Alzheimer Pathology in Parkinson's Disease Related to Antimuscarinic Drugs," *Annals of Neurology*, Aug. 2003.

TWO: Midwestern Medicine Show

38   **Alvin Straight**: His story was told in *The Straight Story*, a 1999 film directed by David Lynch. A short biography of Straight can be found at *The Des Moines Register*'s website (desmoinesregister.com).

40   **number of children . . . taking prescription sleeping pills**: Statistic is from Medco Health Solutions press release of Oct. 17, 2005.

40   **spending as much . . . as McDonald's**: Andrew Pollack, "With New Sleeping Pill, New Acceptability?" *The New York Times*, Dec. 17, 2004.

40   **"night after night after night"**: Ad for Lunesta that appeared in *Psychiatric Annals* in 2005.

40   **rarely be prescribed for more than ten days**: The FDA approved Ambien only for the "short-term treatment" of insomnia. Also see Sandra G. Boodman, "You May Want to Sleep on It," *The Washington Post*, Jan. 18, 2005.

40   **"I work for a pharmaceutical company"**: My notes from Hillmer's talk, "Insomnia: Should You Lose Sleep Over It?," June 20, 2005, at the Buena Vista Regional Medical Center.

42   **People over the age of sixty-five**: See Glass et al., "Sedative Hypnotics in Older People with Insomnia: Meta-Analysis of Risks and Benefits," *BMJ*, Nov. 11, 2005. Also see David Armstrong, "Sleep Aids May Do Little for Elderly," *The Wall Street Journal*, Dec. 6, 2005.

43   **I could try Ambien . . . for free**: Ad in *MediZine Healthy Living*, Second Quarter 2005.

43   **Sitting on the board of . . . Heart Association**: According to an article entitled "Heart Association," in the *Sioux City Journal* on Aug. 22, 2006, the new president of the Siouxland American Heart Association was a sales rep for AstraZeneca who specialized in "cardiac care." Also on the board was an employee of Schering-Plough. AstraZeneca's Crestor and Schering's Zetia were among the most heavily promoted cardiovascular medicines in 2006.

44   **storybook . . . to promote its antidepressant**: See more on the book, *Kids Like Me*, in chapter 3.

44   **"What you don't know could kill you"**: Ad from Sanofi warning about blood clots. Appeared in *Parade* magazine, Feb. 13, 2005. The company sells the drug Lovenox.

44   **"All it may take is the formation of one clot"**: Ad for Plavix in *MediZine*, Second Quarter 2005.

45   **"The purpose of publicity"**: John Berger, *Ways of Seeing* (London: British Broadcasting Corporation, 1972).

45   **"invasion of one's mind"**: George Orwell, "Politics and the English Language," an essay written Apr. 1946.

45   **seven of the ten biggest advertisers**: Brian Steinberg and Christopher Lawton, "TV News Outlets Revamp Web Sites," *The Wall Street Journal*, July 19, 2005.

46   **35 percent . . . said an ad had prompted them to ask their doctors**: Weissman et al., "Consumers' Reports on the Health Effects of Direct-to-Consumer Drug Advertising," *Health Affairs*, Feb. 26, 2003.

46   **More often than not doctors gave these patients the prescriptions**: Slide presentation called "Verispan's Promotion Review—2004," available at amponline.org. Accessed 2006.

46   **In a study in 2005**: Kravitz et al., "Influence of Patients' Requests for Direct-to-Consumer Advertised Antidepressants," *JAMA*, Apr. 27, 2005.

46   **spend 25 percent . . . of their revenues on promotion**: The companies don't reveal much about their marketing costs, except for reporting their total spending on promotion and administration in their financial statements. Some drug companies spend nearly 50 percent of their sales on selling and administrative costs. For example, Warner-Lambert spent 47 percent of its sales on these costs in 1998, according to its annual financial statements. A consultant working for the Medicare program found the companies spent an average of 31 percent of their revenues on selling and administrative costs in 2001. See "Health Care Industry Market Update: Pharmaceuticals," Jan. 10, 2003, Centers for Medicare & Medicaid Services. These numbers may be understated because some promotional costs are being reported as research expenses. See more in chapter 5.

47   **"The vast majority of drugs"**: Steve Connor, "Glaxo Chief: Our Drugs Do Not Work on Most Patients," *The Independent*, Dec. 8, 2003.

47   **medicines worked in as few as 25 percent**: Spear et al., "Clinical Application of Pharmacogenetics," *Trends in Molecular Medicine*, May 2001.

47   **"If you look across"**: From "The End of Trial and Error," an interview with Mara G. Aspinall, *The Wharton Healthcare Leadership Exchange*, a magazine published by Wharton School of Business, Feb. 2006.

48   **Razadyne**: Until 2006 the drug was known by the brand name Reminyl. Its generic chemical name is galantamine.

48   **average improvement of just 2.7 points:** Jacqueline Birks, "Cholinesterase In-
      hibitors for Alzheimer's Disease," an abstract of study published in July 2006 by
      the U.K.-based Cochrane Collaboration. Available at cochrane.org.

48   **patients had died while taking Razadyne:** Letter sent to doctors by Ortho-
      McNeil Pharmaceuticals on March 31, 2005.

48   **patients taking Aricept died:** "Eisai Reports Results from Latest Donepezil
      Study in Vascular Dementia," corporate press release, March 16, 2006.

49   **"So you compare it to nothing?":** Transcript of the exchange between Dr.
      Straus and Dr. Nicholson included in Stephen S. Hall, "The Claritin Effect, Pre-
      scription for Profit," *The New York Times Magazine*, March 11, 2001.

49   **"until the cows come home":** Comment by Dr. Paul Leber at the FDA's
      Psychopharmacological Drugs Advisory Committee meeting of Nov. 19, 1990.
      Included in David Healy, *Let Them Eat Prozac* (Toronto: James Lorimer & Com-
      pany, 2003).

49   **In more than half these studies:** Khan et al., "Are Placebo Controls Necessary
      to Test New Antidepressants and Anxiolytics?," *International Journal of Neuro-
      psychopharmacology*, Sept. 2002.

50   **"We didn't want to create a cute character":** Brian Steinberg, "Novartis
      Brings Back 'Digger' to TV Spots for Lamisil Drug," *The Wall Street Journal*,
      March 22, 2004.

51   **only 38 percent of patients were cured:** The results of the clinical trials are
      listed in the FDA-approved package label or "prescribing information" for the
      drug available at lamisil.com. Accessed July 2006.

52   **Elidel . . . Superman-like character:** Pictured at elidel.com in 2005.

52   **Eczema Beast:** Ad available at protopic.com in 2005.

52   **creams . . . could cause cancer:** FDA Public Health Advisory on Elidel and
      Protopic, March 10, 2005.

53   **giving teens seven free music downloads:** Described at differin.com in Feb.
      2007 and in Public Citizen's "Testimony Before the Senate Special Committee
      on Aging on the Impact of Direct-to-Consumer Drug Advertising on Seniors'
      Health and Health Care Costs," Sept. 29, 2005.

53   **girls create their own melodic ring tones:** From promotion of Alesse called
      "Meet the Alesse Girls!" at muchmusic.com. Accessed Apr. 2006. The site included
      many games for girls, including one in which they could decorate their virtual
      bedrooms and another in which they could take the "Personality Power Test."

53   **play is a child's number one need:** James U. McNeal, *The Kids Market: Myths
      and Realities* (Ithaca, N.Y.: Paramount Market Publishing, 1999), p. 160.

53   **"My research suggests":** Ibid., p. 202.

53 "This ad works wonders": From "Ad Agency Review 2004," *Medical Marketing & Media*, July 2004.

53 a puppy called Max: "Getting the Maximum," published on pmlive.com, website of *Pharmaceutical Marketing* magazine, Jan. 7, 2005.

53 a magic dragon named Spot: Online version of storybook entitled *Adventures with Max and Spot*, available at learningaboutgrowth.com. Accessed Sept. 2006.

53 created Spot to be the embodiment of . . . Saizen: Saizen case study described on website of the CPR Group, a Fleishman-Hillard Company. See cprworldwide.com. Accessed Sept. 2006.

54 Magic Foundation: History and corporate pharmaceutical sponsors accessed from the group's website, magicfoundation.org, Sept. 2005.

54 measured the height of children: The screenings in public schools by the Magic Foundation and by the Human Growth Foundation led to an investigation by the Federal Trade Commission. See Rick Weiss, "Are Short Kids 'Sick'?," *The Washington Post*, March 15, 1994. Also see Ralph T. King, Jr., "Profit Prescription: In Marketing of Drugs, Genentech Tests Limits of What Is Acceptable," *The Wall Street Journal*, Jan. 11, 1995.

55 "I was short": "Me and My Growth Hormone," *The Magic Foundation Magazine*, 2004. The foundation said the story was "contributed anonymously by an affected child."

55 National Depression Screening Day: Dr. Douglas Jacobs, a Harvard professor and consultant to at least one pharmaceutical company, helped create National Depression Screening Day in 1991. In 2005 he was the executive director of Screening for Mental Health, Inc., the group that promoted the screenings. The group boasted it had become the largest provider of mental health screening in the United States, testing more than two hundred thousand Americans for mental illness each year. A careful look at the group's website, mentalhealthscreening .org, finds that the screenings were funded by five drug companies, all sellers of antidepressants. See background information at mentalhealthscreening.org. Accessed Oct. 2005. The group says its primary goal is to find and help people who may be on the verge of committing suicide. In 2004, however, a panel of experts brought together by the federal government warned that there was a lack of evidence that such screenings decreased suicide attempts or actually helped people more than hurt them. The experts said they could find no studies that looked at the possible harm caused by the screenings, which includes prescribing antidepressants to people who do not need them. See U.S. Preventive Services Task Force, *Screening for Suicide Risk: Recommendation and Rationale*, May 2004, Agency for Healthcare Research and Quality. Available at ahrq.gov.

55 "I got more anxious": Katie Melson, "Are You Depressed?," *Iowa State Daily*, Oct. 8, 2003.

55   **Central College . . . published the results:** See *CampusTown*, a newsletter for the Central College community, Nov. 17, 2004.

56   **Wyeth . . . hired Cara Kahn:** Paul Glader, "Maker of Depression Drug Plans Forums at Colleges," *The Wall Street Journal*, Oct. 10, 2002.

56   **screenings at . . . Hy-Vee supermarket:** Article in *The Bulletin*, a biweekly newsletter of Mercy Medical Center in Des Moines, Sept. 27, 2002.

56   **more than 25 percent of those quizzed:** Shelly Greenfield et al., "Treatment for Depression Following the 1996 National Depression Screening Day," *American Journal of Psychiatry*, Nov. 2000.

57   **"Gone are the days":** Quote is from Teri P. Cox, the senior managing partner of Cox Communications Partners, "Forging Alliances: Advocacy Partners," published in a supplement to *Pharmaceutical Executive*, Sept. 2002.

57   **Council for Leadership on Thrombosis:** Described in press release from Aventis, "Medical Experts Unite to Raise Awareness of Risk, Threat of Blood Clots," Feb. 14, 2002.

57   **Pfizer helped pay for a conference:** See "UI to host conference on health care and young women," University of Iowa news release, Nov. 5, 2003. Also see agenda for the conference entitled "Romance, Risks, & Reason," held on Dec. 5 and 6, 2003, at the Holiday Inn in Coralville, Iowa.

57   **The company was trying to show in studies:** For example, see study the company paid for that tested whether Zoloft helped women with bulimia. Sloan et al., "Efficacy of Sertraline for Bulimia Nervosa," *International Journal of Eating Disorders*, accepted for publication Sept. 23, 2003.

57   **"We know that men":** Quote from Janice Lipsky, Pfizer's marketing director, in Mike Hembree, "Martin a Winner for Viagra: Pfizer Says NASCAR Gives Its Blue Pill a Good Push," *The Greenville News*, Oct. 16, 2003.

58   **major bass fishing competitions:** See press release, "New BASS Sponsor Cialis Showcases Interactive Presence in Augusta," March 2, 2005.

58   **In Tennessee, when kids went online:** Cialis was promoted at tnbass.com. Accessed Oct. 25, 2005. That website was linked to cialis.com, which included detailed descriptions of sexual stimulation.

59   **Crestor Charity Challenge:** Described in *Tour 2005 Up Close*, a PGA magazine distributed during the golf tournament.

59   **"Physicians must tell their patients the truth":** "The Statin Wars: Why AstraZeneca Must Retreat," *The Lancet*, Oct. 25, 2003.

59   **Cialis . . . gone blind:** Side effects listed in the Cialis "Prescribing Instructions," last revised June 5, 2007.

60   **had forty of its "agents" roam the stands:** Doug Campbell, "Nascar: We're Sticking with RJR," *The Business Journal of the Greater Triad Area*, Apr. 28, 2000.

60   RJR also erected driving simulators: Barry Meier, "The Media Business: A
      Controversy on Tobacco Road," *The New York Times*, Dec. 4, 1997.

60   "With tobacco, you can't": Larry Woody, "The End of Tobacco Road:
      NASCAR Will End the 31-Year Winston Era," *Auto Racing Digest*, Dec. 2003.

61   fans were screened for depression: "GlaxoSmithKline and Joe Gibbs Racing
      Join Forces in the 'Racing for Life' Health Screening Program at Bristol," press
      release, March 23, 2004. Accessed at joegibbsracing.com. Also see similar dis-
      ease screening of race fans by Pfizer called "Tune-up for Life." Described in
      "Gentlemen . . . Start Your Engines," *Effective Clinical Practice*, March–Apr.
      2002.

61   "I cried last week": Mark Martin's guestbook on markmartin.org. Accessed in
      2005.

61   Pfizer . . . inside churches: See Pfizer press release dated July 9, 2004, which
      describes Senior Rx Savings Weekend.

62   screen members of urban African American churches: "Pfizer Joins Forces
      with Unite for Sight for a National 'Glaucoma and You' Church Tour in January,"
      press release, Jan. 2006. Available at uniteforsight.org.

62   The magazine's publisher aggressively courted: See press release, "Guide-
      posts Magazine opens its 2.6 million circulation to advertising for first time in
      55 years," June 2000. Also see guidepostsmedia.com. Accessed Sept. 2005.

62   "The healing purple pill": Ad for Nexium in *Guideposts*, June 2005.

63   "I would hinder God": Paul D. Meier, ed., *Blue Genes* (Carol Stream, Ill.:
      Tyndale, 2005).

63   conference for industry executives: "Rethinking Patient Compliance," a
      meeting scheduled for Nov. 14 and 15, 2005, at the Crowne Plaza Philadelphia
      Hotel and organized by the Strategic Research Institute.

63   building giant databases . . . on physicians: Lou Sawaya, "Know Your Physi-
      cians: The Importance of Profiles," *Pharmaceutical Representative* magazine.
      Published online at pharmrep.com, Sept. 2002.

63   paid physicians or pharmacies . . . review their patient files: See more on
      how Warner-Lambert did this in chapter 7.

63   purchase the information from consulting firms: For one description of this
      tactic, see Jere Doyle, "Alternative Media: How to Capture Your Target Con-
      sumers' Profile Data Online," *Pharmaceutical Executive*, Feb. 1, 2006.

63   more than fifty-five million Americans: Taryn Foniri, "Patient-Level Data and
      Primary Market Research: A Powerful Combination," *Product Management To-
      day*, June 2005. Also see Jean-Patrick Tsang, "Patient Data Comes of Age," *Phar-
      maceutical Executive*, May 1, 2003. The overall process of collecting personal

data on consumers is known in the drug industry and other industries as customer relationship management or CRM.

64   **names and addresses . . . easy to obtain:** Some firms accumulate the names of
patients and their diseases and then sell this information. For example, a consultant wrote in 1997 that a two-step process called patient mapping consisted
of first purchasing a database with names of patients and their diseases and
then calling them for more information. Kenneth A. March, "A Blueprint for
Consumer-Driven Marketing," *Medical Marketing & Media*, March 1997.

64   **relationship marketing:** For an explanation, see Ilyssa Levins, "One-on-One
Relationship Marketing Comes of Age," *Medical Marketing & Media*, June 1998.

64   **"profiled and active":** From Amy Valley and Kim Ramko, "The Customer: A
Single View," *Pharmaceutical Executive* magazine's *PE Product Management*,
Feb. 1, 2002.

64   *Sesame Street:* Information was obtained from everydaykidz.com as well as
from sesameworkshop.org in Aug. 2006. Also see "Pointers for Parents: Sesame
Workshop and EveryDayKidz.com Teaming Up to Educate Parents and Kids
About Asthma," an article by North American Precis Syndicate, which distrib-
utes feature stories for corporations. Accessed at napsnet.com in Aug. 2006.

64   **Serono, a Swiss company:** This describes the website created by Serono for
children called coollearnings.com. Accessed Aug. 2006.

65   **like a dinner "date":** Described in David L. Stern, "E-Marketing at the Tipping
Point," *Pharmaceutical Executive*, Feb. 2, 2006.

65   **Xenicare program:** Described in article entitled "Tailored Support," available
on micromass.com. Accessed Apr. 2006.

65   **ranked the physicians . . . lifetime prescribing potential:** Described in an article by Martin DeWitt and Joel Krauss of the Executive Advisory Group. "Getting Market-Focused Results in the Pharmaceutical Industry," *PharmaVOICE*,
March 2003.

65   **"Segment physicians according to their value":** David Lefkowitz, "How to
Target Top Prescribers," *Pharmaceutical Executive*, Feb. 2003.

65   **one invitation, embossed in silver ink:** Said the presentation at the dinner on
June 30, 2005, would be "Irritable Bowel Syndrome: Here and Now." At the time
Salix was trying to expand the market for its antibiotic called Xifaxan by getting
doctors to try it in patients suffering from irritable bowel syndrome, a use not approved by the FDA.

66   **Linn Street Café:** Menu and wine list accessed through linnstreetcafe.com,
Aug. 2005.

66   **82 percent of the physicians:** According to statistics for April 2003 collected
by Verispan, a consulting group. Statistics were included in slides from a presen-

tation by Kelly Sborlini of Verispan on Jan. 21, 2004, to the Healthcare Marketing & Communications Council.

66   **a strip club . . . called Woody's:** See decision in *Stephanie A. Carr v. Schering-Plough* in Iowa's Unemployment Insurance Services Division, May 26, 2005. Her testimony was first reported in Clark Kauffman, "Drug Makers Wine and Dine Doctors for Business," *The Des Moines Register*, June 20, 2005.

66   **the nation has rules and laws:** In 1960, Congress passed a law banning radio broadcasters from taking cash or anything of value in exchange for playing specific songs. Federal judges must publicly disclose any gift valued at more than $250. Stockbrokers cannot give gifts valued at more than one hundred dollars, according to the rules of the National Association of Securities Dealers.

67   **between 65 percent and 80 percent of the cost:** According to the Accreditation Council for Continuing Medical Education, the total cost of these courses in 2005 was $1.7 billion. To pay for these courses, the pharmaceutical industry and other commercial ventures provided $1.1 billion. In addition, the companies and other organizations paid $236 million to advertise and exhibit at the events, further reducing the cost to physicians.

68   **academy had charged . . . a thousand dollars:** "Exhibitor Prospectus: Annual CME Forum for Family Physicians," Iowa Academy of Family Physicians, 2005.

68   **Dr. William Osler said in a speech:** William Osler, "The Importance of Postgraduate Study," *The Lancet*, July 14, 1900. Also see a history of continuing medical education in Adrienne Rosof and William Felch, eds., *Continuing Medical Education: A Primer* (New York: Praeger, 1992).

69   **"Very often doctors are more influenced":** Interview aired as part of "Science for Sale?" a segment appearing on *NOW with Bill Moyers* on PBS on Nov. 22, 2002. The story was reported by Walt Bogdanich and Melody Petersen for *The New York Times*. Transcript available at pbs.org.

69   **summer educational event:** Described in article entitled "Summer Seminar" on the website of the Iowa Academy of Family Physicians (iaafp.org). Accessed in 2005.

69   **bring their whole families to ski:** Described in brochure for the Twenty-fifth Annual Otolaryngology Late Winter Symposium, organized by physicians at the University of Nebraska Medical Center.

69   **Dermatologists . . . in Miami's South Beach:** Described in program agenda of the South Beach Symposium, organized by the Florida Society of Dermatology and Dermatologic Surgery, and held Feb. 12 to 15, 2004, at the Loews Miami Beach Hotel. The doctors could receive twenty-eight hours of continuing education credit.

70   **occupational health nurses:** Brochure for Sixth Annual Occupational Health Nursing Conference on Nov. 12, 2004, in Dubuque.

70   **pharmacists . . . at the CR Chop House:** Dinner on May 19, 2005, described
      at website for the Iowa Pharmacy Association (iarx.org), 2005.

70   **Iowa Physician Assistant Society:** From minutes of board of directors meet-
      ing, available at group's website (iapasociety.org). Accessed 2005.

71   **$65,000 grants:** The university encouraged its faculty to apply for these grants,
      which were listed on the *Grant Bulletin* website at uiowa.edu in 2006.

71   **Research Day:** The agenda and description of this event, held Feb. 20,
      2003, were included on the department of internal medicine's website at
      healthcare.uiowa.edu. The website shows a photo of Bart Brown from Pfizer
      handing a check to pay for the activities to the university's Dr. Peter Densen.

71   **mobile clinic:** Pfizer provided a thirty-thousand-dollar grant to the university
      to buy and refurbish a bus as a traveling clinic. See university news release,
      "Students to Unveil Mobile Clinic Bus," Apr. 19, 2004.

71   **director of the university's hospital:** Donna Katen-Bahensky listed her mem-
      bership on the advisory board of Pfizer Health Solutions in her 2005 profile on
      the hospital's website at uihealthcare.com.

71   **"a bad academic":** See Phil Davidson, "Official Lauds Irate Scientists," *The
      Daily Iowan*, Feb. 20, 2003.

71   **other state employees were banned:** The state's gift law is described in Iowa
      Code, Chapter 68B. Accessed May 2006.

71   **some professors had to report any annual payment:** The university's conflict
      of interest rules are described in its *Operations Manual*, Chapter 18. Accessed on-
      line May 2006.

71   **kept these reports secret:** In May 2006, I asked the university for the financial
      disclosure reports that had been filed by ten professors. These reports were
      meant to disclose payments the professors had received from drugmakers and
      other companies. The university's press office referred me to the Clinical Trials
      Office, which referred me to Dr. Richard Hichwa, the university's Conflicts of
      Interest Officer. Dr. Hichwa did not return any of the many messages that I left
      on his e-mail and voice mail. I then filed a request for the documents under the
      state's public records law (Iowa Code, Chapter 22). This request went to Marc
      Mills, the university's general counsel. Within days, Mr. Mills denied my request
      for the disclosure forms. He said the documents were "confidential personnel in-
      formation" that was exempt from disclosure under the law.

72   **"creating wealth":** From notes to speech and slide presentation entitled
      "Roadmap to the Future: Shaping a Common Agenda," by Dr. Jean Robillard.
      These notes were included on website listing faculty meetings at medicine
      .uiowa.edu. Accessed May 2006.

72 **"a large population of potential research participants":** See website used by the school's Clinical Trials Office to describe its operations to industry (research.uiowa.edu/cto/companies/resources.html). Accessed May 2006.

72 **Iowans . . . made good study subjects:** Jim Pollock, "More Iowans Taking Part in Clinical Trials," *The Des Moines Business Record*, Apr. 9, 2006.

72 **136 scientists managing clinical trials:** From an overview of the University of Iowa's clinical trials at centerwatch.com. Accessed May 2006.

72 **standard written contracts with . . . companies:** The university had master agreements with sixteen companies, according to the Clinical Trials Office website in May 2006.

72 **Drug companies were asking for waivers:** See Mark Sidel, "Report for the 2004–05 Academic Year," University of Iowa Research Council.

72 **the university . . . did not promise to pay:** Described at Clinical Trials Office website, research.uiowa.edu/cto/invest-coord/contract-types.html. Accessed May 2006.

73 **rules for professors who worked for the industry:** See university's *Operations Manual*, Chapter 18. Accessed online May 2006.

73 **Dr. Jennifer Robinson . . . "conflicts of interest":** Disclosed at biocritique.com, May 2006.

74 **She made this disclosure:** See Wanner et al., "Atorvastatin in Patients with Type 2 Diabetes Mellitus Undergoing Hemodialysis," *NEJM*, July 21, 2005. Dr. Robinson wrote a letter to the journal to comment on this study, which was published Oct. 27, 2005, with a reply from the original article's authors. In an interview in Oct. 2007, Dr. Robinson said Pfizer did not ask her to write the letter. She estimated that a quarter of her annual income came from ten drug companies. "I'm not really beholden to anybody," she said. "You should be more worried about those who work for just one company."

74 **the Bayer Corporation paid:** This study and many others were performed by the College of Public Health's Lipid Research Clinic, which Dr. Robinson directed in 2006. The Baycol study is described in Insull et al., "Efficacy and Safety of Cerivastatin 0.8 mg in Patients with Hypercholesterolaemia: The Pivotal Placebo-Controlled Clinical Trial," *The Journal of International Medical Research*, Spring 2000.

74 **take Baycol off the market:** Melody Petersen and Alex Berenson, "Papers Indicate That Bayer Knew of Dangers of Its Cholesterol Drug," *The New York Times*, Feb. 22, 2003.

75 **Dr. Vincent Traynelis:** Internal document from Medtronic dated Sept. 19, 2002, and entitled "MSD Consultants (fully executed Agreements)." MSD stands for Medtronic Sofamor Danek, the company's subsidiary that focuses on selling devices for spinal surgery. The list includes the names of seventy-nine physicians

whom Medtronic called "consultants" and the "annual amount" they were to receive. The top paid surgeon, according to the list, was Dr. Thomas Zdeblick, from the University of Wisconsin, who was to receive four hundred thousand dollars.

75   **Novartis quoted . . . Dr. Satish Rao:** See press release from Novartis, "Zelnorm Safety and Efficacy Demonstrated in Largest Studies Ever Conducted in Chronic Constipation," May 19, 2004.

75   **Dr. Rao disclosed that he worked as a consultant and speaker:** His disclosure was made at mdnetguide.com for a program titled "Case-Based Medicine Teaching Series: Functional Gastrointestinal Disorders—Part 3 of 4." Originally released Sept. 2004. Accessed from website, May 2006.

75   **European Union had twice turned down:** See press release issued by European Medicines Agency, March 24, 2006.

76   **"He is Dr. Zelnorm":** Interview with Dr. Abramson, June 24, 2005.

76   **FDA demanded in July 2007:** The government first ordered Zelnorm to be removed from the market. See government press release, "FDA Announces Discontinued Marketing of GI Drug, Zelnorm, for Safety Reasons," March 30, 2007. Later the agency agreed it could be sold on a restricted basis to certain women. See "Zelnorm Available Under Restricted Use," FDA Consumer Update, July 27, 2007.

77   **"can work beautifully":** My notes from talk by Dr. Reed on June 30, 2005, at the Jordan Creek Town Center.

78   **half the patients taking Imitrex:** Clinical trials are described in Imitrex Prescribing Information, June 2006.

78   **the triptans' possible side effects:** Described in Imitrex Prescribing Instructions, June 2006.

78   **withdrawal headaches lasting four days:** See Katsarava et al., "Clinical Features of Withdrawal Headache Following Overuse of Triptans and Other Headache Drugs," *Neurology,* 2001.

78   **in 2004 she gave a talk:** In October 2004, Dr. Reed gave a talk about treating herpes at a conference of the Iowa Physician Assistant Society held at the Cedar Rapids Marriott. Her talk was paid for by a grant from GlaxoSmithKline, which sells Valtrex, a drug for herpes. Conference agenda available at iapasociety.org. Accessed 2005.

78   **one that GlaxoSmithKline had paid for:** Dixie L. Harms, of Family Medicine of Urbandale, gave an online seminar paid for by GlaxoSmithKline. The seminar, "Case in Review: Effective Management of Your Migraine Patient," was available at the website CE-Today. It was published July 2005. Accessed at ceoncd.com, Sept. 2006.

79   **One of the other doctors:** Dr. Barbara L. Hodne, of Family Medicine of Urbandale, disclosed that she received money from GlaxoSmithKline, Pfizer, Novartis, and Forest in a presentation called "Is it GERD or NERD?," available at pri-med.com in 2005.

THREE: Chemical Imbalance

81   "It was the ADHD": Interview with Patrick Hurley, June 24, 2005.

84   **each Iowan now picked up fourteen prescriptions:** Statistics for 2005 from statehealthfacts.org, a website maintained by the Kaiser Family Foundation.

84   **"I don't know what to do":** Brian Morelli, "State Offers Info on New Drug Plan," *The Iowa City Press-Citizen*, Nov. 8, 2005.

84   **average number of prescriptions . . . increased by 28 percent:** In 2000 the average number of prescriptions per capita in Iowa was 10.87. By 2005 the number had increased to 13.9 prescriptions. Statistics are from the Kaiser Family Foundation and are available at statehealthfacts.org.

84   **"If I have an important test":** Drew Kerr and Scott Rieckens, "Speeding Past Test Stress," *The Daily Iowan*, Dec. 12, 2005.

85   **"The way medications get used":** Interview with Gene Lutz, July 1, 2005.

85   **Two-thirds of the day care centers:** Sinkovits et al., "Medication Administration in Day Care Centers for Children," *Journal of the American Pharmaceutical Association*, June 25, 2003.

85   **25 percent of the school's students:** Susan M. Hegland, "Children Medicated for ADHD in the Early Grades: Who Are They?," available at public.iastate.edu. Accessed 2005.

85   **"Putting children on Ritalin":** Interview with Susan Hegland, 2005.

86   **"Hey dude":** From blog at classadrivers.com. Accessed March 21, 2006.

86   **64 percent of their total sales:** Walgreens's Form 10-K for year ended Aug. 31, 2005.

86   **Walgreens opened drugstores in America:** According to a corporate press release dated Jan. 4, 2006, Walgreens had 5,080 drugstores at the end of 2005, an increase of 366 stores from the year before. According to a Domino's press release, the pizza chain opened its five thousandth store in the United States in Jan. 2006.

87   **Iowa's more rural areas:** See Russ Oechslin, "Walgreens Sets Spencer Plans," *Sioux City Journal*, Aug. 5, 2006.

87   **construct one in just three days:** Medicap, the pharmacy franchise company, promised to erect a pharmacy, with preengineered parts, in three days. Described at medicap.com. Accessed 2005.

87   **Dozens of supermarkets:** According to the Iowa Board of Pharmacy Examiners, the number of pharmacies in Iowa increased from 927 in 1990 to 944 in 2006. That small increase is misleading, however, because many small independent pharmacies in Iowa have closed and been replaced by chain pharmacies like Walgreens as well as by pharmacies in supermarkets or in big retail stores like Wal-Mart. These new pharmacies fill more prescriptions each day on aver-

age than the independent pharmacies. According to a presentation by Walgreens executives in June 2006, the chain's pharmacists filled about 280 prescriptions every day in each store while an independent pharmacy filled on average just 110 prescriptions each day.

89   **five thousand per hour:** The rate Medco could fill prescriptions is from Merck's *Annual Report 2000*.

89   **McDonaldization:** George Ritzer, *The McDonaldization of Society* (Thousand Oaks, Calif.: Pine Forge Press, 2000).

89   **forty-two flavors:** Described at flavorx.com. Accessed Oct. 2005.

90   **The heartburn drug Tagamet:** The drug is one of dozens of medicines included on the list known as the Beers Criteria. Doctors are warned against prescribing these medicines to people over the age of sixty-five.

90   **Congress had tried to protect Americans:** This became law with the Durham-Humphrey Amendment of 1951, which amended the Federal Food, Drug, and Cosmetic Act of 1938.

91   **Almost 14 percent of the Iowans covered:** *The Wellmark Report: An Analysis of Prescription Drug Use in Iowa and South Dakota*, 2003.

92   **nine written questions about their mood:** See a description of the introduction of this screening program in Iowa in Zlatko Anguelov, "Depression Disease Management Program," *Currents*, a newsletter published by University of Iowa Health Care, Winter 2000. Accessed Oct. 2005 at uihealthcare.com. Wellmark was still distributing the Pfizer-developed depression questionnaire in 2007, according to its website.

92   **Wellmark said doctors should give the quiz:** The "targeted population" for the depression screening is described in "Treatment of Major Depression in Primary Care: Clinical Practice Guideline," a document Wellmark referred physicians to on its website (wellmark.com). Accessed June 2007.

92   **Pfizer . . . had paid to create the questionnaire:** PRIME-MD was developed by Dr. Robert L. Spitzer of the New York State Psychiatric Institute, working under a grant from Pfizer. The PRIME-MD questionnaire and program were trademarked by Pfizer. See press release from Pfizer, "Study Published in JAMA Finds First Patient-Administered Questionnaire for Mental Health Disorders 85 Percent Effective in Diagnosis," Nov. 11, 1999. Also see Spitzer et al., "Validation and Utility of a Self-Report Version of Prime-MD," *JAMA*, Nov. 10, 1999.

92   **two-question test:** Kroenke et al., "The Patient Health Questionnaire-2," *Medical Care*, Nov. 2003.

92   **quarter of patients diagnosed:** For example, see Kinkman, et al., "False Positives, False Negatives, and the Validity of the Diagnosis of Major Depression in Primary Care," *Archives of Family Medicine*, Sept. 1998.

92   questionnaire in two rural clinics: Bergus et al., "The Limited Effect of Screen-
     ing for Depressive Symptoms with the PHQ-9 in Rural Family Practices," *The Jour-
     nal of Rural Health*, Fall 2005.

92   "We found that the same thing": E-mail from Dr. Bergus, Oct. 15, 2007.

93   startling 369 percent rise in just three years: "Medco Study Reveals Pediatric
     Spending Spike on Drugs to Treat Behavioral Problems," press release from
     Medco Health Solutions, May 17, 2004.

93   "'Okay,' the mother said": Overheard while waiting outside a doctor's office in
     Iowa in 2005. At the time, Lexapro was not approved for use in children.

94   "Our system is broken": Interview with Dr. Sharon Collins, June 23, 2005.

95   "We're seeing kids on three, four, five": Interviews with Dr. Jeffrey Lobas on
     May 15, 2005, and July 7, 2005.

96   session for physicians on how to treat: "ADHD and Other Disruptive
     Behaviors in Preschool Children: Challenges in Diagnosis and Treatment,"
     Pediatric Academic Societies' 2005 Annual Meeting, Washington Convention
     Center, May 15, 2005.

97   five times as many prescriptions for Ritalin . . . in 1996: Farasat Bokhari et
     al., "An Analysis of the Significant Variation in Psychostimulant Use Across the
     U.S.," *Pharmacoepidemiology and Drug Safety*, published online June 25, 2004.

97   almost 10 percent of all ten-year-old boys: According to testimony at an FDA
     meeting on Feb. 9, 2006, and described in Steven E. Nissen, "ADHD Drugs and
     Cardiovascular Risk," *NEJM,* Apr. 6, 2006.

97   as does Iowa as a whole: In Iowa the rate of children medicated for attention
     problems increased by 17 percent between 2001 and 2003, according to an
     analysis of prescription data by Wellmark, the state's largest health insurer. The
     prescriptions varied radically on the basis of the community where the child lived.
     The highest rates were in Iowa City and Cedar Rapids, where 6.5 percent of all
     children were taking Ritalin or a similar drug. See *The Wellmark Report: An
     Analysis of Prescription Drug Use in Iowa and South Dakota (Tenth in a Special
     Series),* June 2004. These two Iowa cities were also shown to have a very high
     rate of stimulant use in Bokhari's study in 2004.

97   Other states with high numbers of medicated children: Statement of Ter-
     rance Woodworth, deputy director, Office of Diversion Control, Drug Enforce-
     ment Administration, before the House Committee on Education and the
     Workforce, May 16, 2000.

97   IMPACT OF ATTENTION DEFICIT-HYPERACTIVITY: *School Health Services News-
     letter*, May 2002, available at state.ia.us/educate.

98   fivefold increase from just four years earlier: Bhatara et al., "Trends in Com-
     bined Pharmacotherapy with Stimulants for Children," *Psychiatric Services*,
     March 2002.

98   Many of the disorders described: Duncan Double, "The Limits of Psychiatry,"
      BMJ, Apr. 13, 2002.

99   Critics of the *DSM* have argued: See Alix Spiegel, "The Dictionary of Disorder:
      How One Man Revolutionized Psychiatry," *The New Yorker*, Jan. 3, 2005.

99   a drug called Tofranil: See David Healy, *Let Them Eat Prozac* (Toronto: James
      Lorimer & Co., 2003), pp. 20 and 35.

99   "making us all crazy": Stuart A. Kirk, "Are We All Going Mad, or Are the
      Experts Crazy?," *Los Angeles Times*, Aug. 14, 2005.

99   compulsive shopping disorder: Transcript of news story, "Dr. Jack Gorman
      Discusses Two New Studies Presented at the American Psychiatric Association
      Convention," ABC News: *Good Morning America*, May 9, 2001.

100   Dr. Gorman was also a consultant: These drug companies are listed in Barlow
      et al., "Cognitive-Behavioral Therapy, Imipramine or Their Combination for
      Panic Disorder," *JAMA*, May 17, 2000.

100   The flurry of publicity caused: "American Psychiatric Association Issues
      Statement on Compulsive Shopping," press release, Aug. 18, 2003.

100   In Iowa about 70 percent: Statistic from Iowa State University press release,
      "Child Care Industry Vital to Iowa's Business Climate, Future Workforce,"
      Apr. 28, 2005.

100   A study in 2004 found: Christakis et al., "Early Television Exposure and Sub-
      sequent Attentional Problems in Children," *Pediatrics*, Apr. 2004.

101   a program called TeenScreen: Eve Bender, "Groups Want Depression Screen-
      ing to Be Part of School Examinations," *Psychiatric News*, Apr. 4, 2003.

101   Shaffer . . . has worked as a consultant: He disclosed that he was a consult-
      ant to Roche, Wyeth, and GlaxoSmithKline in "Preliminary Report of the Task
      Force on SSRIs and Suicidal Behavior in Youth," American College of Neuropsy-
      chopharmacology, Jan. 21, 2004. He has also disclosed that Solvay has paid for
      his work. For example, see D. Shaffer and L. Craft, "Methods of Adolescent Sui-
      cide Prevention," *Journal of Clinical Psychiatry*, 1999.

101   21 percent of American children: Shaffer et al., "The NIMH Diagnostic
      Interview Schedule for Children Version 2.3 (DISC-2.3): Description, Accept-
      ability, Prevalence Rates, and Performance in the MECA Study," *Journal of the
      American Academy of Child and Adolescent Psychiatry*, July 1996.

101   studies had not been able to prove: U.S. Preventive Services Task Force,
      Screening for Suicide Risk: Recommendation and Rationale, May 2004, Agency
      for Healthcare Research and Quality, Rockville, Md. Available at ahrq.gov.

101   The pharmaceutical industry had long been involved: Press release from
      American Foundation for Suicide Prevention entitled "Adolescent Angst . . . or

Something More Serious?" Also see Jim Rosack, "Suicide Prevention Advocates Emphasize New Strategies," *Psychiatric News*, Apr. 7, 2000.

101 **at least seven school districts in Iowa:** From teenscreen.org. Accessed June 2007.

102 **"If you ask a sixteen-year-old":** Interview with Pam Wheeler, May 2005.

102 **Child Health Month:** Described in Winter 2002 newsletter of the Iowa Chapter of the American Academy of Pediatrics. Details of the event are also described in "Health Reports: Child Health Month Encourages Asking for Help," an article published Oct. 8, 2001, online at uihealthcare.com. Accessed June 2007.

102 **a storybook it published:** Constance H. Foster, *Kids Like Me*, published by Solvay Pharmaceuticals in 1997. I found the storybook in a library maintained by a state-funded agency in Iowa that works with the public schools on mental health issues and employs many of the school psychologists. In the winter of 2001 the agency's staff recommended the book to parents and students. See "5-Star PEC Library Materials," an article in *Let's Connect!*, a newsletter of Area Education Agency 6, Winter 2001.

103 **"Zoloft may help correct":** From "Patient Summary of Information About Zoloft," published by Pfizer, Oct. 2000.

103 **an elaborate museum exhibit:** "Brain: The World Inside Your Head," described at Pfizer.com/brain. Accessed July 20, 2005. The Iowa Science Teachers Section of the Iowa Academy of Science included a link to the virtual tour of the Pfizer exhibition on its website, which was aimed at helping teachers find useful information for their students. See ists.pls.uni.edu/links/biology.

104 **"Science Made Simple":** From concerta.net. Accessed Nov. 2005.

104 **"They make the child 'normal'":** Larry B. Silver, *ADHD: Attention Deficit-Hyperactivity Disorder and Learning Disabilities: Booklet for the Classroom Teacher*, published by Novartis in 1997.

104 **At an event for children:** Notes from my visit to Jordan Creek Town Center in July 2005. The children's event was called Rock in Prevention.

105 **drugs for the brain and central nervous system:** "Nervous Breakdown: A Detailed Analysis of the Neurology Market," UBS Warburg, June 2001.

105 **"I spent the first several years":** Quote from Dr. David Burns is from Lacasse and Gomory, "Is Graduate Social Work Education Promoting a Critical Approach to Mental Health Practice?," *Journal of Social Work Education*, 2003. Also see Lacasse and Leo, "Serotonin and Depression: A Disconnect Between the Advertisements and the Scientific Literature," *PLoS Medicine*, Dec. 2005.

105 **"It may surprise you":** Elliot S. Valenstein, *Blaming the Brain: The Truth About Drugs and Mental Health* (New York: Free Press, 1998), p. 4.

106　**"We have hunted"**: Kenneth S. Kendler, "Toward a Philosophical Structure for Psychiatry," *American Journal of Psychiatry*, March 2005.

106　**"no data to indicate"**: This is from the document the scientists distributed to the public on the final day of the conference, after weighing the scientific evidence. The paper is entitled "National Institutes of Health Consensus Development Conference Statement, Diagnosis and Treatment of Attention Deficit Hyperactivity Disorder (ADHD), Nov. 16–18, 1998." Later, the panel's official statement was edited to say, "There is no independent valid test for ADHD. Although research has suggested a central nervous system basis for ADHD, further research is necessary to firmly establish ADHD as a brain disorder."

106　**"The assumption that the ADHD"**: William B. Carey, "Is ADHD a Valid Disorder," in *Attention Deficit Hyperactivity Disorder: State of the Science*, ed. Jensen and Cooper (Kingston, N.J.: Civic Research Institute, 2002).

106　**"Look at Peter's eyes"**: Interview with Sandy Koppen, June 23, 2005.

107　**can have an effect similar to cocaine**: *Drugs of Abuse*, 2005 edition, Drug Enforcement Administration, U.S. Department of Justice.

107　**The drug's label warns**: Package insert or label for Dexedrine, published by GlaxoSmithKline, Jan. 2002.

108　**long list of side effects**: Package insert for Paxil, published by GlaxoSmithKline, Sept. 2005.

108　**"I was out of it all the time"**: Interview with Peter Koppen, July 29, 2005.

FOUR: The Early Years

115　**Take the pharmaceutical giant Merck**: Other American companies led by physicians, scientists, or men with scientific training in the early to mid-twentieth century included Abbott Laboratories, Eli Lilly & Company, and the Upjohn Company. Dr. Ernest H. Volwiler served as the president of Abbott Laboratories in the 1950s. Dr. Volwiler rose through the company's ranks after becoming a pioneer in the field of anesthetic medicine and developing a breakthrough drug used in surgery called Pentothal. Earlier Dr. Alfred S. Burdick, a former medical school professor, had served as president of Abbott Laboratories. The Upjohn Company was founded by W. E. Upjohn, a physician trained at the University of Michigan. The company was later led by his descendants, among them E. Gifford Upjohn, who was also trained as a physician. Eli Lilly & Company was founded by Colonel Eli Lilly, a pharmaceutical chemist. His descendants who eventually ran the company included Josiah K. Lilly and Eli Lilly II, both trained at the Philadelphia College of Pharmacy.

115　**"medicine is for the people"**: Transcript of speech by George W. Merck at the Medical College of Virginia at Richmond, Dec. 1, 1950. Obtained from online archive at merck.com, July 2006.

116   companies had little interest in science: Some of the best descriptions of this
      early history of the industry have been by John P. Swann in *Academic Scientists and
      the Pharmaceutical Industry* (Baltimore: Johns Hopkins University Press, 1988),
      James Harvey Young in *The Medical Messiahs* (Princeton, N.J.: Princeton Uni-
      versity Press, 1992), and Philip J. Hilts in *Protecting America's Health* (New York:
      Alfred A. Knopf, 2003).

116   "It is well known": Quote by John Abel included in John Parascandola, "The
      'Preposterous Provision'": The American Society for Pharmacology and Experi-
      mental Therapeutics' Ban on Industrial Pharmacologists, 1908–1941," in *Pill
      Peddlers: Essays on the History of the Pharmaceutical Industry* (American Institute
      of the History of Pharmacy, 1990).

116   "How could old Max": Sinclair Lewis, *Arrowsmith* (New York: Harcourt Brace,
      1925).

116   "It is only from laboratories free": Quoted in James Harvey Young, "Public
      Policy and Drug Innovation," *Pharmacy in History*, 1982.

117   George Merck vowed: See chapter on Merck Sharp & Dohme in *Pharmaceu-
      tical Company Histories,* vol. 1, ed. Gary L. Nelson (Bismarck, N.D.: Woodbine
      Publishing, 1985).

117   promised to keep their new laboratories: Described in John P. Swann, "Uni-
      versities, Industry, and the Rise of Biomedical Collaboration in America," *Pill
      Peddlers.*

117   "not only willing, but eager and anxious": Clowes quoted in Swann's essay in
      Pill Peddlers.

117   George Merck changed his mind: Hilts, p. 103.

118   "university-like atmosphere": Quote by Waksman in Nelson, p. 86.

118   He convinced George Merck: Nelson, p. 86. Also see Steve Ainsworth, "Strep-
      tomycin—Arrogance and Anger," *The Pharmaceutical Journal*, Feb. 25, 2006.

118   "anyone could concoct": Hilts, p. 75.

118   a sweet-tasting syrup: For one account of this tragedy, see Paul M. Wax,
      "Elixirs, Diluents, and the Passage of the 1938 Federal Food, Drug and Cosmetic
      Act," *Annals of Internal Medicine*, March 15, 1995.

119   "The most amazing thing": Quote is from "Fatal Remedy," *Time*, Nov. 1, 1937.

119   some fifty-eight thousand scientists: Hilts, p. 93.

119   "one of the major events": Young, *Medical Messiahs*, chapter 12.

119   More truly effective drugs: Hilts, p. 105.

120   "This has been the best year": Brown quoted in "Rx for Health," *Time*,
      Dec. 16, 1957.

120   *The Saturday Evening Post*: Young, *Medical Messiahs*, chapter 12.

121 **"Americans have come to believe":** Quoted in ibid.

121 **The rate . . . slowed:** Among the writers who have looked at this period are James Le Fanu, *The Rise and Fall of Modern Medicine* (New York: Carroll & Graf, 1999), and Edward S. Golub, *The Limits of Medicine* (Chicago: University of Chicago Press, 1997).

122 **the companies lobbied successfully:** Hilts, p. 121.

123 **hearing . . . held by Senator Estes Kefauver:** One of the best descriptions of these hearings is by Richard Harris, *The Real Voice* (New York: Macmillan, 1964).

123 **"I think more than half":** Ibid., p. 79.

124 **"a matter of inadequate income":** Brown's quote is from transcripts of "Administered Prices in the Drug Industry: Hearings Before the Subcommittee on Antitrust and Monopoly of the Committee on the Judiciary," U.S. Senate, Dec. 7 to 12, 1959.

124 **"we can't put two sick people":** Harris, p. 64.

124 **Dr. E. Gifford Upjohn . . . testified:** "The Double Image," *Time*, Dec. 21, 1959.

125 **"not as good":** Lasagna quoted in ibid.

125 **"structural roulette":** Walter Modell's article in *Clinical Pharmacology and Therapeutics* is quoted in "Too Many Drugs," *Time*, May 26, 1961.

125 **a drug manufacturer in Cincinnati:** Some of the best chroniclers of this tragedy as it happened were journalists from *The Sunday Times* of London. See *The Sunday Times* Insight Team's *Suffer the Children* (New York: Viking Press, 1979). A more recent retelling of the thalidomide disaster is by Hilts in *Protecting America's Health*.

126 **Vick Chemical Company:** In October 1960 this company became known as Richardson-Merrell.

126 **"completely safe":** Insight Team, p. 29.

126 **"especially well-suited for calming":** Chemie Grünenthal ad for thalidomide, quoted in "Sleeping Pill Nightmare," *Time*, Feb. 23, 1962.

126 **"selling them on Kevadon":** Insight Team, p. 73.

127 **Frances O. Kelsey:** Her story was first told in a front-page article, Morton Mintz, "Heroine of FDA Keeps Bad Drug Off Market," *The Washington Post*, July 15, 1962.

128 **deformities in some eight thousand infants:** Hilts, p. 158.

128 **delivered three deformed babies:** Insight Team, p. 83.

129 **"They wrenched some of us":** Harold A. Clymer, "The Economic and Regulatory Climate: U.S. and Overseas Trends," in *Drug Development and Marketing: A Conference Sponsored by the Center for Health Policy Research of the American Enterprise Institute* (Washington, D.C.: American Enterprise Institute, 1975).

129 **funded mostly by . . . industry:** Information accessed from the website maintained by the Tufts Center for the Study of Drug Development, csdd.tufts.edu, in July 2006. The center says it works independently from the companies that fund the majority of its operations.

130 **A wide-ranging group of critics:** For example, see Public Citizen, "Rx R&D Myths: The Case Against the Drug Industry's R&D 'Scare Card.'" Report accessed at citizen.org, July 2006. Also see Merrill Goozner, *The $800 Million Pill* (Berkeley, Calif.: University of California Press, 2004), and Marcia Angell, *The Truth About the Drug Companies* (New York: Random House, 2004).

130 **Taxol was discovered by scientists:** See "Technology Transfer: NIH–Private Sector Partnership in the Development of Taxol," U.S. Government Accounting Office, June 2003.

130 **of the nation's twenty-one most important drugs:** "The Benefits of Medical Research and the Role of the NIH," Joint Economic Committee of Congress, May 2000.

131 **Bristol-Myers paid money to Armstrong's cancer charity:** See transcript of the Dec. 14, 1999, conference call among Armstrong, Bristol-Myers's public relations staff, and the media. Accessed at cycleofhope.org, July 2006.

131 **credited the company with saving his life:** Armstrong explained his financial partnership with Bristol-Myers this way: "This is a company, had they not been in existence, had these drugs not been in existence, I wouldn't be alive. That's the bottom line. There is no way around it. Twenty years ago, when these drugs weren't around, 90% of the people who had this illness died. Now, that the drugs are here and Bristol-Myers is here, 95% of the kids live." Transcript of conference call with the media, Dec. 14, 1999.

131 **"This miracle is brought to you":** Transcript of conference call, Dec. 14, 1999.

131 **Bristol-Myers . . . did not *discover* them:** According to Armstrong's charity (livestrong.org, accessed July 2006), the cyclist received one round of BEP chemotherapy (Bleomycin, Etoposide, and Platinol) and three rounds of VIP (Etoposide, Ifosfamide, and Platinol). Bristol-Myers sold Bleomycin, Ifosfamide, and Platinol, which is the brand name for cisplatin. Bleomycin was discovered by a Japanese institute. Ifosfamide was discovered by a German company. Cisplatin was discovered by scientists at Michigan State. The U.S. government had a major role in paying for the clinical trials needed to show that each of these drugs worked against cancer. For a good analysis of who discovered cancer medicines and who paid for the required clinical trials, see "Federally Funded Pharmaceutical Inventions," testimony before the Senate's Special Committee on the Aging by Ralph Nader and James Love, Feb. 24, 1993.

131 **decade-long legal battle:** See "Contractor Scrutiny by U.S. Curbed," *The New York Times*, Apr. 20, 1983.

FIVE: An Awakening: The Age of the Blockbuster

133   **Dr. James W. Black:** Much of this story comes from Dr. Black's autobiography, which was published by the Nobel Foundation in Stockholm, Sweden, *Les Prix Nobel 1988*, ed. Tore Frangsmyr. Accessed in July 2006 at nobelprize.org.

133   **largely self-taught:** "Sir James Black: Learning by Doing," *Molecular Interventions*, June 2004.

133   **proved to his teacher:** Alan Taylor, "Or Is This Our National Hero?," *Sunday Herald*, Jan. 25, 2004.

134   **had not been able to get ICI interested:** Viviane Quirke, "Putting Theory into Practice: James Black, Receptor Theory and the Development of the Beta-Blockers at ICI, 1958–1978," *Medical History*, Jan. 2006.

135   **A hot topic of discussion:** "How Much of the Stomach Should Be Cut Out?" *Time*, Jan. 3, 1964.

135   **tested more than seven hundred chemical compounds:** M. Michael Wolfe and Thomas J. Nesi, *Heartburn: Extinguishing the Fire Inside* (New York: W. W. Norton, 1997), p. 80.

135   **"inherently toxic":** Ibid., p. 82.

135   **tweaking the chemical structure:** Lawrence K. Altman, "Ulcer Cases and Surgery Decline; Drug Seems to Control Severity of Illness," *The New York Times*, July 28, 1981.

136   **decline in the number of ulcer surgeries:** The pharmaceutical industry attributes this decline to Tagamet and similar drugs, but the drugs cannot take full credit. The rate of peptic ulcers had been falling even before the drugs were introduced. Between 1960 and 1972 the rate had fallen 50 percent. Such a fast decline implies that the ulcers were caused by an infectious agent. This was later proved by Dr. Barry Marshall. See Le Fanu, p. 153.

136   **fifteen million . . . had taken Tagamet:** Altman, *The New York Times*, July 28, 1981.

136   **follow along behind Dr. Black:** Interview of Sir David Jack, former research director at a division of Glaxo, with Dr. Max Blythe on March 24, 1997. Dr. Jack said Glaxo began work on an ulcer drug in 1972 after he listened to a lecture by Dr. Black. Interview is part of the Medical Sciences Video Archive of Oxford Brookes University Library. Excerpts available at brookes.ac.uk/schools/lifesci/medical.

137   **Dr. Jack later explained that . . . Zantac:** Matthew Lynn, "Prudence and the Pill Pusher," *The Independent*, Nov. 3, 1991.

137   **analysts on Wall Street were not impressed:** "British Drug Maker Hopes It Has Found Its Own Tagamet," *The New York Times*, Nov. 26, 1981.

137 **Rather than set Zantac's price:** "Glaxo Wellcome: A Marketing Council Case Study: From Product-Based Company to Customer-Driven Organization." The council's website is marketingcouncil.org. Accessed 2004. Also explained in Brian O'Reilly, "Drugmakers Under Attack," *Fortune*, July 29, 1991.

137 **Glaxo used the extra money:** See examples of these studies in McIsaac et al., "Ranitidine and cimetidine in the healing of duodenal ulcer," *Alimentary Pharmacology & Therapeutics*, Oct. 1987.

138 **contracting to use hundreds:** Richard Wright, "How Zantac Became the Best-Selling Drug in History," *Journal of Health Care Marketing*, Winter 1996.

138 **make heartburn into an acute and chronic "disorder":** Vince Parry, "The Art of Branding a Condition," *Medical Marketing & Media*, May 2003.

138 **they reduced simply to GERD:** Ibid.

138 **Gallup Organization:** "Frequent Antacid Users Prevalent, Says Gallup Survey," press release from Glaxo, March 31, 1988.

138 **recruited the actress Nancy Walker:** Robert Cross, "Comedian's Fare Gets Last Laugh on Heartburn," *Chicago Tribune*, Aug. 25, 1988.

139 **Glaxo Institute for Digestive Health:** Parry, May 2003. Also see description at institute's website, gidh.com. Accessed July 2006.

139 **runner's reflux:** William Stockton, "On Your Own: Heartburn for Fun and Profit: A Saga," *The New York Times*, May 22, 1989.

139 **the company hired a sculptor:** "Glaxo's Expanding Galaxy," *The Economist*, Nov. 23, 2001.

139 **"I can tell you quite frankly":** Matthew Lynn, Nov. 3, 1991.

140 **"There was an awakening":** Brian O'Reilly, "Drugmakers Under Attack," *Fortune*, July 29, 1991.

140 **blockbuster model:** For just one description of the process, see Christopher Bogan and David Wang, "Launching a Blockbuster: The Making and Marketing of Megabrands," *Pharmaceutical Executive*, Aug. 20, 2000

140 **The pharmaceutical companies now spend:** An analysis in 2003 by A. T. Kearney, a consulting firm, found that the typical American industrial company spent about 17 percent of its revenues on selling and on general and administrative expenses. Pharmaceutical companies, however, spent on average at almost twice that rate, allocating about 33 percent of their revenues to those costs. See "Preparing Now for Business in a Post-Blockbuster Era," a slide presentation by Christopher White, vice president, A. T. Kearney, at the Economist Pharmaceuticals Roundtable, Nov. 19, 2003.

140 **must spend as much as $1 billion:** AstraZeneca executives quoted in "The Trend Toward Megabrands," written by consultants at IMS Health, Feb. 1, 2000. Accessed at imshealth.com, Oct. 2004.

141 **industry's own hiring statistics:** Numbers for 1995 were 49,409 employees in research and development and 55,348 employees in marketing. Stats for 1995 and 2000 are from "Table 18: Domestic U.S. Employment, Ethical Pharmaceuticals, Research-Based Pharmaceutical Companies, 1990 to 2000," in *Pharmaceutical Industry Profile 2001*, Pharmaceutical Research and Manufacturers of America, Washington, D.C.

141 **Scientists had begun to lose their power:** Steven N. Wiggins, "The Pharmaceutical Research and Development Decision Process," in *Drugs and Health: A Conference Sponsored by the American Enterprise Institute for Public Policy Research*, 1981. The conference was held in Washington, D.C., on Nov. 15 and 16, 1979.

142 **"In the beginning":** Pierre Simon interview is from David Healy, *The Psychopharmacologists III* (London: Hodder Arnold, 2000).

142 **about 16 percent . . . new and significant:** My calculation from data available on the FDA's website at fda.gov/cder/rdmt/pstable.htm.

142 **"We've seen the rise":** Quote by Matthew Emmens in "Viewpoint: In Your Own Words," *Pharmaceutical Executive*, Aug. 2006.

142 **"has become quite stale":** Duncan Moore, "Pharmaceuticals—Interesting Times in a Cyclical Industry," in *IP Value 2006: Building and Enforcing Intellectual Property Value* (Globe White Page Ltd., 2006). Available at buildingip value.com.

143 **"financial-engineering vehicles":** Speech by Dr. Erling Refsum on Feb. 8, 2002, at Life Sciences: An Industry in Transition, a conference at the University of Michigan. Video of speech available at zli.bus.umich.edu. Accessed June 2007.

143 **"We sometimes joke":** Quoted in Sharon Reier, "Blockbuster Drugs: Take the Hype in Small Doses," *International Herald Tribune*, March 1, 2003.

143 **Barry Marshall:** See Terence Monmaney, "Marshall's Hunch," *The New Yorker*, Oct. 10, 2005. Also see Le Fanu, p. 147.

144 **"If the drug companies":** Lawrence K. Altman, "Nobel Came After Years of Battling the System," *The New York Times*, Oct. 11, 2005.

145 **about 5 percent of ulcer patients:** From the public information campaign the Centers for Disease Control began in 1997. Available at cdc.gov/ulcer/history.

145 **In December 1990:** See transcript of "Advertising, Marketing and Promotional Practices of the Pharmaceutical Industry: Hearing Before the Committee on Labor and Human Resources," U.S. Senate, Dec. 11 and 12, 1990.

151 **"Victory in these":** Kessler et al., "Therapeutic-Class Wars: Drug Promotion in a Competitive Marketplace," *NEJM*, Nov. 17, 1994.

152 **"help promote greater consumer awareness":** Dr. Friedman quoted in government news release, "FDA to Review Standards for All Direct-to-Consumer Rx

Drug Promotion: New Guidance for Prescription Drug TV and Radio Ads First Step," Aug. 8, 1997.

152 **Friedman resigned the next year:** Dr. Friedman left the FDA on June 14, 1999, according to the written announcement by Dr. Henney. Searle's drug Celebrex was approved on Dec. 31, 1998.

153 **That sum was far more:** News release from TNS Media Intelligence and Competitive Media Reporting, "1999 Ad Spending: GM, Cable Networks and the Internet are the Winners," March 29, 2000.

153 **Joan Lunden:** Schering-Plough news release, "Joan Lunden Teams Up with Schering Corporation to Fight Seasonal Allergy Symptoms," July 7, 1998.

153 **sales of antihistamines soared:** See "Factors Affecting the Growth of Prescription Drugs Expenditures," an issue brief by the National Institute of Health Care Management Foundation, July 1999.

153 **like the "edutainment":** Beth Miller, "Consumer Tactics Could Give Rx Ads a Shot in the Arm," *Medical Marketing & Media*, May 1999.

153 **"Viagra changed pharmaceuticals":** Kelly quoted in David Goetzl, "Ad Age Marketer of the Year: Pfizer; What Next After Viagra, Lipitor and Celebrex?," *Ad Age*, Dec. 10, 2001.

153 **name that evoked energy:** "Viagra Case Study" described by Interbrand Wood Healthcare, a consulting firm hired by Pfizer to create the Viagra name. See interbrandwood.com. Accessed July 2002. Also see "As Potent as Its Moniker; The Names of Pills Matter," *The Economist*, Jan. 18, 2003.

154 **Viagra . . . most recognizable brand names:** Paul Norman, "What's the Prescription for a Perfect Name?," *European Pharmaceutical Executive*, Oct. 1, 2003.

154 **consumer-marketing machine:** Melody Petersen, "What's Black and White and Sells Medicine?," *The New York Times*, Aug. 27, 2000.

154 **candy cone . . . hog-judging contest:** See Samuel Mines, *Pfizer: An Informal History* (New York: Pfizer, 1978).

155 **In 1947:** Pfizer Annual Financial Statements for 1947 and 1997.

155 **"*Today* show to *Sesame Street*":** *The Face of Opportunity*, a brochure printed by Pfizer in 2002.

155 **CRAM:** Petersen, Aug. 27, 2000.

155 **Marketing infused every aspect of a drug's development at Pfizer:** This is from my interviews with Pfizer executives in Aug. 2000. "We start with the researchers working side by side with marketing from the very beginning," said Patrick Kelly, one of the company's top marketing executives. Dr. John F. Niblack, Pfizer's top scientist, said the company had formalized the process of

marketers' directing decisions in the lab in the 1980s. "We try to make sure that research is not developing something that no one particularly wants," he said.

156 **"We'll spend as much":** Interview with William Steere, Aug. 2000.

156 **seven of the eight experimental drugs:** Goldman Sachs, the investment bank, was tracking these eight experimental drugs in Pfizer's pipeline, according to a report by James Kelly on Jan. 22, 2004: Dynestat, Spiriva, Caduet, Pregabalin, Indiplon, Macugen, Daxas, and Exubera.

156 **Serono soared by two billion:** David Stievater, "Joint Marketing Deals Reward Pharma Industry," *The Boston Globe*, Sept. 8, 2002.

157 **most profitable drug company in the world:** No other drug company earned more than Pfizer in profits in 2001. See "Fortune 500," *Fortune*, Apr. 2002.

157 **"perfect time to leave":** Melody Petersen, "Pfizer Chief to Retire, Leaving Successor Hard Act to Follow," *The New York Times*, Aug. 11, 2000.

157 **leaving with a pension:** Estimates of pension and value of stock and options are mine on the basis of information in Pfizer's Proxy Statement dated March 8, 2001.

157 **lifetime use of a car:** Described in Pfizer's annual proxy statements. In some years, including 2004 and 2005, Steere voluntarily paid for the cost of the transportation Pfizer provided.

158 **brochure . . . by Ethical Strategies:** Picked up from a booth at the Pharmaceutical Marketing Congress, held Sept. 30 to Oct. 2, 2002, at the Wyndham Franklin Plaza Hotel in Philadelphia.

159 **MegaDouble plan:** My notes from attending the meeting on Sept. 28, 2000.

159 **"Everyone in the industry knows":** Letter written by Peter R. Dolan in *World*, a magazine published by Bristol-Myers, Dec. 2000.

160 **"We have one fundamental objective":** Quote by Rick Lane in "Leadership to Get Us There," ibid.

160 **Opportunity Seeking Blockbusters:** Described in "Facing the Tough Questions: Answers About Our Future from the Company's Senior Leadership Team," *World*, June 2000.

160 **"If you look at":** Rick Lane quote in "Leadership to Get Us There," *World*, Dec. 2000.

161 **only thirteen of them:** Pecoul et al., "Access to Essential Drugs in Poor Countries: A Lost Battle?," *JAMA*, Jan. 27, 1999.

161 **abandoned efforts to discover . . . antibiotics:** "Bad Bugs, No Drugs," a report by the Infectious Diseases Society of America, July 2004.

162 **"it has to feed on whales":** Solomon's letter published in Forest Laboratories *Annual Report* of 2002.

162 **at least twenty prescription drugs:** See list of sixteen drugs removed from market between 1975 and 2000 in Lasser et al., "Timing of New Black Box Warnings and Withdrawals for Prescription Medications," *JAMA*, May 1, 2002. Omitted from that list were Redux and Pondimin, two diet drugs, which were removed in 1997. Between 2000 and 2005 four more drugs were withdrawn, including Bextra, Vioxx, Baycol, and Raplon.

162 **more than 10 percent were either:** Lasser et al.

162 **single class of new medicines . . . killed fifty thousand:** This tragedy involved the heart drugs Tambocor and Enkaid. The case is detailed in Thomas Moore, *Deadly Medicine* (New York: Simon & Schuster, 1995).

163 **There was something about Baycol:** These details come from internal corporate documents offered as evidence by plaintiffs in litigation against Bayer in 2003. Also see Melody Petersen and Alex Berenson, "Papers Indicate that Bayer Knew of Dangers of Its Cholesterol Drug," *The New York Times*, Feb. 22, 2003, and Melody Petersen, "Bayer Official Offers Defense in Texas Trial of Drug Suit," *The New York Times*, March 1, 2003.

163 **Within a hundred days:** Psaty et al., "Potential for Conflict of Interest in the Evaluation of Suspected Adverse Drug Reactions," *JAMA*, Dec. 1, 2004.

165 **doctors ignored these labels:** Raymond L. Woosley, "Drug Labeling Revisions—Guaranteed to Fail?," *JAMA*, Dec. 20, 2000.

166 **Dorothy Hamill and Bruce Jenner:** Melody Petersen, "Pushing Pills with Piles of Money," *The New York Times*, Oct. 5, 2000.

166 **"I just—I felt old":** Transcript of the *Larry King Live* show, Aug. 29, 2000.

167 **"It's something you can take":** Bart Conner quoted in Michael Haederle, "Hard Landing: Used to Competing Through Pain, a Former Olympic Gymnast Learns to Live with Osteoarthritis," *People*, Aug. 7, 2000.

168 **news stories . . . about the new "superaspirins":** For example, see Jerome Groopman, "Super Aspirin," *The New Yorker*, June 15, 1998, as well as Gina Kolata, "Drug Makers Say New Painkillers Work Without Side Effects," *The New York Times*, Nov. 11, 1998.

168 **sixteen thousand Americans with arthritis:** Wolfe et al., "Gastrointestinal Toxicity of Nonsteroidal Anti-inflammatory Drugs," *NEJM*, June 17, 1999.

169 **"I just can't wait":** Internal e-mail from Alise Reicin to her colleagues on Feb. 25, 1997, 10:39 p.m. This document and others were posted on a website (saferdrugsnow.org) in 2005 by a group of lawyers involved in litigation against Merck.

169 **excluded most patients with serious heart disease:** The researchers excluded from the trial most patients who suffered heart problems and were recommended to take aspirin to reduce their risk of heart attack. Only 4 percent of the

patients in the trial had heart problems serious enough to require aspirin treatment. The researchers also selected for the trial mostly women, who as a group suffer fewer heart attacks than men. Almost 80 percent of the patients in the trial were women with an average age of fifty-eight. See Bombardier et al., "Comparison of Upper Gastrointestinal Toxicity of Rofecoxib and Naproxen in Patients with Rheumatoid Arthritis," *NEJM*, Nov. 23, 2000.

169 **"clearly there":** Internal e-mail sent by Dr. Edward Scolnick to Dr. Reicin and other Merck executives on March 9, 2000, 6:18 p.m.

170 **the new study, VIGOR:** Bombardier et al., Nov. 23, 2000.

170 **Merck now had an explanation:** For years after the VIGOR study was published in 2000, the company's official position was that naproxen had an ability to protect the heart. Executives made this argument in press releases and in statements to the FDA. In 2002, researchers said they had found that naproxen did have a cardioprotective effect. See Rahme et al., "Association Between Naproxen Use and Protection Against Acute Myocardial Infarction," *Archives of Internal Medicine*, May 27, 2002. But other scientists concluded the potential benefit from naproxen could not have explained all the additional heart attacks in patients taking Vioxx in the VIGOR study. See Juni et al., "Risk of Cardiovascular Events and Rofecoxib: Cumulative Meta-analysis," *The Lancet*, Dec. 4, 2004. Those researchers said that Vioxx should have been withdrawn several years earlier than it ultimately was.

170 **Merck spent $160 million to advertise Vioxx:** "Prescription Drugs and Mass Media Advertising, 2000," a report by the National Institute for Health Care Management Research and Education Foundation, Nov. 2001.

171 **nine thousand dinners, meetings:** Joanna Breitstein, "Spending Hits a Wall," *Pharmaceutical Executive*, Sept. 2002.

171 **hired so many . . . rheumatologists:** Merck regularly paid fifteen hundred dollars to doctors giving a lecture, according to an internal corporate document that explained its "Business Management HEL Programs." It also paid doctors two thousand dollars to be a "visiting consultant" for a day. This document and others were obtained in an investigation led by Representative Henry Waxman in 2005. Many of these documents are available to the public at a website maintained by the University of California, San Francisco (dida.library.ucsf.edu).

171 **the way they shook hands:** Internal Merck document called "Professional Presence," a guide for sales reps.

171 **Obstacle Response Guide:** Described in internal Merck memo, "Bulletin for Vioxx: New Obstacle Response," dated May 1, 2000. Memo is addressed to "all field personnel with responsibility for Vioxx."

171 **Cardiovascular Card:** This was a Merck document entitled "In Response to Your Questions: Cardiovascular System: Clinical Profile in Osteoarthritis Stud-

ies." This document was described in an investigation of Merck's sales practices by Representative Henry Waxman and his staff. See Waxman's "The Marketing of Vioxx to Physicians," a memo sent to the Democratic members of the Government Reform Committee, May 5, 2005. Available at www.oversight.house.gov.

171 **mingling of numbers that the FDA had warned was not appropriate:** Waxman memo of May 5, 2005, p. 18.

172 **Dodge Ball Vioxx:** Internal document created by Merck, later used as evidence in lawsuits against the company.

172 **In an article:** Mukherjee, Nissen, and Topol, "Risk of Cardiovascular Events Associated with Selective COX-2 Inhibitors," *JAMA*, Aug. 22, 2001.

172 **doctors at Vanderbilt University:** Ray et al., "Cox-2 Selective Non-steroidal Anti-inflammatory Drugs and Risk of Serious Coronary Heart Disease," *The Lancet*, Oct. 5, 2002.

six: Ghostwriters and Secret Studies

174 **"important advance":** Novartis press release, "FDA Grants Marketing Clearance for Ritalin LA," June 6, 2002.

174 **A "key challenge" in selling Ritalin LA:** "Regaining Leadership in a Market," a slide presentation by Novartis executives at a meeting of the Healthcare Marketing & Communications Council on Apr. 16, 2003. Slides available at hmc-council.org. Accessed Aug. 2004.

176 **"We would like to help draft":** Transcript of conference call on Sept. 13, 2002. Parts of this transcript were included in Melody Petersen, "Madison Avenue Plays Growing Role in Drug Research," *The New York Times*, Nov. 11, 2002. It was also part of a segment appearing on *NOW with Bill Moyers* on PBS on Nov. 22, 2002. The story was reported by Walt Bogdanich and Melody Petersen for *The New York Times*. When I asked them about the call, Markowitz and Patrick told me that IntraMed did not dictate what their paper said. "No figure, no table, anything goes in without our approval," Markowitz told me. Jed Beitler, the chairman of the division at WPP that includes IntraMed, told me that his firm does not ghostwrite articles but only makes "editorial suggestions." He said, "The doctors are the ultimate writers." Novartis executives said the article was not intended to conclude that one product was better than the others but was a review of the available medications in which the authors could suggest theoretical advantages.

177 **disinterestedness was one of "the norms" of science:** R. K. Merton, "Science and Technology in a Democratic Order," *Journal of Legal and Political Sociology*, 1942. This was later published as "Science and Democratic Social Structure," in Robert K. Merton, *Social Theory and Social Structure* (New York: Free Press,

1968). Also see a discussion of Dr. Merton's work in Sheldon Krimsky, *Science in the Private Interest* (Lanham, Md.: Rowman & Littlefield, 2003).

177   **"Could you patent the sun?"**:   Exchange included in David M. Oshinsky, *Polio: An American Story* (New York: Oxford University Press, 2005). Oshinsky also describes how Salk later did try to commercialize other discoveries, including an AIDS vaccine. He founded a company called Immune Response Corporation to develop that vaccine. When the company went public in 1990, Dr. Salk's shares were worth more than three million dollars.

178   **"For most industrial scientists"**:   John Ziman, "Why Must Scientists Become More Ethically Sensitive Than They Used to Be?," *Science*, Dec. 4, 1998.

178   **changes swept through campuses:**   Krimsky, p. 29.

178   **first patent to be placed on a living organism:**   *Diamond v. Chakrabarty*, 447 U.S. 303 (1980).

179   **helped start 1,633 new companies:**   "Licensing Survey FY 1991–FY 1995," Association of University Technology Managers. Accessed at autm.net in 2007.

179   **researchers at Stanford:**   Rogers et al., "Assessing the Effectiveness of Technology Transfer Offices at U.S. Research Universities, *The Journal of the Association of University Technology Managers*, 2000.

179   **husband-and-wife team from Denmark:**   Helle Krogh Johansen and Peter C. Gøtzsche, "Problems in the Design and Reporting of Trials of Antifungal Agents Encountered During Meta-analysis," *JAMA*, Nov. 10, 1999.

182   **"When the patients agreed to take part"**:   Drummond Rennie, "Fair Conduct and Fair Reporting of Clinical Trials," *JAMA*, Nov. 10, 1999. Rennie asked Pfizer to respond to the findings by Gøtzsche and Johansen, but the company declined. Seven months later the company changed its mind. In a letter to the journal, it said it had changed some of its research practices to reduce the chance that trials were reported multiple times. The company said it agreed with the Danes' assertion that *oral* doses of amphotericin B and nystatin did not have a role in the treatment of serious fungal infections. It also said that at the time the Diflucan trials were planned in the 1980s and early 1990s, the medical community had believed that a study of these oral doses was warranted, a statement that Gøtzsche and Johansen disputed. It later became clear that Pfizer scientists had learned little from the experience. In 2006, Johansen, Gøtzsche, and another scientist reported that they had uncovered similar disturbing inconsistencies in trials of Pfizer's new antifungal drug called Vfend. The company had again designed the trials in a way that made Vfend appear better than it really was. See Jorgensen et al., "Flaws in Design, Analysis and Interpretation of Pfizer's Antifungal Trials of Voriconazole and Uncritical Subsequent Quotations," *Trials*, Jan. 19, 2006.

183 **"awash with money"**: Drummond Rennie, "Acceptance Address: Puking and Mewling, Then Sitting in Slippers, Then Drooling," *Science Editor*, Sept.–Oct. 2001.

184 **"the blending of science and marketing"**: A transcript of this discussion was published as a special report, "When Worlds Collide: The Unleashed Power of Marketing/R&D Collaboration," in *Pharmaceutical Executive*, Sept. 2002.

184 **the marketers were standing beside the scientists**: See explanation of why Wyeth-Ayerst moved its marketers into its research laboratories in article by Cavan Redmond, the company's senior vice president of global strategic marketing, "Branding: Change & Challenge," *Pharmaceutical Executive*, Sept. 1, 2001. He said the company's marketers were involved even before the company began testing the drug in human volunteers—that is, at Phase 0, when it was still in the test tube and being studied only in animals.

184 **An essential part of this strategy was . . . publication planning**: The industry regularly held conferences on how better to use this marketing technique. For example, a two-day conference held in Philadelphia in Dec. 2006 was called Second Annual Forum on Strategic Publication Planning. The event's brochure said that drug companies greatly benefited when they got research published in a medical journal. "It's an automatic validation unmatched by any other medium," the brochure said.

185 **increased spending on what they called research and development**: For example, the pharmaceutical companies regularly include the cost of clinical studies done after a drug is approved in their research and development costs, even though the studies were done to expand sales of an existing product and were often suggested by marketers. This is described in chapter 4 of *Science and Engineering Indicators 2006*, published by the National Science Foundation.

185 **the companies' share . . . 62 percent**: Bekelman et al., "Scope and Impact of Financial Conflicts of Interest in Biomedical Research," *JAMA*, Jan. 22, 2003.

185 **behind the scenes . . . executives who called the shots**: This was clear, for example, in Pfizer's trials of Diflucan, which are described in this chapter. It was also apparent in Merck's trial of Vioxx, described in chapter 5.

186 **IntraMed . . . opened its doors for business in 1974**: From sudler.com, Nov. 2006.

186 **"simple, magical strategies"**: Ibid.

186 **lay the groundwork for rapid prescribing**: Joseph Brown, "Sudler & Hennessey," *Med Ad News*, Apr. 1, 2000.

186 **skilled in the development of key messages**: Ibid.

186 **Axis . . . "brand the science"**: According to the firm's website in Nov. 2006, one of its "strategic services" was to "brand the science." See axis-healthcare.com. The firm had many subsidiaries, including Fusion Medical Education, which ex-

plained on its website that the goal of its strategic medical writing services was "to drive product prescriptions."

186   **"highly sophisticated publication plan"**: This was one of the client cases that Excerpta Medica described on its website (excerptamedica.com), May 2002.

187   **names of the firms . . . rarely appeared**: Infrequently the marketing firms will disclose their involvement in helping write the article in a line in the manuscript. For example, the work of IntraMed's division Imprint Publication Science was disclosed in a 2006 article in this way: "The author thanks Imprint Publication Science, NY, for editorial support." The article also said it had been paid for through "an unrestricted educational grant" from GlaxoSmithKline. See Alan B. Ettinger, "Psychotropic Effects of Antiepileptic Drugs," *Neurology*, Dec. 2006. By 2007 such disclosures were still rare, however. The editors at the best journals attempt to stop ghostwriting by requiring that all contributors to an article be named, but the firms work around such requirements by having the academic authors submit the manuscripts for publication.

187   **An internal document**: "Worldwide Publications Status Update: Zoloft, Prepared by Current Medical Directions, Jan. 29, 1999." This document is available at a website created by Dr. David Healy (healyprozac.com).

188   **They found fifty-five articles**: David Healy and Dinah Cattell, "Interface Between Authorship, Industry and Science in the Domain of Therapeutics," *British Journal of Psychiatry*, 2003.

188   **"look fishy"**: Memo to Bonnie Rossello from Sandra Stahl at Ruder Finn on June 5, 1997. This was part of a number of documents made public in lawsuits against SmithKline, the maker of Paxil.

189   **phone call from . . . Edelman**: Troyen A. Brennan, "Sounding Board: Buying Editorials," *NEJM*, Sept. 8, 1994.

189   **Revenues earned from medical writing**: Karyn Korieth, "Medical Writing Market Appreciation," *The CenterWatch Monthly*, July 2004. The article says that drug companies began regularly employing medical writers only in the last decade.

189   **Complete Healthcare**: Details described at the firm's website (chcinc.com), Nov. 2006.

190   **"your words in someone else's mouth"**: Merrill Rose, "Activism in the 90s: Changing Roles for Public Relations," *Public Relations Quarterly*, 1991. For more on public relations in America, see Sheldon Rampton and John Stauber, *Trust Us, We're Experts* (New York: Tarcher Putnam, 2001).

191   **"Deploy third parties"**: Maxine Taylor, "Practical Guide: Public Relations Part 3: What Is Crisis Management?," published Feb. 1, 2002, at PMLive.com, a website that features content from *Pharmaceutical Marketing* magazine.

191   **a copy of an invoice:** Documents were made public in a class-action lawsuit
        filed against Wyeth, the diet pill manufacturer. Also see Charles Ornstein, "Fen-
        phen Maker Accused of Funding Journal Articles," *The Dallas Morning News*,
        May 23, 1999.

192   **largest annual gathering of . . . psychiatrists:** Meeting of the American Psy-
        chiatric Association in Atlanta in 2005.

193   **"The evidence is strong":** Richard Smith, "Medical Journals Are an Extension
        of the Marketing Arm of Pharmaceutical Companies," *PLoS Medicine*, May 17,
        2005.

193   **"Far more dominant":** Graham Dukes, "Development of the Pharmaceutical
        Industry: How, Why and When Corruption Came In," a paper presented at the
        Eleventh International Anti-Corruption Conference, held in Seoul, South Ko-
        rea, May 25 to 28, 2003.

193   **Forest Laboratories were in a bind:** Melody Petersen, "Madison Avenue Plays
        Growing Role in Drug Research," *The New York Times*, Nov. 22, 2002.

194   **All three trials came back:** Described in Gorman et al., "Efficacy Comparison
        of Escitalopram and Citalopram in the Treatment of Major Depressive Disorder:
        Pooled Analysis of Placebo-Controlled Trials," *CNS Spectrums*, Apr. 2002.

194   **"compulsive shopping disorder":** See chapter 3.

194   **provided sound bites for television news:** Press release, "FDA Approves Treat-
        ment for Generalized Anxiety Disorder," Apr. 17, 2001. The release describes a
        video news segment with sound bites from Gorman that television news stations
        were asked to put on the air.

195   **Forest paid Medworks Media:** Interviews with Forest executives in fall of
        2002.

195   **"provocative findings":** Gorman et al., Apr. 2002.

195   **press releases quoting Professor Gorman:** For example, see "Results of Sev-
        eral Clinical Trials of Escitalopram, Citalopram and Placebo and Pooled Analy-
        ses of These Trials to Be Presented Today at American Psychiatric Association
        Meeting," May 9, 2001, and "Pre-Clinical Data Sheds Light on the Potency of
        Lexapro," June 24, 2002.

196   **sales representatives . . . offering free massages:** Kerry Dooley, "Forest Labs
        Says Celexa Successor Effective, Faster," Bloomberg News, May 9, 2001.

196   **dinner was held at Daniel:** Described in July 11, 2002, letter sent to Dr.
        Brown by Forest Laboratories, as well as the menu printed on parchment by the
        restaurant, which welcomed the "Celexa/Lexapro Advisory Board Meeting" on
        Aug. 27, 2002.

196 **"I think it's disgusting"**: Interview with Dr. Brown in the summer of 2002. His comments first appeared in the article I wrote for the *Times* that appeared Nov. 22, 2002.

197 **Lexapro was no better**: "Escitalopram (Lexapro) for Depression," *The Medical Letter*, Sept. 30, 2002. Also see Staffan Svensson and Peter R. Mansfield, "Escitalopram: Superior to Citalopram or a Chiral Chimera?," *Psychotherapy and Psychosomatics*, Jan.–Feb. 2004.

197 **"an instant success"**: Corey Davis et al., "Forest Laboratories Inc.: Lexapro Blastoff! Raising Estimates," report from J. P. Morgan, Sept. 11, 2002.

197 **advertising firms . . . owned or had large investments**: Interpublic's Torre Lazur McCann bought a CRO called Target Research in 2002. Omnicom owned a minority stake in Scirex in 2002, and it later acquired the entire company. WPP's CommonHealth formed a joint venture through its HLS Clinical Systems division with a CRO called Advanced Biologics. This is described in Steve Zisson, "Pace of CRO Acquisitions Accelerates," *The CenterWatch Monthly*, July 2002. In 2002 WWP's Sudler & Hennessey also owned a CRO called Medicina Domani Pharma. See Frank Scussa, "Sudler & Hennessey," *Med Ad News*, Apr. 1, 2002. In 2006 a company called inVentiv Health owned a firm that performed clinical drug trials as well as several large advertising agencies. InVentiv explained in its 2005 annual report that it had expertise not just in pharmaceutical advertising but in all aspects of the clinical research process, from designing the study to recruiting patients.

198 **"closer to the test tube"**: From press release, "Scirex Launches $20 Million Strategic Partnership with Diversified Agency Services (DAS) An Omnicom Group, Inc. Company," Nov. 29, 1999.

198 **"We provide services that go"**: This interview with Joe Torre aired as part of "Science for Sale?," a segment appearing on *NOW with Bill Moyers* on PBS, Nov. 22, 2002. The story was reported by Walt Bogdanich and Melody Petersen for *The New York Times*. Transcript available at pbs.org.

199 **"an excess of serious adverse events, including death"**: This is from the unredacted written review by the FDA medical officer who was considering whether to approve Bextra to treat acute pain. The consumer group Public Citizen filed a lawsuit against the FDA to gain access to these documents. The group then wrote about what it found in the papers. See "Lawsuit Reveals Serious Safety Problems with the Nonsteroidal Anti-inflammatory Drug (NSAID) Valdecoxib (Bextra)," *Health Letter*, Public Citizen's Health Research Group, Sept. 2004.

199 **Pharmacia had paid the Scirex scientists**: Daniels, et al., "The Analgesic Efficacy of Valdecoxib vs. Oxycodone/Acetaminophen After Oral Surgery," *Journal of the American Dental Association*, May 2002.

199 **Three scientists who later reviewed the Scirex study**: In 2002, I had three scientists not affiliated with Pharmacia review the study for an article I was re-

searching. See Petersen, "Madison Avenue Plays Growing Role in Drug Research," *The New York Times*, Nov. 11, 2002.

200 **FDA demanded that Pfizer:** "FDA announces series of changes to the class of marketed non-steroidal anti-inflammatory drugs," government press release, Apr. 7, 2005.

200 **the tobacco industry hired academic scientists:** For example, see Joaquin Barnoya and Stanton A. Glantz, "The Tobacco Industry's Worldwide ETS Consultants Project: European and Asian Components," *The European Journal of Public Health*, 2006.

200 **tobacco companies secretly began:** Hong and Bero, "How the Tobacco Industry Responded to an Influential Study of the Health Effects of Secondhand Smoke," *BMJ*, Dec. 14, 2002.

201 **They simply kept that evidence locked up:** See Aug. 16, 2006, ruling by U.S. District Judge Gladys Kessler that the tobacco industry had engaged in a decades-long racketeering scheme to keep the public from knowing the dangers of tobacco. She wrote: "Even though Defendants have known internally about addiction for decades, they have endeavored to keep the extensive research and data they had accumulated out of the public domain and out of the hands of the public health community by denying that such data existed." The ruling, which spans more than sixteen hundred pages, details the tobacco industry's actions to manipulate what scientific data were published. *U.S. v. Philip Morris et al.*, Civil Action No. 99-2496, U.S. District Court for the District of Columbia.

201 **"There are no plans to publish":** Internal document from SmithKline entitled "Seroxat/Paxil Adolescent Depression: Position Piece on the Phase III Clinical Studies." This document was first reported on by the BBC in a story on Feb. 3, 2004, titled "GSK Knew Seroxat Wasn't 'Effective' on Children."

201 **"This paper will not be published":** Interoffice memo dated July 28, 1997, that describes the minutes from a meeting of the Nifedeipine/Cerivastatin Publication Committee. Part of documents that were later made public in lawsuits filed against Bayer.

202 **"Stein has been quite vocal":** Interoffice memo dated Dec. 1, 1999, that describes the minutes from a meeting of the Cerivastatin Communication Committee.

202 **"Please note that the findings are preliminary":** E-mail from Leonard Jokubaitis to other executives on Aug. 28, 1998. This was later made public in litigation against the company.

202 **"a unique" drug:** The "Propulsid Core Message" was included in an internal newsletter for sales reps called *The Propulsid Link*, issue dated May 1999.

202 **"watched in amazement as Shamu":** From article titled "Taking the Show on the Road," *The Propulsid Link*, May 1999.

203 **three hundred reports that the drug:** Deaths and injuries were described on a slide created by executives for a presentation they gave to the FDA on Oct. 15, 1999.

203 **"your nighttime heartburn medicine":** From a slide FDA officials presented to executives at a private meeting on March 27, 1998. Both the slide and minutes written by executives at that meeting were later made public in litigation.

203 **executive named Darryl Kurland:** Copy of message sent by Kurland to Alan F. Joslyn, Sept. 16, 1998.

204 **learning to "manage the FDA":** This was discussed by executives in a memo entitled "Propulsid Lessons Learned," which was written after the company agreed to stop promoting the drug.

204 **"stand in front of world":** From notes written by hand on the agenda for the "Propulsid AC Planning Meeting" of Feb. 15, 2000. This document is available at a website created by lawyers involved in litigation against Johnson & Johnson (saferdrugsnow.org). Accessed 2006.

204 **The executives announced the company:** The company continued to make the drug available to a few patients in a limited access program. See "Janssen Pharmaceutica Stops Marketing Cisapride in the U.S.," an FDA Talk Paper, March 23, 2000.

204 **More than a hundred . . . had died:** Described in an Apr. 11, 2000, letter from Public Citizen to Jane Henney, the commissioner of the FDA. The letter was based on death reports the consumer group had received from the FDA.

204 **The attorney general sued the company:** *The People of the State of New York, by Eliot Spitzer v. GlaxoSmithKline,* filed on June 2, 2004, in the State Supreme Court in Manhattan.

205 **"cutting-edge" research:** Internal memo to "All Sales Representatives Selling Paxil" from Zachary Hawkins, Aug. 16, 2001.

205 **at least 50 percent . . . never been published:** Kay Dickersin and Drummond Rennie, "Registering Clinical Trials," *JAMA,* July 23, 2003.

205 **one of thirty-seven experiments:** MacLean et al., "How Useful Are Unpublished Data from the Food and Drug Administration in Meta-analysis," *Journal of Clinical Epidemiology,* Jan. 2003.

206 **"The right to search for truth":** Einstein's words are engraved on his memorial at the National Academy of Sciences building in Washington.

206 **a fraction of . . . interventions:** For example, see David M. Eddy, "Evidence-Based Medicine: A Unified Approach," *Health Affairs,* Jan.–Feb., 2005.

206 **"most claimed research findings are false":** John P. A. Ioannidis, "Why Most Published Research Findings Are False," *PLoS Medicine,* Aug. 2005.

206   "most studied of any drug for children": For example, Regina Moran, executive director of public relations at Novartis, used this phrase in Warren R. Ross, "Ritalin's Revival," *Medical Marketing & Media*, Aug. 2003.

206   Ritalin Man: Novartis created these toys in the 1970s. A model is planned to be on display at the Advertising Icon Museum in Kansas City when it opens in 2008. The museum has photos of some of its exhibits, including the Ritalin Man, available at toymuseum.com. Accessed June 2007.

207   many of the scientists and physicians: Most studies of stimulants have been paid for either by the government or by the drug manufacturers. Most studies funded by the government were not done independently from the manufacturers, however. The government selected scientists who often had significant financial ties to the industry to lead those trials.

207   meetings to develop these doctors into a faculty of advocates: A common marketing tactic in the industry is to hold meetings for doctors at which they learn about a new product and are trained to give speeches about it to their peers. In the transcript of the call involving IntraMed on Sept. 13, 2002, Shane Schaffer, the Novartis executive, referred to these events as "faculty development meetings." He said he had spoken with Dr. Markowitz at one of these events, which the company had held in Chicago.

207   boasted about . . . launching Ritalin LA: "Regaining Leadership in a Market," slide presentation by Novartis Pharmaceuticals Corporation at the Healthcare Marketing & Communications Council meeting of Apr. 16, 2003. The presentation was also the subject of an article by William R. Ross, "Ritalin's Revival," *Medical Marketing & Media*, Aug. 2003.

207   National Association of School Nurses: *Straight Talk About Responsible Treatment: S.T.A.R.T. Now: A Reference Guide for Teens with ADHD,* Novartis Pharmaceuticals, 2002. Also see June 4, 2002, press release from Novartis about its partnership with the National Association of School Nurses.

208   Beethoven . . . Bell . . . Einstein: Those writing the brochure for Novartis referenced this claim to a website, www.adhdrelief.com/famous, which sells a nutritional supplement for those diagnosed with ADHD. The site's creators had listed the names of more than a hundred famous people, from Tom Cruise to Leonardo de Vinci, and were asking members of the public to e-mail them with more names of people they believed suffered from ADHD. The list included short notes on why the person was thought to have the disorder. Abraham Lincoln, for example, was said to have ADHD because he "entered the Black Hawk War as a captain and came out a private." Accessed June 2007.

208   pink-colored plastic binder: Dorsey Griffith, "ADHD in Girls Comes in Focus," *The Sacramento Bee*, Oct. 27, 2002.

208   **survey . . . with the help of Dr. Patricia Quinn:** Described in Novartis press release, "Nationwide Survey of More than 3,000 People Uncovers Gender Differences in ADHD," Aug. 19, 2002.

208   **Dr. Quinn told the many journalists:** She spoke to many journalists who had received the company's press releases. See, for example, Janice Billingsley, "Girls with Attention-Deficit Disorder Need Attention," *HealthDay*, Aug. 23, 2002.

209   **Oregon researchers combed through the medical literature:** Described in their final report. See *Drug Class Review on Pharmacologic Treatment for ADHD*, Oregon Evidence-Based Practice Center, Oregon Health & Science University, May 2006. Available at ohsu.edu/epc.

209   **Celltech Pharmaceuticals had paid:** This study was published as Greenhill et al., "A Double-Blind, Placebo-Controlled Study of Modified Release Methylphenidate in Children with Attention-Deficit/Hyperactivity Disorder," *Pediatrics*, March 2002. The researchers had added even more bias to the trial by excluding any children who had tried methylphenidate in the past but stopped taking it because it did not ease their symptoms or they suffered side effects. This gave the researchers a pool of young volunteers who were more likely to have good results with Metadate. See what the Oregon researchers said about the bias in this trial in an appendix to their final report called "Evidence Tables."

210   **questioned the design of the study:** Described in the FDA Medical Review of Ritalin LA, application number 21-284, which was written by Dr. Andrew Mosholder.

210   **published in a medical journal in 2003:** Biederman et al., "Efficacy and Safety of Ritalin LA, a New, Once Daily, Extended-Release Dosage Form of Methylphenidate, in Children with Attention Deficit Hyperactivity Disorder," *Pediatric Drugs*, 2003.

210   **In 2006 he disclosed:** See list in Biederman and Faraone, "The Effects of Attention-Deficit/Hyperactivity Disorder on Employment and Household Income," published on Medscape General Medicine, July 18, 2006, and available at medscape.com.

211   **"helped to support the notion":** See "An Interview with Dr. Joseph Biederman," *ESI Special Topics*, July 2005. Online at esi-topics.com.

211   **the company didn't completely know:** The prescribing instructions for Ritalin state, "The mode of action in man is not completely understood, but Ritalin presumably activates the brain stem arousal system and cortex to produce its stimulant effect. There is neither specific evidence which clearly establishes the mechanism whereby Ritalin produces its mental and behavioral effects in children, nor conclusive evidence regarding how these effects relate to the condition of the central nervous system." This version of prescribing instructions is dated Feb. 2006. Obtained from novartis.com in March 2006.

SEVEN: "Neurontin for Everything"

This chapter is based largely on my interviews with David Franklin, as well as thousands of pages of internal corporate documents, transcripts, depositions, and other papers that were part of the case, *United States of America, ex rel. David Franklin v. Pfizer and Parke-Davis, a division of Warner-Lambert Company.* This case, Civil Action No. 96-11651-PBS, was filed in U.S. District Court in Boston, Massachusetts, in 1996 and settled in 2004. Many of these documents are available in an online archive maintained by the University of California, San Francisco. See dida.library.ucsf.edu.

212   **sat on the Continental jetliner:** E-mail from Franklin, March 19, 2007.

213   **He had sent his résumé:** Volume 3 of Deposition of David Franklin, Sept. 14, 2000.

214   **"There is some question":** Disclosure of Information by Relator David P. Franklin, a document filed in U.S. District Court.

214   **Michael Valentino:** Volume 3 of Deposition.

215   **"lots of yeses":** Ibid.

216   **"I didn't really believe it":** E-mail from Franklin, March 19, 2007.

216   **Fenway Park:** Ibid.

216   **sight of blood:** Interview with Franklin, March 11, 2003.

217   **"the perfect fit":** E-mail from Franklin, March 19, 2007.

218   **a series of internal meetings:** Relator's Separate Statement of Disputed Material Facts, May 27, 2003.

218   **5 to 10 percent of the epilepsy patients . . . got worse:** "Parke-Davis' Neurontin Recommended for Approval as 'Add-on' Therapy for Refractory Seizures in Epilepsy," *The Pink Sheet*, Dec. 21, 1992.

218   **$500 million:** Relator's Separate Statement of Disputed Material Facts.

218   **internal wish list:** The conditions the executives talked about are listed in an internal memo dated Oct. 25, 1995, by Francie Kivel on the subject of "Reporting of Neurontin Indication Publications Analysis."

219   **rumor or anecdotal reports:** Disclosure of Information, p. 7.

219   **Executives at the highest levels:** These men are listed in internal corporate documents as members of the New Product Committee, which planned how the company would promote Neurontin to treat migraines and other off-label conditions. This was also described in a Sept. 16, 2002, court deposition given by John Boris, a Warner-Lambert executive. Boris explained that the New Products Committee was "a decision-making body of senior management."

219   **memo written by John T. Boris:** "Neurontin Marketing Assessment," July 31, 1996. This was Exhibit #31 to Relator's Separate Statement of Disputed Material Facts.

220 **It was founded in the 1860s:** See brief history of Warner-Lambert and Parke-Davis provided at pfizer.com.

220 **the marketing of cocaine:** Steven B. Karch, *A Brief History of Cocaine* (Boca Raton, Fla.: Taylor & Francis, 2006), p. 58.

221 **Dr. Sigmund Freud:** *Cocaine: 1977,* ed. Robert C. Petersen and Richard C. Stillman, NIDA Research Monograph #13, May 1977.

221 **"should have a great future":** Karch, p. 106.

221 **first days at Parke-Davis:** E-mail from David Franklin, March 19, 2007.

222 **told him to call on pediatricians:** Franklin describes this in detail in his lawsuit. For example, see Disclosure of Information. Also see Volume 3 of Deposition of David Franklin.

223 **laugh when they saw the slide:** Disclosure of Information, p. 21. Franklin explained that the company often updated the slide with new conditions that it claimed Neurontin could treat. It was updated so often, he said, that it was kept in a different format from the rest of the slides he was given to show physicians.

223 **"I'm embarrassed to show you":** This is Franklin's recollection of Magistro's speech. See Disclosure of Information, p. 21.

224 **"That's where we need to be":** This is Franklin's recollection of Ford's speech. See Disclosure of Information, p. 11.

224 **"adequate and well-controlled investigations":** Federal Food, Drug, and Cosmetic Act (21 U.S.C. 355).

225 **drugs for schizophrenia to patients with Alzheimer's:** The danger of this off-label use has been widely reported. For example, see Benedict Carey, "Drugs to Curb Agitation Are Said to Be Ineffective for Alzheimer's," *The New York Times,* Oct. 12, 2006.

225 **Tambocor and Enkaid:** Thomas J. Moore, *Deadly Medicine* (New York: Simon & Schuster, 1995).

225 **more than 90 percent of the prescriptions written for some drugs:** For example, the FDA said in 2006 that 94 percent of the prescriptions for Gabitril, a drug approved for epilepsy, were off label. The government also said it was receiving reports that the drug was causing seizures in these patients. See Flowers et al., "Seizure Activity and Off-Label Use of Tiagabine," *NEJM,* Feb. 16, 2006.

225 **avoid writing things down:** Disclosure of Information, p. 7.

226 **"don't leave a paper trail":** Disclosure of Information, p. 30.

227 **the employee operating the video camera:** Disclosure of Information, p. 9.

227 **precision marketing reports:** Disclosure of Information, p. 14.

228 **average bonus . . . more than . . . salary:** For example, in 2001, the average annual salary for a sales rep selling the painkiller OxyContin for Purdue Pharma

was $55,000, while the average annual bonus was $71,500. The highest annual sales bonus that year for an OxyContin rep was $240,000. See "OxyContin Abuse and Diversion," U.S. General Accounting Office, Dec. 2003.

228 **"What we need to do is"**: Transcript of voice mail message that was recorded by Franklin.

229 **Cline Davis . . . sat on the committee**: Deposition given by John M. Knoop, Sept. 25, 2002.

229 **Neurontin War Games**: See "Neurontin War Games," an internal document written by Cline Davis & Mann and dated Apr. 3, 1996.

230 **meeting held at the Château Elan**: Event is described in internal document titled "Consultants Meeting, Château Elan, Aug. 1–5, 1996."

230 **paid each of them $750**: Handwritten notes of an unnamed executive dated Apr. 23, 1996, and supported by other evidence in the lawsuit filed by Franklin.

230 **"$3mm investment"**: Handwritten notes dated Apr. 23, 1996.

230 **agreed to promote Neurontin for experimental uses**: For example, see memo from Clare Cheng of Cline Davis & Mann to Parke-Davis, July 18, 1996.

230 **prepared the slides and lecture notes**: For example, see "Parke-Davis Neurontin Monotherapy Task Force Training Meeting," a document written by Bina O'Brien of Proworx and dated Feb. 27, 1997.

230 **"Good morning, everyone"**: Transcript of speeches made at "Advances in Anticonvulsants," a regional consultants' meeting, at Jupiter Beach, Florida, Apr. 1996. The meeting's attendee list includes the names of seventy-five physicians, almost all of them from the northeastern United States.

231 **One . . . was held at the Ritz-Carlton**: "Neurology Update: Anticonvulsants: A Regional Consultants Meeting, May 10–11, 1996, Schedule of Events."

231 **"The problem with Neurontin"**: Transcript of speech by Dr. Longmire at the Ritz-Carlton in Boston on May 11, 1996. Years later Dr. Longmire claimed he did not know that Parke-Davis had involved him in an illegal marketing scheme. He claimed that his speeches were based on what he had actually found in his research and observed in his patients. He said that he had asked Parke-Davis executives before he gave the speeches whether it was legal and ethical to talk about how Neurontin could be used for off-label uses. He said he was assured by executives that the talks were legal.

232 **wrote more prescriptions for Neurontin when they got home**: Described in "Relator's Opposition to Defendants' Motion for Summary Judgment."

232 **"You'd like to think"**: E-mail from David Franklin, March 24, 2007.

233 **"counteract a possible 'negative' presentation"**: Internal memo dated June 24, 1997, from Bina O'Brien and Jennifer Guilmette of Proworx to Allen Crook and Vic Delimata of Parke-Davis.

234 **Bayliss drafted a letter:** Copy of a draft of a letter written by John Bayliss of IntraMed and addressed to Dr. John M. Pellock. The draft letter is dated Sept. 23,
1996. It was sent to Kim Keppler at Parke-Davis along with a memo from Bayliss
dated Sept. 24, 1996.

234 **wrote to executives at Parke-Davis:** From document prepared by Medical Education Systems, "Grant Request: Scientific Article Series in Support of
Epilepsy Education," Dec. 12, 1996.

235 **"DRAFT COMPLETED":** From document faxed by Medical Education
Systems on Oct. 29, 1997, and entitled "Articles on Antiepileptic Drug Use in
Epilepsy and Other Disorders."

235 **delivered boxes of them to Franklin:** Volume I of Franklin Deposition, given
on Sept. 12, 2000.

235 **paid one physician more than $300,000:** Franklin's lawyers accumulated the
payments made to physicians in a database. The top-paid speaker was Dr. B. J.
Wilder, who earned $307,958 at speaking events between Jan. 1994 and Nov.
1997. See list of these payments in Relator's Separate Statement of Disputed
Material Facts, May 27, 2003, p. 47.

235 **"I was here on the beach":** Transcript of speeches made at Advances in Anticonvulsants, a regional consultants' meeting, at Jupiter Beach, Florida, in Apr.
1996.

236 **pay $303,600 to publish his book:** Letter from Dr. Ilo Leppik to Allen Crook
at Parke-Davis, Nov. 18, 1996. Dr. Leppik told me in an interview in 2002
that he did not believe his book was "a marketing vehicle" for the drug company.
He said the book described the use of all epilepsy medicines and not just
Neurontin.

236 **"a great Neurontin believer":** Relator's Separate Statement of Disputed Material Facts, p. 49.

236 **Dr. Wilder asked the company:** Letter written by B. J. Wilder, president,
Epilepsy Research Foundation of Florida, Inc., to Edda Guerrero, at Parke-
Davis, Apr. 29, 1996.

236 **"influence physicians from the bottom up":** The company's targeting of medical residents is described in an internal memo, "Business Strategies to Penetrate
the Hospital Segment of the Northeast Customer Business Unit," undated.

237 **earn fifty dollars for each patient's record:** Disclosure of Information, p. 20.

237 **STEPS trial:** Plan to pay more than a thousand doctors is described in internal
document titled "Epilepsy Awareness & Support Exchange," undated. Also see
the description of how doctors began writing higher doses of the drug in "Neurontin 1997 Situation Analysis," May 24, 1996.

237 **selected the consultants on the basis of their potential:** Disclosure of Information, p. 19.

238 **"Hotel too cold inside":** From "Program Evaluation" for Atlantic City event held June 26 to 28, 1998.

238 **"Hired car":** From "Program Evaluation" for event at Helmsley Park Lane Hotel, June 12 to 14, 1998.

239 **sales rep . . . in the examination room:** Disclosure of Information, p. 19, and transcript of voice mail message by Steve Bitman, recorded by Franklin in 1996.

240 **Double vision was also a sign:** According to the FDA-approved prescribing instructions, patients who overdose on Neurontin suffer from double vision. The instructions also list blurred vision as a frequent side effect of the drug.

241 **FDA was receiving hundreds of reports:** Obtained through a request made under the federal Freedom of Information Act.

241 **"My principle exposure":** Comments by physicians were collected in "Low Use of Neurontin Among Neurologists," a report by Curtis and Prinz Incorporated, Sept. 10, 1996.

241 **"slow adopters":** Memo by J. Rizzo to J. Knoop, dated Sept. 17, 1996.

242 **"You keep telling me":** My interview with David Franklin, March 11, 2003.

242 **They threw tantrums:** Lee et al., "Behavioral Side Effects of Gabapentin in Children," *Epilepsia*, Jan. 1996.

242 **"I froze":** E-mail from David Franklin, March 24, 2007.

242 **"it's such a small number of kids":** This is a description of the conversation as Franklin remembered it and as was documented in the lawsuit he brought against the company. See Disclosure of Information, p. 16.

243 **Magistro . . . told him he should leave quietly:** Interview with Franklin, March 11, 2003.

243 **lawyers began calling him:** E-mail from Franklin, March 24, 2007.

243 **"I was completely stressed out":** Volume 3 of Deposition of Franklin.

243 **False Claims Act:** See history of this law at taf.org, a website created by Taxpayers Against Fraud, a group that helps whistle-blowers.

245 **nearly 90 percent of Neurontin prescriptions:** Relator's Separate Statement of Disputed Material Facts, May 27, 2003.

245 **Injury reports . . . to the FDA:** Obtained under the federal Freedom of Information Act.

246 **Neurontin worked no better than a sugar pill:** Sporn et al., "A Double-Blind, Placebo-Controlled Trial of Gabapentin Augmentation of Fluoxetine for Treatment of Obsessive-Compulsive Disorder," abstract of poster presented at NIH's New Clinical Drug Evaluation Unit meeting in 2001.

246 **given Neurontin for mania:** Wehner et al., "Gabapentin Associated Mania: A Retrospective, Naturalistic Review," abstract of poster presented at NIH's New Clinical Drug Evaluation Unit meeting in 2001.

246 **"being used like water":** My interview with Dr. Sporn in 2002.

246 **Dr. Alicia Mack:** "Examination of the Evidence for Off-label Use of Gabapentin," *Journal of Managed Care Pharmacy*, Nov.–Dec. 2003.

246 **trained to tell physicians . . . bipolar disorder:** Disclosure of Information, p. 22.

247 **completed the study by 1998:** Snigdha Prakash, "Drug Company Marketing Promotion in the Name of Education," *All Things Considered*, National Public Radio, Jan. 16, 2003.

247 **did not publish the results until September 2000:** Pande et al., "Gabapentin in Bipolar Disorder: A Placebo-Controlled Trial of Adjunctive Therapy," *Bipolar Disorders*, Sept. 2000.

247 **The corporate lawyers argued:** In depositions, Phil Magistro and John Ford testified they had never instructed Franklin or anyone else at Warner-Lambert to give false or misleading information to physicians in an attempt to sell Neurontin. Lisa Kellett, who worked as a medical liaison like Franklin, testified that she had never lied to a physician about Neurontin. Their depositions are summarized in "Defendants' statement pursuant to Local Civil Rule 56.1 of Material Facts as to which there are no genuine issues to be tried," Apr. 14, 2003.

247 **Franklin lost hope:** E-mail from Franklin, March 24, 2007.

248 **quickly sealing the records:** For example, Eli Lilly agreed to pay seven hundred million dollars to a large group of patients who claimed they had been harmed by a drug called Zyprexa but then required the patients and their lawyers not to talk about the evidence that had been uncovered in the case. Under the protective order, all internal corporate documents that had been filed in court were returned to Eli Lilly. See "Confidential Master Settlement Agreement," which was filed with the company's Form 10-Q on Sept. 30, 2005. For a good discussion of secrecy in court proceedings, see Richard Zitrin and Carol M. Langford, *The Moral Compass of the American Lawyer* (New York: Ballantine Books, 1999).

248 **lawyers had wrongly stamped "confidential":** Melody Petersen, "Documents Show Effort to Promote Unproven Drug," *The New York Times*, Oct. 29, 2002.

248 **experts estimated that 90 percent:** Julie Schmit, "Drugmaker Admitted Fraud, but Sales Flourish," *USA Today*, Aug. 16, 2004.

249 **ten billion dollars the company had earned:** Accumulated sales of Neurontin from Pfizer's press releases and financial reports.

249 **paid for 151,434 dinners:** Statistics are from "How to Maximize Your Marketing Mix," a presentation to the Ontario Pharmaceutical Marketing Association

by Jim Dougherty, McGraw-Hill Healthcare Information Group, June 6, 2005. Dougherty attributed the data on the number of meetings to Verispan's 2004 Physicians Meeting and Event Audit.

249 **180 separate investigations:** Described in testimony by James W. Moorman, the president of Taxpayers Against Fraud, before the House Committee on Oversight and Government Reform, Feb. 9, 2007.

249 **"We are not seeing isolated instances":** Testimony of Ronald J. Tenpas before the House Committee on Oversight and Government Reform, Feb. 9, 2007.

250 **they can be expected to harm others:** J. Scott Armstrong, "Social Irresponsibility in Management," *Journal of Business Research*, Sept. 1977.

251 **gifts as small as a cup of coffee:** Katz et al., "All Gifts Large and Small," *The American Journal of Bioethics*, Summer 2003.

251 **started to receive letters:** E-mail from Franklin, March 24, 2007.

252 **purchased a small school:** E-mail from Franklin, June 14, 2007.

252 **"encouraging doctors to experiment":** Interview with Franklin, March 11, 2003.

EIGHT: Altered State

255 **water samples were laced with Tagamet:** Kolpin et al., "Urban Contribution of Pharmaceuticals and Other Organic Wastewater Contaminants to Streams During Differing Flow Conditions," *Science of the Total Environment*, July 2004.

256 **"That just floored me":** Interview with Dana Kolpin, Dec. 2005.

256 **nationwide study:** Kolpin et al., "Pharmaceuticals, Hormones and Other Organic Wastewater Contaminants in U.S. Streams, 1999–2000: A National Reconnaissance," *Environmental Science & Technology*, 2002.

257 **bass on the Potomac River:** Vicki S. Blazer, "Intersex in Bass 'Emerging' Contaminant Issues," presentation at the Chesapeake Bay Commission, Nov. 10, 2006.

257 **mosquito fish . . . became uncoordinated:** Black et al., "Endocrine Effects of Selective Serotonin Reuptake Inhibitors (SSRIs) on Aquatic Organisms," abstract presented at U.S. EPA Meeting on Pharmaceuticals in the Environment, Aug. 23 to 25, 2005.

258 **South Asian farmers had begun:** Oaks et al., "Diclofenac Residues as the Cause of Vulture Population Decline in Pakistan," *Nature*, Feb. 12, 2004. Also see James Gorman, "A Drug Used for Cattle Is Said to Be Killing Vultures," *The New York Times*, Jan. 29, 2004.

258 **wild dogs . . . rat population:** Swan et al., "Removing the Threat of Diclofenac to Critically Endangered Asian Vultures," *PLoS Biology*, March 2006.

259   **McCombs Middle School:** "Student Suspended for Handing Out Prescription Drug," Channel 8 KCCI Des Moines, March 11, 2005.

259   **"We're a society":** Interview with Jean Phillips, May 5, 2005.

259   **girls . . . in Lynnwood, Washington:** Katherine Schiffner, "Prescription Drug Sends Seven Girls to Hospital," *Herald* (Everett, Wash.), March 12, 2005.

260   **teenagers trading . . . painkillers on a school bus:** Frank Wiget, "Teens Bring Pills to School," *Gary Post-Tribune*, March 17, 2005.

260   **assistant principal . . . stealing tablets of Adderall:** Ann Schimke, "Ex-principal Who Used Student's Drugs Is Charged," *The Ann Arbor News*, March 17, 2005.

261   **number of Americans . . . nearly doubled:** Press release, National Center on Addiction and Substance Abuse, "New CASA Report: Controlled Prescription Drug Abuse at Epidemic Level," July 7, 2005.

263   **seventy-five thousand American teenagers and young adults:** Kroutil et al., "Nonmedical Use of Prescription Stimulants in the United States," *Drug and Alcohol Dependence*, Sept. 15, 2006. Also see Shankar Vedantam, "Millions Have Misused ADHD Stimulant Drugs, Study Says," *The Washington Post*, Feb. 25, 2006.

263   **Dr. Arthur M. Sackler:** Barry Meier and Melody Petersen, "Sales of Painkiller Grew Rapidly, But Success Brought a High Cost," *The New York Times*, March 5, 2001.

263   **inducted into the . . . Medical Advertising Hall of Fame:** Sackler's biography is available at mahf.com.

264   **The main message of Purdue's campaign:** Federal investigators published a report on the marketing of OxyContin in 2003. See "Prescription Drugs: Oxy-Contin Abuse and Diversion and Efforts to Address the Problem," report to congressional requesters, U.S. General Accounting Office, Dec. 2003.

264   **for everything from back pain to arthritis:** Purdue's Internal Budget Plans for the marketing of OxyContin for 1996 to 2002.

264   **"myths and misconceptions":** Purdue's 2001 budget plan for marketing Oxy-Contin.

265   **"targets" were obstetricians:** Ibid.

265   **increase the use . . . by elderly:** Purdue's 2000 budget plan for marketing Oxy-Contin.

265   **in dozens of rural towns . . . middle and upper classes:** Dozens of news stories, beginning in 2000, documented the growing abuse of OxyContin and other prescription painkillers in towns in Kentucky, West Virginia, Virginia, Ohio, and Maine. For example, see Meier and Petersen, March 5, 2001. At the same time, researchers have noted that many abusers of prescription narcotics are white

and middle class. For example, see release from Wright State University School of Medicine, "Research Studies Document a New Path to Heroin Use," Feb. 26, 2003.

265 **the state's largest insurer noticed:** Press release from Wellmark, "Iowa Ranks Lower than the Nation in Use of Narcotic Rx Drugs but Narcotic Spending by Wellmark Members Jumps 350 Percent over Five Years," Sept. 1, 2004.

265 **Chelly Griffith:** Ms. Griffith's experience with OxyContin was included in a Citizen Petition of Jan. 23, 2004, that Richard Blumenthal, the attorney general of Connecticut, sent to the FDA. Also see Wendy Weiskircher, "Pain Pill Addict Hopes to Spare Others," *The Des Moines Register*, Nov. 10, 2002.

266 **Barry Miedema:** See "State Champion Basketball Coach Sentenced for Stealing Drugs," *Sioux City Journal*, Aug. 18, 2005. Also see Lynn Campbell, "Teacher Who Fought Addiction May Return," *The Des Moines Register*, March 4, 2006.

266 **Ryan Ray Wichhart:** See stories by Jeff Abell, "Wichhart Mental State Disputed," *The Hawk Eye*, May 4, 2006, and "Mertens' Death Was by Strangulation," *The Hawk Eye*, Dec. 7, 2005.

266 **Rush Limbaugh:** James Barron, "In Show, Limbaugh Tells of a Pill Habit; Plans to Enter Clinic," *The New York Times*, Oct. 11, 2003. Also see Jeff Leeds, "In Legal Deal, Limbaugh Surrenders in Drug Case," *The New York Times*, Apr. 29, 2006.

267 **"national epidemic" of deaths from accidental overdoses:** Paulozzi et al., "Increasing Deaths from Opioid Analgesics in the United States," *Pharmacoepidemiology and Drug Safety*, Sept. 2006.

267 **check for fifty thousand dollars:** Press release from Purdue, "$50,000 Purdue Pharma Prize for Pain Research Awarded to Professor Gerald Gebhart," Apr. 30, 2004.

267 **in Grand Cayman:** Agenda for Spring Pain Research Conference, Apr. 25 to 30, 2004.

268 **American Pain Society . . . had received:** These corporate donors and some of their grants are listed on the society's website (ampainsoc.org). Accessed July 2007. Also see report by the U.S. General Accounting Office, Dec. 2003.

268 **doctors should not hesitate:** For example, see "The Use of Opioids for the Treatment of Chronic Pain: A Consensus Statement from the American Academy of Pain Medicine and American Pain Society." Accessed at the society's website, May 2006. Dr. Gebhardt said in an interview in Oct. 2007 that academic scientists—not employees of Purdue—had selected him to receive the $50,000 award based on his past research efforts. He said he had never had a contract to work for Purdue. He said he believed that some of the ways that Purdue marketed OxyContin were "reprehensible." He added that the American

Pain Society was no different from dozens of other societies of physicians who readily accept money from pharmaceutical manufacturers.

268 **David Brennan:** Reported by academics at the Wharton School of the University of Pennsylvania, which organized the Feb. 2005 conference at which he spoke. See "The Price of Progress: Can Drug Companies Make Medicines More Affordable?," Knowledge@Wharton, a website maintained by the university. Published online Apr. 6, 2005. Accessed at knowledge.wharton.upenn.edu, Apr. 2006.

268 **median-priced home:** In Iowa the median-priced home in 2005 was $129,560, according to the Iowa Association of Realtors.

268 **a drug called Avastin:** These extraordinary prices have been widely reported by news media. See, for example, Alex Berenson, "A Cancer Drug Shows Promise, at a Price That Many Can't Pay," *The New York Times*, Feb. 15, 2006; Amy Dockser Marcus, "Price Becomes Factor in Cancer Treatment," *The Wall Street Journal*, Sept. 7, 2004; and Geeta Anand, "A Biotech Drug Extends a Life, but at What Price?," *The Wall Street Journal*, Nov. 16, 2005.

269 **"Our savings, everything":** Interview with Janice Clausen, July 3, 2007. The Clausens' story was first told in "Couple's Saga Makes Case for Health Reform," an editorial by *The Des Moines Register*, Jan. 28, 2007.

269 **"a pretty thin line":** Interview with Wendy Sontag, May 2006.

270 **Avastin . . . lived about four or five months longer:** Robert J. Mayer, "Two Steps Forward in the Treatment of Colorectal Cancer," *NEJM*, June 3, 2004.

270 **Tarceva . . . twelve days longer:** Denise Gellene, "FDA Weighs Days of Survival," *Los Angeles Times*, Nov. 2, 2005.

270 **Iressa . . . was doing nothing:** Theresa Agovino, "National Cancer Institute Halts Drug Trial," Associated Press, Apr. 19, 2005. Also see Raja Mishra, "Smart Drug for Lung Cancer May Be Pulled from Market," *The Boston Globe*, Apr. 5, 2005.

270 **"I can't accept that":** "Podcast: The Future of the Pharmaceutical Industry, According to Former Merck CEO Roy Vagelos," Apr. 17, 2006, Knowledge@Wharton. Accessed at knowledge.wharton.upenn.edu, 2007.

270 **several times that of inflation:** From 1994 to 2005 the prices of medicines purchased at drugstores increased an average of 8.3 percent every year, more than triple the average annual inflation rate of 2.5 percent. See "Prescription Drug Trends," Kaiser Family Foundation, June 2006.

271 **Iowans paid more for the medicines:** Iowans spent $1,955,852,687 on prescriptions picked up at retail pharmacies in 2004, according to statistics from the Kaiser Family Foundation that are available at statehealthfacts.org. I compared this amount with the annual sales by other types of businesses that

were reported to the state's Department of Revenue for the fiscal year ending March 31, 2005. See "Iowa Retail Sales & Use Tax Report."

271 **drugs were accounting for an ever-greater share:** Cynthia Smith, "Retail Prescription Drug Spending in the National Health Accounts," *Health Affairs*, Jan.–Feb. 2004.

271 **spent nearly $2 trillion:** Catlin, et al., "National Health Spending in 2005: The Slowdown Continues," *Health Affairs*, Jan.–Feb. 2007.

271 **General Motors:** Statistics included in Lee Hawkins, Jr., "As GM Battles Surging Costs Workers' Health Becomes Issue," *The Wall Street Journal*, Apr. 7, 2005.

272 **Real incomes for many . . . starting to decline:** Between 1999–2000 and 2003–2004, there was a 6 percent decline in the real median household income in Iowa from $45,774 to $43,004, according to an analysis of U.S. Census statistics. The early figure was adjusted for inflation so that both amounts are in 2004 dollars. See "The State of Working Iowa 2005," the Iowa Policy Project.

272 **$500-million-dollar-a-year drag:** Anne Kinzel, "What a Drag It Is . . . The Economic Impacts of Rising Health Insurance Premiums," Iowa State Department of Public Health, July 2004.

272 **Tyson Foods accepted a new contract:** Press release from Tyson Foods, "Tyson Cherokee Workers Ratify New Contract," Oct. 7, 2004.

272 **$11,500 for a family of four:** "Employer Health Benefits: 2006 Summary of Findings," Kaiser Family Foundation.

272 **many companies had stopped providing health:** In Iowa, 65.4 percent of Iowans had employment-based health coverage in 2003, down from 69.7 percent in 2000. Statistics are from an Aug. 2004 news release, "Health Care Coverage Falling Off for Iowans," from the Iowa Policy Project. The release cites Iowa data from the U.S. Census Bureau.

273 **Nearly 16 percent . . . without health insurance:** Numbers are from U.S. Census Bureau, "Table HI-4. Health Insurance Coverage Status and Type of Coverage by State."

273 **as many as eighteen thousand uninsured:** See "Insuring America's Health: Principles and Recommendations," by Committee on the Consequences of Uninsurance, Institute of Medicine, 2004.

273 **medical bills . . . send them into bankruptcy:** Himmelstein et al., "Market-Watch: Illness and Injury as Contributors to Bankruptcy," *Health Affairs*, Feb. 2, 2005.

273 **George Hatzigiannakis:** Interview with Hatzigiannakis, Sept. 2006. His story first appeared in *The Des Moines Register*, Apr. 3, 2005, in an editorial, "Let Anyone Buy Health Care."

274   **a savings account of $200,000:** News release from Fidelity Investments, "Fidelity Estimates $200,000 Now Needed to Cover Retiree Health Care Costs," March 6, 2006.

274   **biggest boom in hospital construction:** Dennis Cauchon and Julie Appleby, "Hospital Building Booms in 'Burbs," *USA Today*, Jan. 3, 2006.

274   **a few doctors made more than two million dollars:** Tony Leys, "$2 Million a Year Salaries for 2 Waterloo Doctors Under Fire," *The Des Moines Register*, May 26, 2005. According to the Census Bureau, the median household income in Iowa in 2005 was $43,609.

275   **Topamax . . . for *weight loss*:** These are actual cases discussed in *The DUR Digest*, the quarterly newsletter of the Iowa Medicaid Drug Utilization Review Commission, or described in the minutes of the commission's meetings. Both are available at iadur.org.

275   **A dozen or more drug salespeople:** For instance, according to the minutes of the Iowa Medicaid Drug Utilization Review Commission Meeting of Nov. 2, 2005, in attendance were twenty-three employees of various drug companies.

275   **states spent more to pay the medical bills:** In 2004 states spent 22.3 percent of their budgets on Medicaid, while they spent 21.4 percent on elementary and secondary education. See "2004 State Expenditure Report," National Association of State Budget Officers.

276   **health care consumed about a *third*:** See testimony by Virginia governor Mark Warner and Arkansas governor Mike Huckabee on Medicaid reform before the Senate Finance Committee, June 15, 2005.

276   **raise taxes and cut services:** See, for example, Sarah Lueck, "Surging Costs for Medicaid Ravage State, Federal Budgets," *The Wall Street Journal*, Feb. 7, 2005.

276   **Medicaid had surged:** See "Medicaid Update," by Iowa Legislative Services Agency, Dec. 19, 2003.

276   **officials took hundreds of millions:** See "Medicaid Funding Growth: FY 2005 Through FY 2007," by Iowa Legislative Services Agency, Nov. 17, 2004.

276   **Iowa's three public universities:** See "Iowa's State Fiscal Crisis and Its Impact on Education," by Iowa Fiscal Partnership, Nov. 2004.

276   **"used to pride itself":** "Work to Ease Student Debt," an editorial in *The Des Moines Register*, Apr. 10, 2006.

277   **5 percent of the federal budget:** Jon Resnick, "The Long and Winding Road Ahead: Medicare Part D, Post 2006," an article published by Cambridge Pharma Consultancy, a unit of IMS.

277   **more than 45 percent of the nation's health care:** Catlin et al., "National Health Spending in 2005: The Slowdown Continues," *Health Affairs*, Jan.–Feb. 2007.

277 **America is expected to spend 20 percent of all it produces on health care:** Borger et al., "Health Spending Projections Through 2015: Changes on the Horizon," *Health Affairs*, 2006.

277 **"empty place in my heart":** Interview by Dave Franzman for KCRG-TV 9 on Dec. 8, 2003.

277 **four Iowa children had died:** See Tony Leys, "Flu Struck Early, Then Fizzled," *The Des Moines Register*, March 2, 2004.

278 **Dr. Charles Grose wrote:** "Influenza and Failure of Rocephin Therapy," an article in the newsletter of the Iowa chapter of the American Academy of Pediatrics, Winter 2003–2004.

278 **75 percent had been given an antibiotic:** See Hong et al., "Association of Amoxicillin Use During Early Childhood with Developmental Tooth Enamel Defects," *Archives of Pediatric and Adolescent Medicine*, Oct. 2005.

278 **taking antibiotics increases a person's risk:** For example, see Gonzales et al., "Principles of Appropriate Antibiotic Use for Treatment of Acute Respiratory Tract Infections in Adults," *Annals of Internal Medicine*, March 20, 2001.

279 **A study in Atlanta:** Hofmann et al., "The Prevalence of Drug-Resistant Streptococcus pneumoniae in Atlanta," *NEJM*, Aug. 24, 1995.

279 **patients taking . . . broad-spectrum:** G. G. Rao, "Risk Factors for the Spread of Antibiotic-Resistant Bacteria," *Drugs*, March 1998. Also see Malhotra-Kumar et al., "Effect of azithromycin and clarithromycin therapy on pharyngeal carriage of macrolide-resistant streptococci in healthy volunteers, *The Lancet*, Feb. 10, 2007.

279 **Dr. Richard Besser:** Quoted in Eliza Bussey, "CDC Warns About Overuse of Antibiotics," Reuters, May 9, 2000.

279 **THREATENS TO REVERSE MEDICAL PROGRESS:** From press release issued by the World Health Organization, June 12, 2000.

280 **marketers at Pfizer had outdone:** Melody Petersen, "What's Black and White and Sells Medicine?," *The New York Times*, Aug. 27, 2000.

280 **advertisements . . . *Sesame Street*:** Described in Brooke Shelby Biggs, "Sesame Street Meets Madison Avenue," *Mother Jones*, March 30, 2001.

281 **Sesame Street Sweepstakes:** Described in "Sweepstakes Mixes Education and Fun on Way to Sesame Street," an article from the archive at napsnet.com. Accessed March 2006.

281 **"We used something kids love":** Interview with Pat Kelly, Aug. 2000.

281 **most ear infections go away without drugs:** "Questions and Answers on Acute Otitis Media," American Academy of Pediatrics and American Academy of Family Physicians, available at aap.org. Accessed Sept. 2006.

281 **federal government warned physicians:** Dowell et al., "Acute Otitis Media:
     Management and Surveillance in an Era of Pneumococcal Resistance," *Pediatric
     Infectious Disease Journal*, Jan. 1999.

281 **soared by 35 percent in Iowa:** "The Wellmark Report: An Analysis of Prescrip-
     tion Drug Use in Iowa and South Dakota (Sixth in a Special Series)," no date.
     Accessed at Wellmark.com, March 2006.

282 **"prescribed like water":** As quoted in press release from Wellmark, "Broad-
     Spectrum Antibiotic Use Exceeds National Rate for Iowa Youth," Sept. 3, 2003.

282 **private school in Pittsburgh:** Martin et al., "Erythromycin-Resistant Group A
     Streptococci in Schoolchildren in Pittsburgh," *NEJM*, Apr. 18, 2002.

282 **Iowa government officials weren't trying to track:** Interview with Dr. Patricia
     Quinlisk, Iowa Department of Public Health, Aug. 2005.

283 **estimate that ninety thousand Americans:** "The Problem of Antimicrobial Re-
     sistance," National Institute of Allergy and Infectious Diseases, Apr. 2006, avail-
     able at niaid.nih.gov.

283 **children from Minnesota and North Dakota:** "Four Pediatric Deaths from
     Community-Acquired Methicillin-Resistant *Staphylococcus aureus*—Minnesota
     and North Dakota 1997–1999," Morbidity and Mortality Weekly Report,
     Aug. 20, 1999.

284 **high school wrestlers:** From an update in Dec. 2001 from the Center for Acute
     Disease Epidemiology, Iowa Department of Public Health.

284 **St. Louis Rams:** Kazakova et al., "A Clone of Methicillin-Resistant *Staphylo-
     coccus aureus* Among Professional Football Players," *NEJM*, Feb. 3, 2005.

284 **flesh-eating bacteria:** Miller et al., "Necrotizing Fasciitis Caused by Community-
     Associated Methicillin-Resistant *Staphylococcus aureus* in Los Angeles," *NEJM*,
     Apr. 7, 2005.

284 **two million Americans have MRSA:** Kuehnert et al., "Prevalence of *Staphylo-
     coccus aureus* Nasal Colonization in the United States, 2001–2002," *Journal of
     Infectious Diseases*, Jan. 15, 2006.

284 **This particular strain:** Robinson et al., "Re-emergence of Early Pandemic
     Staphylococcus aureus as a Community-Acquired Methicillin-Resistant Clone,"
     The Lancet, Apr. 2, 2005. Also see Clara Penn, "Pandemic Bug Returns as Com-
     munity MRSA Strain," *New Scientist*, Apr. 1, 2005.

285 **Centers for Disease Control warned:** "CDC to Monitor Children's Flu Com-
     plications," Associated Press, Dec. 9, 2003. Also see Centers for Disease Con-
     trol and Prevention, "Update: Influenza-Associated Deaths Reported Among
     Children Aged <18 Years—United States, 2003–04 Influenza Season," *Morbidity
     and Mortality Weekly Report*, Dec. 19, 2003.

285 **Specialist Dustin Colby:** Elizabeth Owens, "Guard Accident Probe Continues," *The Des Moines Register*, Aug. 29, 2004; "Pain-killers Implicated in Soldier's Fatal Crash," Associated Press, Nov. 13, 2004; "Officials: Prescription Drugs Could Be Factor in Deaths of Soldier, Sergeant, Mother Defends Son's Memory," KCCI Channel 8, Nov. 12, 2004; Bert Dalmer, "Official Doubts Pain Pills Caused Guard Accident," *The Des Moines Register*, Nov. 20, 2004; William Petroski, "Guard: Drugs Slowed Soldier's Reaction Time," *The Des Moines Register*, Feb. 5, 2005. Also see press release from the Iowa National Guard, Feb. 4, 2005.

286 **one simulated driving test:** Linnoila et al., "Effects of Diazepam and Codeine, Alone and in Combination with Alcohol, on Simulated Driving," *Clinical Pharmacology and Therapeutics*, 1973. This study is cited in Ray et al., "Medications and the Older Driver," *Clinics in Geriatric Medicine*, May 1993.

286 **The government does not know:** See letter by Jim Hall, the chairman of the National Transportation Safety Board, to Rodney E. Slater, U.S. Secretary of Transportation, Jan. 13, 2000.

287 **sixteen thousand motor vehicle accidents:** Ray et al., "Psychoactive Drugs and the Risk of Injurious Motor Vehicle Crashes in Elderly Drivers, *American Journal of Epidemiology*, Oct. 1, 1992.

287 **Some medications are worse than alcohol:** For one example, see Weiler et al., "Effects of Fexofenadine, Diphenhydramine and Alcohol on Driving Performance," *Annals of Internal Medicine*, March 7, 2000.

287 **A group of physicians in New York:** Frucht et al., "Falling Asleep at the Wheel: Motor Vehicle Mishaps in Persons Taking Pramipexole and Ropinirole," *Neurology*, June 1999. Also see "Parkinson's Patients Face Sleep Danger," BBC News, June 10, 1999.

287 **same drugs in 2005:** Avorn et al., "Sudden Uncontrollable Somnolence and Medication Use in Parkinson's Disease," *Archives of Neurology*, Aug. 2005.

288 **people taking Ambien:** Described in slide presentations given by toxicologists at the Wisconsin State Lab of Hygiene. See "Zolpidem Impaired Drivers in Wisconsin: A Six Year Retrospective," a presentation by William R. Johnson at the Society of Forensic Toxicologists, Oct. 2005, and "Ambien: Drives Like a Dream?" by Laura J. Liddicoat and Patrick Harding at the American Academy of Forensic Sciences meeting, Feb. 23, 2006.

288 **Nicholas Little:** Facts described in decision by Court of Appeals of Iowa in *State of Iowa v. Nicholas Little*, Dec. 21, 2005. Mr. Little appealed his conviction of operating while intoxicated. He argued that he should not be charged because he had a prescription for the drugs. He also argued that the medications had rendered him "unconscious" and that he had not intended to operate a motor vehicle. The court denied his request.

290 **"keeps getting higher"**: Interview with Laura Liddicoat, June 2, 2006. Figures for Klonopin cases (136 in 2005) and Valium cases (182 in 2005) are from Liddicoat's presentation, "Ambien: Drives Like a Dream?"

290 **West Virginia**: "Alcohol and Other Drug Use Among Victims of Motor-Vehicle Crashes—West Virginia, 2004–2005," *Morbidity and Mortality Weekly Report,* Dec. 8, 2006.

290 **study of crashes involving . . . trucks**: "Report to Congress on the Large Truck Crash Causation Study," U.S. Department of Transportation, Federal Motor Carrier Safety Administration, March 2006.

291 **"just waking up"**: Interview with Scott Falb, May 24, 2006.

291 **Greyhound bus**: "Highway Accident Report: Greyhound Motorcoach Run-off-the-Road Accident, Burnt Cabins, Pennsylvania, June 20, 1998," National Transportation Safety Board.

291 **killed a thirteen-year-old boy**: Larry King, "Woman Gets Jail for Fatal Accident," *The Philadelphia Inquirer*, Sept. 14, 2004.

291 **Mack semitruck**: "Highway Accident Brief: Single Vehicle Run-off-the-Road and Vault, Pine Bluff, Arkansas, Oct. 13, 1997," National Transportation Safety Board.

291 **The pilot of the ferry**: Anthony M. Destefano, "Pilot Admits He Caused Crash," *Newsday*, Aug. 5, 2004.

292 **"no better than a drunk driver"**: Quoted in William K. Rashbaum and Sewell Chan, "Pilot and Supervisor Sentenced in '03 Staten Island Ferry Crash," *The New York Times*, Jan. 10, 2006.

292 **Some states, like Iowa**: See Iowa Code Section 321J.2, "Operating While Under the Influence of Alcohol or a Drug." Accessed May 2006.

293 **"It's not fair"**: Marsha Dorgan, "Driver Not Guilty of Murder in DUI Crash," *The Napa Valley Register*, Feb. 1, 2006.

293 **Linda Grassi**: Marsha Dorgan, "Manslaughter Conviction Brings 6-month Sentence," *Napa Valley Register*, July 4, 2007.

293 **"not coming off that bus"**: Interview with Betty Pollema, May 2006.

NINE: Deadly Doses

294 **"Well, maybe this will help"**: Interviews with Jerry Houk in Jan. and Feb. 2006.

295 **"billion-dollar blockbuster"**: David Willman, "Rezulin: Fast-Track Approval and Slow Withdrawal," *Los Angeles Times*, Dec. 20, 2000.

295 **Few illnesses are as dramatic**: See William M. Lee, "Acute Liver Failure," *NEJM*, Dec. 16, 1993.

296 **51 percent of the cases of liver failure:** William M. Lee, "Drug-Induced Acute Liver Failure in the United States 2005: Results from the U.S. Acute Liver Failure Study Group," presentation at FDA meeting on Jan. 28, 2005. Available at fda.gov/cder/livertox/presentations2005/William_Lee.ppt. Accessed July 2007.

296 **a letter from Duane Reade:** Letter on Duane Reade letterhead, dated Sept. 5, 2002.

297 **free samples . . . of the antidepressant:** See two articles in *The New York Times* by Adam Liptak, "Free Prozac in the Junk Mail Draws a Lawsuit," July 6, 2002, and "Prozac Mailed Unsolicited to a Teenager in Florida," July 21, 2002.

298 **"My sense is":** Interview with Dr. Mark Graber, Feb. 10, 2006.

299 **as many as 28 percent of all emergency visits:** Tafreshi et al., "Medication-Related Visits to the Emergency Department: A Prospective Study," *Annals of Pharmacotherapy*, Dec. 1999.

299 **Roughly half of Americans ages sixty-five and older:** Kaufman et al., "Recent Patterns of Medication Use in the Ambulatory Adult Population of the United States," *JAMA*, Jan. 16, 2002.

299 **"layer upon layer":** Slide presentation by Jerry Gurwitz, "Optimal Drug Therapy for the Elderly," available at umassmed.edu and accessed June 2006.

299 **seniors more susceptible to the drugs' adverse effects:** Good summary of this problem is included in "Prescription Drugs and the Elderly: Many Still Receive Potentially Harmful Drugs Despite Recent Improvements," U.S. General Accounting Office, July 24, 1995.

300 **"Pretty soon":** Interview with Gloria Fisher, Jan. 25, 2006.

300 **list of dozens of drugs:** Fick et al., "Updating the Beers Criteria for Potentially Inappropriate Medication Use in Older Adults," *Archives of Internal Medicine*, Dec. 8, 2003. A list of these drugs is available at dcri.duke.edu/ccge/curtis/beers.html. Accessed July 2007.

300 **"If you have no idea":** Mark Beers quoted in Joanne Kaldy, "The Evolution of Criteria for Inappropriate Drugs," *Caring for the Ages*, Aug. 2004.

300 **13 percent . . . dangerously inappropriate:** Kelly et al., "Appropriateness of Medication Use in Iowa Medicaid Recipients Residing in Long-Term Care Facilities," *Consultant Pharmacist*, 2000.

300 **almost 18 percent . . . taking medicines that are not safe:** "Prescription Drugs and the Elderly: Many Still Receive Potentially Harmful Drugs Despite Recent Improvements," U.S. General Accounting Office, July 24, 1995.

300 **thirty-two thousand . . . break a hip:** See "Prescription Drugs and the Elderly" by GAO, as well as Ray et al., "Psychotropic Drug Use and the Risk of Hip Fracture," *NEJM*, Feb. 12, 1987.

300 **About 20 percent . . . die:** J. W. Cooper, "Reducing Falls Among Patients in Nursing Homes," *JAMA,* Dec. 3, 1997.

300 **problem appears to be escalating:** "Fatalities and Injuries from Falls Among Older Adults—United States, 1993–2003 and 2001–2005," *Morbidity and Mortality Weekly Report,* Nov. 17, 2006. The increasing deaths correspond with a rise in the number of prescriptions taken by older Americans. One study estimated that the number of prescriptions for each American age sixty-five or older increased from 19.6 in 1992 to 28.5 in 2000 See "Cost Overdose: Growth in Drug Spending for the Elderly, 1992–2010," Families USA, July 2000.

301 **global market for osteoporosis:** See Adis International Limited, "Battling Bone Disease: New Drugs Strengthen the Osteoporosis Market," *Pharmaceutical & Diagnostic Innovation,* Nov. 2004.

301 **Iowa women . . . taking high doses of the sleeping pills:** Gray et al., "Benzodiazepine Use and Physical Performance in Community-Dwelling Older Women," *Journal of the American Geriatric Society,* Nov. 2003.

302 **more than 10 percent . . . had dementia caused by drugs:** J. M. Starr and L. J. Whalley, "Drug-Induced Dementia: Incidence, Management and Prevention," *Drug Safety,* Nov. 1994.

302 **as many as 30 percent . . . from their medications:** Lee et al., "Cardiac 123I-MIBG Scintigraphy in Patients with Drug-Induced Parkinsonism," *Journal of Neurology, Neurosurgery, and Psychiatry,* published online, Aug. 15, 2005.

302 **some doctors in New Jersey:** Avorn et al., "Increased Incidence of Levodopa Therapy Following Metoclopramide Use," *JAMA,* Dec. 13, 1995. Also see Paula A. Rochon and Jerry H. Gurwitz, "Optimising Drug Treatment for Elderly People: The Prescribing Cascade," *BMJ,* Oct. 25, 1997.

302 **Dr. Ryan Carnahan:** Carnahan et al., "The Concurrent Use of Anticholinergics and Cholinesterase Inhibitors: Rare Event or Common Practice?," *The Journal of the American Geriatric Society,* Dec. 2004.

303 **medicines had caused the dementia:** Interview with Dr. Ryan Carnahan, Feb. 2006.

303 **the state's nosologist:** Interview with Jerry McDowell, Jan. 11, 2006.

304 **106,000 Americans had died in 1994:** Lazarou et al., "Incidence of Adverse Drug Reactions in Hospitalized Patients," *JAMA,* Apr. 15, 1998.

304 **five Iowans in 2002 . . . United States in 2002:** Statistics are from the Centers for Disease Control, "Worktable III. Deaths from 358 Selected Causes, by 5-Year Age Groups, Race, and Sex: United States, 2002." Accessed Jan. 2006 at cdc.gov. Robert Anderson at the CDC said in an interview in Oct. 2007 that there were more deaths caused by the adverse effects of medicines that the government had coded in the final statistics to the disease the person was said to be suffering from. He said complications caused by medications were said to be a

factor in 5,494 deaths in 2002, according to the government's analysis of death certificates. This is still only a fraction of the 106,000 Americans estimated to die from the adverse effects of medications each year. Some other deaths caused by prescription drugs are coded on death certificates as "accidental poisoning" by drugs. There were 58 of these deaths in Iowa and 16,394 in the United States in 2002. These deaths are from both prescription drugs and illegal drugs like cocaine and heroin. In 2007, federal researchers reported that these deaths increased by more than 68 percent between 1999 and 2004. They said that most of the increase came from deaths caused by prescription drugs rather than those from heroin or other illegal drugs. See "Unintentional Poisoning Deaths— United States, 1999–2004," *Morbidity and Mortality Weekly Report*, Feb. 9, 2007. Many of these deaths are accidental overdoses. For example, a patient becomes addicted to prescription painkillers and takes too much. Another example is the death of Anna Nicole Smith in Feb. 2007. The medical examiner ruled the former *Playboy* model died of an accidental overdose of a sleeping medication and at least eight other prescription drugs. Such deaths were not included in the 1994 study that estimated that 106,000 Americans died from the adverse effects of drugs taken as prescribed.

305 **"You can see a gunshot wound":** Interview with John Kraemer, Aug. 18, 2005.

306 **articles that instructed physicians:** For example, guidelines published by the National Association of Medical Examiners say that death from "reasonably foreseeable complications of an accepted therapy" should be classified as "natural" deaths. Only when the death is caused by a treatment that is not "reasonable"— for example, if a doctor overdoses a surgery patient with anesthetic—should the death be deemed an "accident." See "A Guide for Manner of Death Classification," National Association of Medical Examiners, Feb. 2002.

306 **"procedure is not the cause of death":** Magrane et al., "Certification of Death by Family Physicians," *American Family Physician*, Oct. 1, 1997.

306 **study by pathologists in Vermont:** Pritt et al., "Death Certificate Errors at an Academic Institution," *Archives of Pathology and Laboratory Medicine*, Nov. 2005.

307 **"If the drugs are at the therapeutic level":** Interview with Dr. Dennis Klein, Aug. 18, 2005.

307 **"They kept calling me":** Interview with Dr. Ljubisa Dragovic, June 17, 2004.

308 **FDA required the manufacturers to warn:** "FDA Directs ADHD Drug Manufacturers to Notify Patients About Cardiovascular Adverse Events and Psychiatric Adverse Events," press release, Feb. 21, 2007.

308 **autopsy rate . . . has plummeted:** See Hoyert et al., "Autopsy Patterns in 2003," Vital and Health Statistics, National Center for Health Statistics, March 2007. Also see Cheryl M. Reichert and Virginia L. Kelly, "Prognosis for the Autopsy," *Health Affairs*, Summer 1985.

309 **40 percent difference . . . cause of death:** George D. Lundberg, *Severed Trust* (New York: Basic Books, 2000), p. 253.

309 **"Medical interventions":** Ibid., p. 8.

309 **"They didn't want the pathologist":** Ibid., p. 252.

309 **Researchers in Norway:** Ebbesen et al., "Drug-Related Deaths in a Department of Internal Medicine," *Archives of Internal Medicine*, Oct. 22, 2001.

310 **In Iowa, doctors and hospitals:** Interview with Kent Nebel, the legal affairs director for the Iowa Board of Medical Examiners, Sept. 15, 2006. Doctors in Iowa must report malpractice settlements to the board, but the public has no access to the information. Also see "Let Patients Know Results," an editorial in *The Des Moines Register*, Sept. 14, 2004, and Tony Leys, "Patients in the Dark on Doctors' Records," *The Des Moines Register*, Dec. 3, 2003.

310 **Many hospitals have avoided:** Joseph T. Hallinan, "Doctor Is Out: Attempt to Track Malpractice Cases Is Often Thwarted," *The Wall Street Journal*, Aug. 27, 2004.

310 **Regulators . . . may get reports of as few as 1 percent:** David A. Kessler, "Introducing MedWatch: A New Approach to Reporting Medication and Device Adverse Effects and Product Problems," *JAMA*, June 2, 1993.

311 **"There's just so much":** Interview with Rosemary Rahm, Dec. 29, 2005.

313 **she discovered a study:** Bombardier et al., "Comparison of Upper Gastrointestinal Toxicity of Rofecoxib and Naproxen in Patients with Rheumatoid Arthritis," *NEJM*, Nov. 23, 2000. Also see a discussion of this study in chapter 5.

314 **Merck pulled Vioxx from pharmacy shelves:** "Merck Announces Voluntary Worldwide Withdrawal of Vioxx," press release sent by Merck, Sept. 30, 2004.

315 **scientist at the FDA testified:** Written testimony of David J. Graham before the Senate Finance Committee, Nov. 18, 2004. Accessed at senate.gov, Feb. 2006.

Epilogue

316 **spend more on medical care than . . . anything else:** See data from U.S. Bureau of Economic Analysis, "Table 2.3.5 Personal Consumption Expenditures by Major Type of Product." According to those figures for 2006, about 17 percent of all goods and services purchased by persons went to medical care. The next highest personal expense was housing, which accounted for 15 percent of personal spending. Personal consumption expenditures, as calculated by the government, are a measure of goods and services purchased by individuals.

316 **not the case in 1980:** See trends in medical and other consumer spending in Reinhardt et al., "U.S. Health Care Spending in an International Context," *Health Affairs*, May–June 2004.

316 **Taxpayers covered nearly half the country's health care:** According to federal statistics, the government paid more than 45 percent of the nation's medical expenses in 2005. See Catlin et al., Jan.–Feb. 2007.

316 **$6,700 for each person:** Catlin et al., "National Health Spending in 2005: The Slowdown Continues," *Health Affairs*, Jan.–Feb. 2007.

316 **By 2015:** Medical costs are expected to make up 20 percent of GDP by 2015 or one dollar of every five dollars that America produces. See Borger et al., "Health Spending Projections Through 2015: Changes on the Horizon," *Health Affairs*, March/Apr. 2006. Medical costs are now double the burden they were in 1980, when they consumed forty-five cents of every five dollars or 9.1 percent of GDP. See Centers of Medicare and Medicaid Services, Office of the Actuary, National Health Statistics.

317 **"good news":** News release from the Pharmaceutical Research and Manufacturers of America, May 23, 2001.

317 **"The current dilemma":** Copy of speech by David Brennan entitled "Revolutionary Discoveries and the State of Healthcare," given at the Detroit Economic Club, March 22, 2004. Accessed at astrazeneca.com, 2006.

317 **medicines were often introduced in other nations:** Discussed in "Testimony on Prescription Drug User Fee Act of 1992 (PDUFA)," by Michael A. Friedman, the lead deputy commissioner of the FDA, before the House Committee on Commerce, Subcommittee on Health and the Environment, Apr. 23, 1997.

317 **research . . . done by academic or government scientists:** In 1980, 32 percent of biomedical research was paid for by the industry. By 2000 the industry's share had grown to 62 percent of total research spending. Bekelman et al., "Scope and Impact of Financial Conflicts of Interest in Biomedical Research," *JAMA*, Jan. 22, 2003.

317 **Between 1980 and 2003:** Source is "Table 2.4.5U Personal Consumption Expenditures by Type of Product," Bureau of Economic Analysis.

318 **written by academics who work as consultants:** For example, the industry often points to studies done by Frank R. Lichtenberg, a professor at the Columbia University Graduate School of Business. Dr. Lichtenberg is a consultant to, or has received grants from, Pfizer, Merck, and other pharmaceutical companies as well as from the American Enterprise Institute.

318 **an expense that may exceed:** See discussion of study by Ernst & Grizzle in the notes to the Introduction.

318 **a list of the longevity:** From OECD Health Data, Oct. 2006. Available at oecd.org.

319 **"Pace yourself":** Quote is from "Heartburn-Friendly Fair Food," available at prilosecotccountry.com. Accessed Aug. 2006.

319   **Obesity can take more than a decade:** Olshansky et al., "A Potential Decline in Life Expectancy in the United States in the 21st Century," *NEJM*, March 17, 2005.

319   **More than 40 percent of American women:** Prescription data for the estrogen drugs is from Hersh et al., "National Use of Postmenopausal Hormone Therapy," *JAMA*, Jan. 7, 2004.

320   **breast cancer had suddenly plummeted in 2003:** The statistics were announced at the San Antonio Breast Cancer Symposium in Dec. 2006 and widely reported in the media. For example, see Gina Kolata, "Breast Cancer Rate Falls in U.S., Study Shows," *The New York Times*, Dec. 14, 2006. Also see Ravdin et al., "The Decrease in Breast-Cancer Incidence in 2003 in the United States," *NEJM*, Apr. 19, 2007.

320   **"has obviously broken down":** Presentation by Dr. Janet Woodcock at the Committee on the Assessment of the U.S. Drug Safety System, the National Academies' Institute of Medicine, June 8, 2005.

320   **More Americans now abuse prescription drugs than they do cocaine:** "Abuse of Prescription Drugs to Surpass Illicit Drug Abuse, says INCB," Press Release No. 4, International Narcotics Control Board, March 1, 2006.

321   **"We call it a sales force":** Interview with Hank McKinnell, Aug. 2000.

321   **drugs for anemia . . . increase the risk of death:** "FDA Public Health Advisory: Erythropoiesis-Stimulating Agents," March 9, 2007.

322   **one of every four people diagnosed with depression:** Wakefield et al., "Extending the Bereavement Exclusion for Major Depression to Other Losses," *Archives of General Psychiatry*, Apr. 2007.

322   **scores of these cases *every day*:** In chapter 9, I cited the 1998 study that estimated that 106,000 Americans died in 1994 from adverse effects of their medications. Yet fewer than 300 deaths were officially attributed to adverse drug reactions in 2002 in the CDC's final mortality statistics. See further discussion in notes to chapter 9.

322   **case of Karen Garcia:** Interviews with Evan Bridwell, program director at KUZZ, May 4, 2007; and with Commander Christopher Speer of the Kern County Sheriff's Coroner Division, Oct. 17, 2007. Also see news release from Kern County Sheriff's Department, Nov. 15, 2006.

324   **Hospitals were once required to do autopsies on at least 20 percent:** Cheryl M. Reichert and Virginia L. Kelly, "Prognosis for the Autopsy," *Health Affairs*, Summer 1985.

324   **"therapeutic complication":** Interview with Dr. James Gill of the New York City Office of the Chief Medical Examiner, Oct. 19, 2007. Also see Gill et al., "Use of 'Therapeutic Complication' as a Manner of Death," *Journal of Forensic Sciences*, Sept. 2006.

325 **companies have failed to submit the reports to the government:** In 2002 the consumer group Public Citizen called for a criminal investigation of Abbott Laboratories after FDA inspectors found the company did not report a death suspected to have been caused by the diet drug Meridia. The inspectors also found Abbott's reports to the government about seven other deaths related to Meridia were either wrong or not supported by source documents the company had collected on the deaths. See FDA inspection report, dated Apr. 3, 2002, and sent to John D. Wolfinger at Abbott.

325 **nearly 95 percent of American physicians:** Campbell et al., "A National Survey of Physician-Industry Relationships," *NEJM*, Apr. 26, 2007.

327 **"You can design":** Interview with David Franklin, March 11, 2003.

327 **what some doctors now call propaganda:** For example, see Giovanni A. Fava, "Financial Conflicts of Interest in Psychiatry," *World Psychiatry*, Feb. 2007.

327 **called for the government to create a national scientific agency:** For example, see Uwe E. Reinhardt, "An Information Infrastructure for the Pharmaceutical Market," *Health Affairs*, Jan.–Feb. 2004.

328 **If you knew a drug worked for only 40 percent:** This is from scientific studies of Zelnorm, a drug for irritable bowel syndrome, which was aggressively promoted by Novartis to women until the FDA demanded its use be sharply restricted in 2007. Studies are described in the label for Zelnorm, dated July 22, 2002.

328 **doctors often don't tell people about the dangers:** In 2004 only 26 percent of patients said they had been told about a drug's risks and given directions on how to use it by their physician, according to an FDA survey. See fda.gov/cder/Offices/ODS/y2ktitle.htm.

330 **"In analysis after analysis":** Interview with Michael Elashoff, May 2004. Also see David Willman, "How a New Policy Led to Seven Deadly Drugs," one of a series of stories that appeared in the *Los Angeles Times* in 2000. The news stories detailed the pharmaceutical industry's influence inside the FDA and later won a Pulitzer Prize.

330 **"completely at odds with the will of Congress":** Letter from Dr. James B. D. Palmer, senior vice president at Glaxo Wellcome, to Heidi M. Jolson, director of the FDA's division of antiviral drug products, March 2, 1999.

331 **case was not an isolated one:** For another example, see a former FDA physician's description of how the agency ignored questions about the safety of an antibiotic called Ketek. David B. Ross, "The FDA and the Case of Ketek," *NEJM*, Apr. 19, 2007.

331 **more than a dozen drugs approved since 1992:**Here is a list of these drugs compiled from the FDA's website: Baycol, Raplon, Lotronex, Propulsid, Rezulin, Raxar, Posicor, Duract, Redux, Bextra, Vioxx, Zelnorm, Serzone, and Trovan.

333   **15 percent of American deaths are caused by inactivity or a poor diet:** Mokdad et al., "Correction: Actual Causes of Death in the United States, 2000," *JAMA*, Jan. 19, 2005.

333   **doctors do little to encourage:** For older adults, see "Prevalence of Health-Care Providers Asking Older Adults About Their Physical Activity Levels—United States, 1998," *Morbidity and Mortality Weekly Report*, May 17, 2002. For children, see "Selected Findings on Child and Adolescent Health Care from the 2004 National Healthcare Quality/Disparities Reports," Agency for Healthcare Research and Quality, March 2005.

333   **people living in the worst smog:** For example, see Bell et al., "Ozone and Short-term Mortality in 95 U.S. Urban Communities, 1987–2000," *JAMA*, Nov. 17, 2004.

334   **banned in other countries:** See, for example, Marla Cone, "U.S. Rules Allow the Sale of Products Others Ban," *Los Angeles Times*, Oct. 8, 2006.

334   **growing number of doctors have refused:** For example, Dr. Bob Goodman, an internist in Manhattan, has created a group called No Free Lunch, which encourages physicians to stop accepting gifts from the drug industry. See nofreelunch.org.

334   **Don't take any drug before you know all the risks:** A good source of independent information on prescription drugs is Public Citizen, the consumer group. See "Ten Rules for Safer Drug Use" at the group's website (worstpills.org). Accessed March 2007.

BIBLIOGRAPHY

Angell, Marcia. *The Truth About the Drug Companies*. New York: Random House, 2004.

Berger, John. *Ways of Seeing*. London: British Broadcasting Corporation, 1972.

Beveridge, W.I.B. *The Art of Scientific Investigation*. New York: Vintage Books, 1950.

Diller, Lawrence H. *Running on Ritalin*. New York: Bantam Books, 1998.

Golub, Edward S. *The Limits of Medicine: How Science Shapes Our Hope for the Cure*. Chicago: University of Chicago Press, 1997.

Goozner, Merrill. *The $800 Million Pill*. Berkeley: University of California Press, 2004.

Harris, Richard. *The Real Voice*. New York: Macmillan, 1964.

Healy, David. *The Antidepressant Era*. Cambridge, Mass.: Harvard University Press, 1998.

———. *The Creation of Psychopharmacology*. Cambridge, Mass.: Harvard University Press, 2002.

———. *Let Them Eat Prozac*. Toronto: James Lorimer & Co., 2003.

———. *The Psychopharmacologists III*. London: Hodder Arnold, 2000.

Hilts, Philip J. *Protecting America's Health: The FDA, Business, and One Hundred Years of Regulation*. New York: Knopf, 2003.

Huxley, Aldous. *Brave New World*. New York: Harper & Brothers, 1932.

Karch, Steven B. *A Brief History of Cocaine*. Boca Raton, Fla.: Taylor & Francis, 2006.

Krimsky, Sheldon. *Science in the Private Interest*. Lanham, Md.: Rowman & Littlefield, 2003.

Kutchins, Herb, and Stuart Kirk. *Making Us Crazy*. New York: Free Press, 1997.

Leach, William. *Land of Desire: Merchants, Power, and the Rise of a New American Culture*. New York: Pantheon, 1993.

Le Fanu, James. *The Rise and Fall of Modern Medicine*. New York: Carroll & Graf, 1999.

Lewis, Sinclair. *Arrowsmith*. New York: Harcourt Brace, 1925.

Liebenau, J., G. Higby, and E. Stroud, eds. *Pill Peddlers: Essays on the History of the Pharmaceutical Industry*. Madison, Wis.: American Institute of the History of Pharmacy, 1990.

Lundberg, George D. *Severed Trust*. New York: Basic Books, 2000.

Mahoney, Tom. *The Merchants of Life*. New York: Harper Brothers, 1959.

McNeal, James U. *The Kids Market: Myths and Realities*. Ithaca, N.Y.: Paramount Market Publishing, 1999.

Meier, Barry. *Pain Killer: A "Wonder" Drug's Trail of Addiction and Death*. New York: Rodale, 2003.

Meier, Paul D., ed. *Blue Genes*. Carol Stream, Ill.: Tyndale, 2005.

Merton, Robert K. *Social Theory and Social Structure*. New York: Free Press, 1968.

Mines, Samuel. *Pfizer: An Informal History*. New York: Pfizer, 1978.

Mintz, Morton. *By Prescription Only*. Boston: Houghton Mifflin, 1967.

——— and Jerry S. Cohen. *Power, Inc.* New York: Viking, 1976.

Moore, Thomas J. *Deadly Medicine*. New York: Simon & Schuster, 1995.

———. *Prescription for Disaster: The Hidden Dangers in Your Medicine Cabinet*. New York: Simon & Schuster, 1998.

Nelson, Gary L., ed. *Pharmaceutical Company Histories*, vol. 1. Bismarck, N.D.: Woodbine Publishing, 1985.

Payer, Lynn. *Disease-Mongers: How Doctors, Drug Companies, and Insurers Are Making You Feel Sick*. New York: John Wiley & Sons, 1992.

Rampton, Sheldon, and John Stauber. *Trust Us, We're Experts*. New York: Tarcher Putnam, 2001.

Ries, Al, and Laura Ries. *The Fall of Advertising and the Rise of PR*. New York: HarperCollins, 2002.

Ritzer, George. *The McDonaldization of Society*. Thousand Oaks, Calif.: Pine Forge Press, 2000.

Romains, Jules. *Knock, ou Le triomphe de la médecine*. Paris: Gallimard, 1924.

Rosof, Adrienne, and William Felch, eds. *Continuing Medical Education: A Primer.* New York: Praeger, 1992.

Shnayerson, Michael, and Mark J. Plotkin. *The Killers Within: The Deadly Rise of Drug-Resistant Bacteria.* New York: Little, Brown, 2002.

Stauber, John, and Sheldon Rampton. *Toxic Sludge Is Good for You!* Monroe, Maine: Common Courage Press, 1995.

Sunday Times Insight Team. *Suffer the Children.* New York: Viking Press, 1979.

Swann, John P. *Academic Scientists and the Pharmaceutical Industry: Cooperative Research in Twentieth-Century America.* Baltimore: Johns Hopkins University Press, 1988.

Valenstein, Elliot S. *Blaming the Brain: The Truth About Drugs and Mental Health.* New York: Free Press, 1998.

Wolfe, M. Michael, and Thomas J. Nesi. *Heartburn: Extinguishing the Fire Inside.* New York: W. W. Norton, 1997.

Young, James Harvey. *The Medical Messiahs: A Social History of Health Quackery in Twentieth-Century America.* Princeton, N.J.: Princeton University Press, 1992.

Zitrin, Richard, and Carol M. Langford. *The Moral Compass of the American Lawyer.* New York: Ballantine Books, 1999.

ACKNOWLEDGMENTS

The writing of this book required the help of so many people that it is not possible to name them all here.

Over the years, I've done hundreds of interviews with corporate executives and employees, Wall Street analysts, physicians, scientists, government regulators, lawmakers, law enforcement officials, and patients. All of them took time out of busy schedules to talk to me, and I'm indebted to each of them.

I have benefited greatly from the work of academics and others who have spent years documenting the pharmaceutical industry's influence on the practice of medicine. I'm especially grateful to the doctors and scientists who talked with me about their concerns. Every doctor and scientist looking objectively and honestly at the medical system deserves the public's greatest respect. It has become clear that they are in the courageous minority. Most of today's medical professionals are content to echo the promotional messages of the industry or simply stay silent, which is no better.

I am deeply thankful to David Franklin and his lawyer, Thomas Greene, who fought hard to unseal corporate documents and make sure the public understands just how far executives have been willing to go in their promotional campaigns, even when it meant putting patients in danger. I am also grateful to the dozens of people, including congressional staff members, patient advocates, librarians, and many others, who brought critical information to my attention, helped me find facts, or explained complex data. While I did much original reporting for this book, I also have been aided by the work of other journalists. Some of the most illuminating news stories were the daily efforts of local newspaper and television journalists, who have recorded what has happened in their communities as the industry succeeds in getting us to take more pills.

My foremost gratitude goes to the families and individuals who bravely agreed to share their personal stories about prescription drugs in the hope they could help others. Among those people are the Koppen family, Jerry Houk, and Rosemary Rahm.

I also owe a great deal to Sarah Crichton for her clear-sighted editorial judgment, as well as to the rest of the staff at Farrar, Straus and Giroux for expertly bringing everything together. My gratitude also goes to Ellis Levine for his valuable legal counsel.

I'm lastingly indebted to Barney Karpfinger, my agent, for his encouragement and friendship, as well as for his perceptive suggestions on the manuscript.

And I want to thank my family and friends, many of whom fed me and offered me their spare bedrooms on my trips through Iowa. More important, they never stopped encouraging me, even when my research and writing dragged on far longer than expected. Richard Blood provided his sharp eye and finely skilled editing touch to some of the book's early pages. And I'm eternally grateful to my husband, Michael, who spent hours reading my first draft and offering knowing advice. Without his support, this book would not have been written.

INDEX

A NOTE ABOUT THE AUTHOR

MELODY PETERSEN wrote about the pharmaceutical industry as a reporter for *The New York Times*. She has also worked at *The Philadelphia Inquirer* and the *San Jose Mercury News*. Her investigative reporting won a Gerald Loeb Award, one of the highest honors in business journalism. She is a former certified public accountant with degrees from the University of Iowa and the University of Maryland. Born and raised in Iowa, she lives with her husband in Los Angeles.